The Complete Guide to
Women's Health

All You Need to Know for a Healthy Life

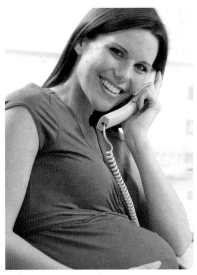 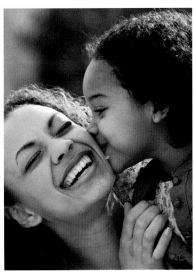 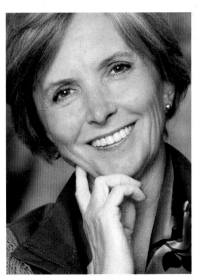

Chief Medical Editor
Sandhya Pruthi, MD, Mayo Clinic

APPLE

First published in the UK in 2010 by Apple Press Ltd

Apple Press Ltd
7 Greenland Street
London NW1 0ND

A Marshall Edition
Conceived, edited and designed by
Marshall Editions Ltd
6 Blundell Street
London N7 9BH

ISBN: 978-1-84543-358-1

10 9 8 7 6 5 4 3 2 1

FOR MARSHALL EDITIONS
Design Schermuly Design
Project Editor Mary Lindsay
Picture Manager Veneta Bullen
Creative Direction Kenneth Carroll
Managing Editor Paul Docherty

Originated in Hong Kong by Modern Age
Printed and bound in Singapore by Star Standard Industries (Pte) Ltd

Front cover photo Corbis/Mina Chapman; **Back cover** (from left to right): Shutterstock/Monkey Business Images; iStock/ Digitalskillet; iStock/Anne Clark; iStock/Randy Plett; **Spine** Shutterstock/Monkey Business Images

NOTE TO OUR READERS
The information in this book should not be substituted for, or used to alter, medical therapy without your doctor's advice. For a specific health problem, consult your doctor for guidance.

The Complete Guide to
omen's Health

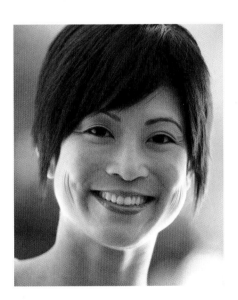

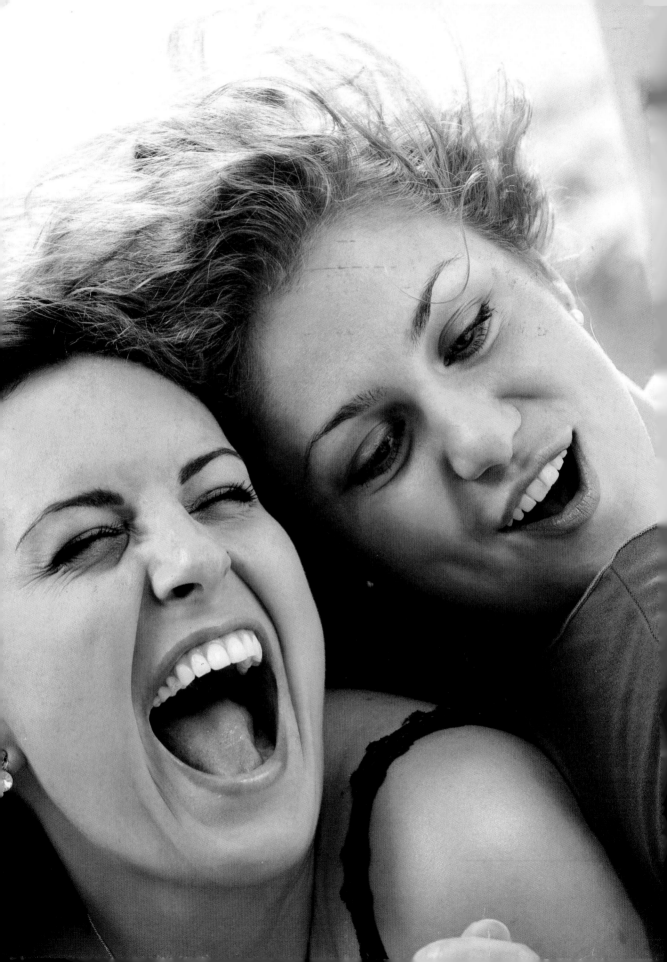

Contents

Introduction

Thanks to an amazing outpouring of medical research on women in recent years, we now have the information we need to keep ourselves healthier than was ever possible before. This research has revealed that women respond differently from men to many illnesses, including stress, depression and heart disease, and their treatments. They also have a natural protection against certain threats to health, such as stress and viruses, that men don't have. That's why this book is different from other health books. The four female doctors who have written it—all practitioners at Mayo Clinic in Rochester, Minnesota—have filtered this new research through the lens of their experience to provide up-to-date, concise information that will enable you to maintain a healthy body and a healthy mind—and to know what to do if things go wrong.

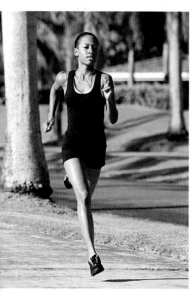

BUILD A HEALTHY BODY
Find an exercise you enjoy so you'll feel good day in and day out.

There is so much information about your health readily available on the Internet and in the media that it can be very challenging to determine what's important and what's accurate. Added to that, opinions differ, and reports on medical theories and treatments can be confusing. Are there risk factors for heart disease that are unique to women? What are the screening recommendations to prevent a variety of cancers? Are some cancers hereditary and others the result of environmental exposures? Many medical topics will make news headlines, but few are given enough space and depth to help us understand what they mean.

The goal of this book is to provide you with the tools for achieving good health by synthesizing and organizing medical information and telling you about the most up-to-date medical advances and the conclusions of the latest research. The book charts the health issues that are important to all women, from early adulthood–focusing on contraceptive choices, pregnancy and reproductive health–through to middle and advanced age–focusing on mental health and heart and musculoskeletal health. It enables you to communicate effectively with your doctor or specialist and take an active part in your mental and physical health and any treatment and recovery you may require.

CONVENTIONAL, COMPLEMENTARY AND ALTERNATIVE MEDICINE

If you are diagnosed with a disorder, you will want to gather information to better understand the causes, risk factors and management and treatment options. This book will keep you well informed about the fundamental facts so you will know what to ask, what to expect and what the aims and outcomes of various treatments may be.

Medications and therapies are improving all the time, and this book offers you the most up-to-date information on what they are and how they are used to treat various medical conditions. It describes conventional medical treatments, such as drugs and radiation, but also includes therapies such as yoga that complement conventional treatment, as well as therapies such as Traditional Chinese Medicine that offer alternatives to conventional medicine.

Whichever treatment options you choose, you should discuss them thoroughly with your family doctor before you use them. There is no one more qualified to help you become the healthy woman you want to be.

HAVING CHILDREN
Watching a child develop from a helpless baby to an independent adult is one of a woman's greatest joys.

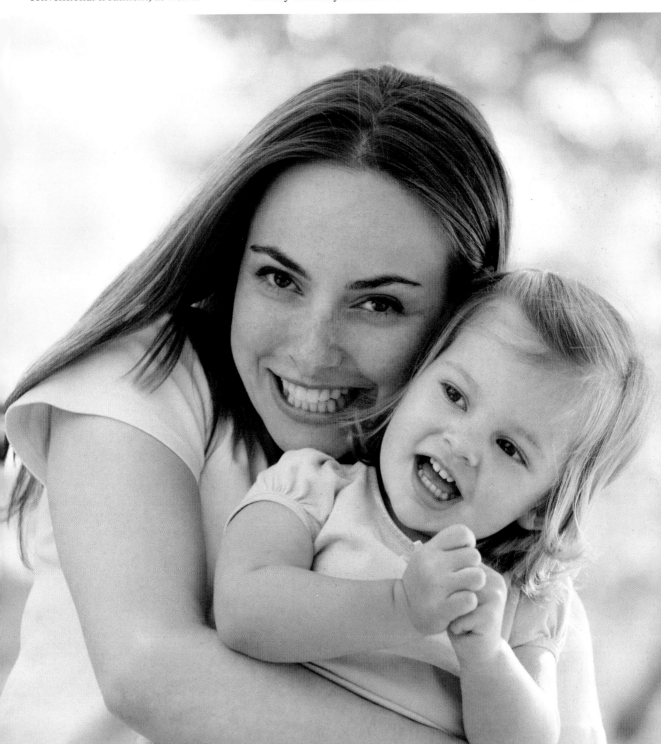

How to use this book

The book is divided into eight chapters, organized to provide easy access to information across the spectrum of health issues. The most up-to-date information is highlighted and key points summarized throughout the book. If you are looking for information on a specific topic, find it by looking at the table of contents on p. 5 or the index at the end of the book.

THE HEALTHY WOMAN

Chapter 1 looks at ways in which you can achieve your optimum good health–allowing for a little indulgence–through diet, exercise, sleep, coming to terms with your looks and asserting your rights in the workplace. It takes an overview of the health issues that may affect you in the seasons of your life and examines how the female body systems, from your bones and muscles to your digestive and immune systems, function in good health.

CHALLENGES TO YOUR HEALTH

Turn to Chapter 2 to read about the health issues and specific disorders that commonly affect the various female body systems and some of the rarer disorders. Each section uses the most up-to-date research to advise on the causes of problems, how to minimize the risks of developing them and just what the treatments and outlook are.

TRY A NEW SPORT
Regularly engaging in sports and other physical activities will help keep you in shape both physically and mentally.

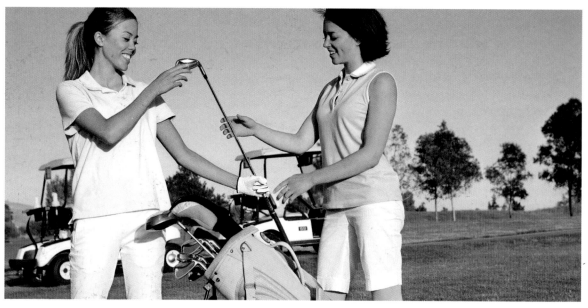

A HEALTHY MIND

Chapter 3 is a thorough overview of mental health conditions, including eating disorders and addictions related to alcohol, smoking and drugs. The latest information about anxiety-related disorders, including obsessions, phobias, post-traumatic stress and stress levels, is also found in this chapter.

CONTRACEPTION, CONCEPTION AND PREGNANCY

Many women are interested in the benefits of the latest contraceptive options. Chapter 4 provides up-to-date information on these and on conception and reproductive and pregnancy problems. It also explains the stages of pregnancy and gives advice on motherhood.

REPRODUCTIVE SYSTEM HEALTH

What are the latest screening guidelines for early detection of breast cancer and cervical cancer? In Chapter 5, read about these guidelines and learn about uterine and ovarian problems that you may encounter during your reproductive years.

SEX AND SEXUALITY

Chapter 6 takes a frank look at your sexual self, discussing ways to discover your own sexuality, relationships, intimacy, fantasy and abuse. The pages on sexual problems steer you through the pain or embarrassment to help you find a sympathetic solution, while a section on sexually transmitted infections (STIs) makes it clear exactly what to do if you suspect you have an STI.

URGENT ILLNESSES

Read Chapter 7 to find out what happens when body systems stop working perfectly. This is the place to learn more about infections and the difference between bacteria and viruses. The emergency first aid section contains essential information to have on hand should there be an accident at home or in your workplace.

HEALING THE BODY

Chapter 8 provides helpful charts that detail tests, tell you which specialists do what, and lists drugs by type and use that are available today to treat a variety of medical conditions. It also includes a complete listing of conventional medical treatments, complementary treatments and alternatives to both.

GIVING BACK
Whether it's volunteering in a community garden or helping children learn to read, as women age, some of them stay happy and healthy by giving back to the communities that have sustained them.

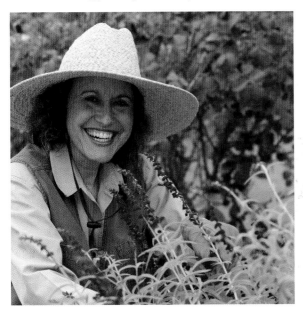

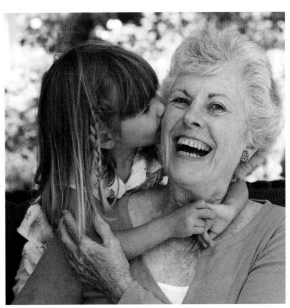

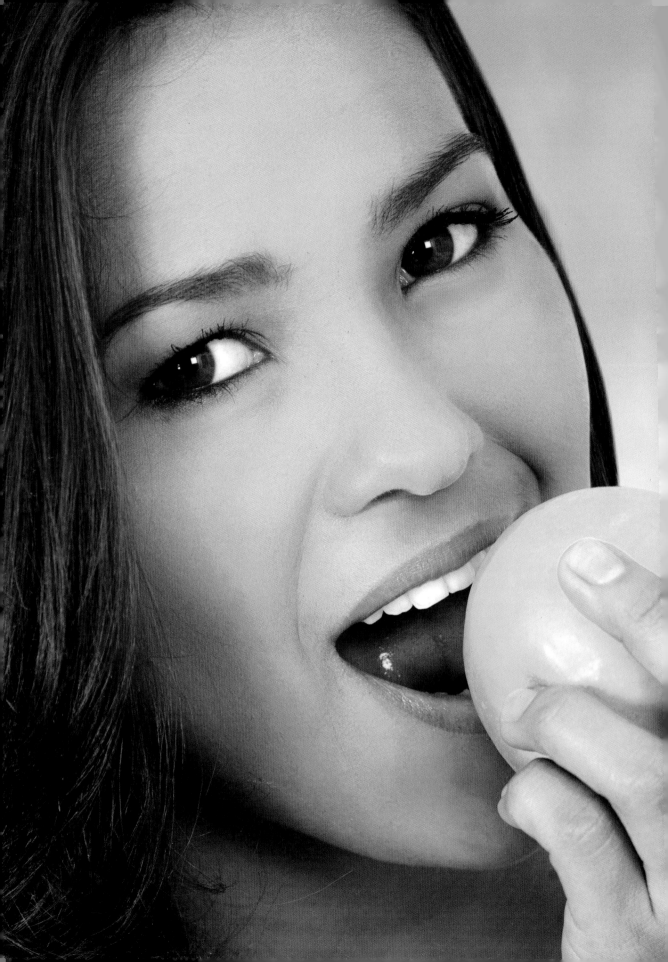

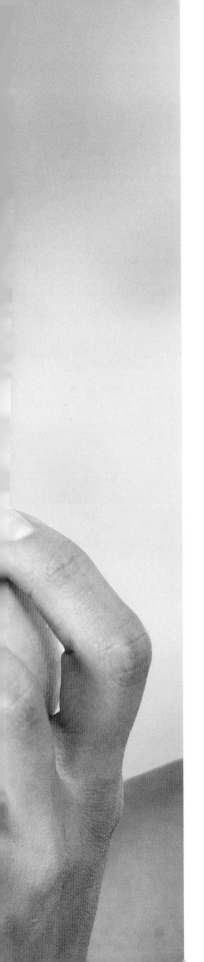

BEING
A WELL
WOMAN

A healthy woman is one who is happy and full of energy. She looks forward to each new day and has the kind of strength that carries her through times of stress. Her life has meaning and purpose. Knowing what factors are needed to achieve and sustain her health is important–and starts with understanding what makes her the way she is and how the workings of her body systems reflect the effects of hormones and genetics.

The Seasons of a Woman's Life

As a woman, you will experience many physical and emotional changes during your lifetime. These are not always clearly defined by age, and one stage of life may blend into another as the seasons do. In fact, you may become aware only in retrospect that there has been a transition. Nevertheless, each stage has its own features and associated health issues.

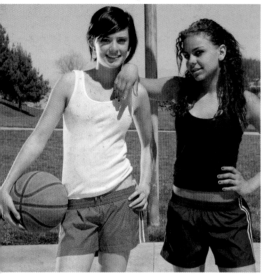

THE EMERGING WOMAN
As you develop from a child into a teenager and then into a young woman, your friends, body, learning and lifestyle will provide a strong base for your future health and achievements.

THE EMERGING WOMAN

When you emerge from adolescence, you move gradually away from your parents' influence and towards greater independence. Taking care of yourself is all within your own hands, and you become ready to take on some of the responsibilities of the adult world. Women not only have to focus on their health and wellness but also have to make decisions about careers, marriage, childbearing and raising a family.

Today, you may be more likely to delay having a child until you reach your late 20s or early 30s, so you can concentrate on your career, studies or travel. You may be reluctant to relinquish your freedom and strive to achieve the same economic independence as your male friends.

As a young adult woman, you can expect to have good health. But this does not mean forgetting to sustain this good health with sound nutrition, exercise and regular health checks with your GP. Your doctor can, for example, give you guidance and counsel you about new screening guidelines for prevention and early detection of cervical cancer.

At this age you may not fully grasp how certain lifestyle behaviours can impact good health and consequently put you at risk for certain diseases. You may spend time at the gym but decide to smoke and drink. You may be tempted to go on crash diets and consume junk food. A hectic social life may mean you also go without sleep on a regular basis and may experiment with illegal drugs.

Early womanhood is also a time when emotional problems can dominate your life, and some may encounter anxiety, depression or eating disorders. You will look to your friends for support, guidance and advice. This is also the time to find a doctor whom you trust and are comfortable with.

You may seek a sexual partner without necessarily having commitment in mind. Indeed, you may have had several sexual partners before you begin a long-term relationship. This has become acceptable behaviour in Western cultures but carries its own risks. You need to be aware of the importance and availability of new contraceptive options, and know the risks of contracting sexually transmitted diseases, such as HIV, herpes, chlamydia and gonorrhoea. Your future wellbeing and happiness could depend on whether or not you practise safe sex.

THE 30-SOMETHING WOMAN

Like many women, you may find that your 30s are a time when your confidence has grown and you feel happy to be yourself, relieved to have left the uncertainties and peer pressures of early adulthood behind. You may be well established in your career and know what you want out of life.

Reliable contraception has made it possible to put parenthood on hold until you and your partner believe the conditions are right. Alternatively, you may decide that you don't want a co-parent and choose to go it alone. If you are considering childbearing, you should be aware of the importance of good health before conception and get your body into peak form before trying to become pregnant. However, you may choose to pursue your career or interests instead of having children, or you may find that a partnership is fulfillment enough without feeling the need for motherhood as well.

Motherhood and work

Most women are able to conceive naturally and have healthy babies who give them great pleasure in the years of nurturing. You may be surprised by the intensity of the love you have for your child; alternatively, bonding with your baby may take time to develop.

Your relationship with your partner, if you have one, will change with the arrival of the baby. It can be enriched by your mutual joy in the child, especially if you parent together and accept equal responsibility. However, the relationship may be put under pressure by the new demands. Relationships with both sets of parents and extended family will also change and need to be balanced.

Equally, if you continue to work, particularly if you have a successful and demanding career, you may find that managing a job and a family is more difficult than you had anticipated, even if you have help at home. Trying to establish a routine that allows you to be a person as well as a mother may be more challenging than you expected.

The woman who has unrealistic expectations of what motherhood involves may feel the loss of freedom that she so much appreciated and may have taken for granted. Some mothers may even experience depression. Prolonged depression after the birth of a baby is frequently caused by hormonal changes. Such depression should not be dismissed merely as "baby blues" and should always be taken seriously.

As a new mother, you may be alarmed by the demands the new baby makes on you. You may not have the support of extended family to turn to at this time and you can feel lonely and depressed. This is a time to make efforts to look to other mothers in your community for company, support and encouragement. Parenting is a time of many challenges and also a time to learn the necessary

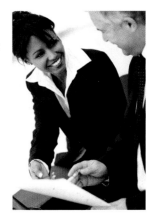

FREEDOM OF CHOICE
Many women choose to delay motherhood, giving them the chance to pursue a career and enjoy a carefree social life.

You may find that your 30s are a time when you feel happy to be yourself.

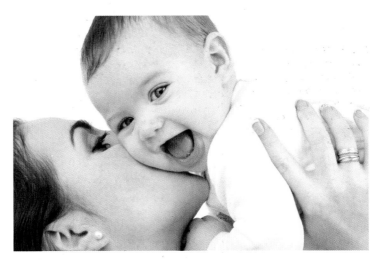

skills to meet the demands of raising children and working as a team with your partner.

Equally, for those without children, career pressures or life stressors can impact wellbeing. This is a time when separation from a partner, family stressors or work challenges can trigger depression and anxiety. If you don't wish to lean on your friends and family, seeing your doctor, a counsellor or psychotherapist can be a great help.

BECOMING A MOTHER
When you have a baby, you probably no longer think of yourself first but rather of the child who gives you a new sense of purpose and direction in life.

13

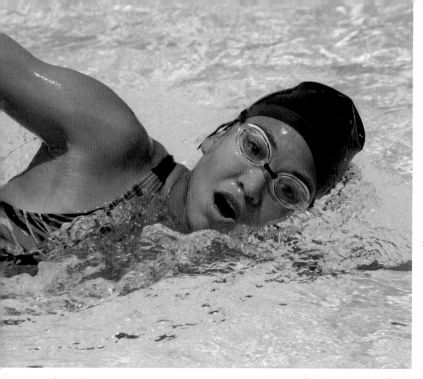

KEEPING FIT
Maintain a healthy weight and calm mind with regular exercise such as swimming.

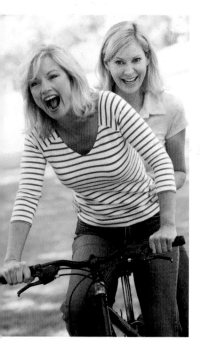

A STIMULATING WOMAN
Discovering new talents, or reviving those that were set aside previously due to lack of time, may lead to new friendships with those who share the same interests.

THE MIDLIFE WOMAN

For most women, the 40s and 50s are a fulfilling stage of life. At work, your career may have been enhanced and opened up more opportunities resulting in more responsibilities. Your personal life may be more settled than the turbulent earlier years, either in a relationship or with single status. It's no wonder studies show that women in their 50s are the happiest.

The 40s can also be a hugely varied time: you may be challenged with child-raising responsibilities, or your children may be becoming more independent, leaving you with time to take up new interests or work opportunities.

By the age of 40, those women who are still interested in childbearing may experience difficulties with getting pregnant. Women learn that in their 40s their biological clock is ticking, and there is approximately a 25 per cent chance every month of getting pregnant.

If motherhood is delayed, the cause may take longer to identify but, while past generations accepted infertility as something they had to live with, modern advances in medical science have provided new options to women who have difficulty conceiving. These techniques–although often costly– range from *in vitro* fertilization (IVF), sometimes using donor eggs or sperm, to finding a surrogate mother to carry and give birth to a child.

At the other end of the scale, you may suffer from the "empty nest syndrome", a feeling of loss when your children leave home. Occupying yourself with new, absorbing interests or taking up a sport may help fill the gap. Bear in mind that their love for you has not necessarily altered because your role in their lives has changed. Adult children can become good friends and confidantes and never really grow out of needing the support of their parents.

Having reared your children and enjoyed watching them become independent through good and not-so-good times may have given you the confidence to take on any challenge that comes your way. Now is your chance to transfer the skills acquired during your years of raising children to enhance your career or branch out and pursue your hobbies or take on the challenge of a new business opportunity.

The middle years do not necessarily bring problems with health, although you may have a tendency to gain weight. Now is the time to deal with those extra pounds and to take note of important screening recommendations such as a mammogram for early detection of breast cancer. It's also time to make sure you get the regular exercise and healthy diet necessary to prevent heart disease.

The menopausal challenge

Menopausal changes can be a time of great joy but you might also be distressed by the range of symptoms as a result of hormonal fluctuations. The end of fertility and no longer worrying about pregnancy can bring great relief. This can have a positive effect on your sex life and your attitude towards embarking on new interests. The passage through the menopausal years will be marked by physical and emotional changes, some of which can be difficult. But sensitivity, a better understanding of the way your body changes, and a knowledge of new options can help you navigate through these tough times. The goal is to focus on wellbeing and good health, which will provide a smooth transition to the "golden" years.

THE OLDER WOMAN

With good health and vitality on your side, you can hope to live life to the fullest for 20 to 30 years after the age of 60. An optimistic approach to life after retirement can allow you to reach new career heights, discover great happiness as a role model to the young, be an inspiration to your children and grandchildren, and provide valued companionship to your friends.

If you understand yourself and focus on ways to reduce risk factors that can compromise your health, inhibit mobility and threaten independence, you are already taking the best steps to help yourself. While medical advances can help–improved surgery provides new joints, such as hip replacements, and can give hearts new life with bypass operations–prevention remains the goal for better health.

Stay on the move

As a woman ages, she can still benefit from addressing factors that are important to maintaining a healthy lifestyle and positive attitude. It is never too late to stop smoking or to cut back on alcohol intake. Now is the time to continue to eat nutritious meals and exercise regularly.

Exercise may need to be modified to suit your state of mobility, but a brisk walk every day keeps both body and mind stimulated. You should consult your doctor about what sort of exercise is suitable for you. Some women find a personal trainer a wonderful resource to determine their optimal exercise plan. Exercising the mind is as important as exercising the body and now is the chance to find ways to be creative and pursue new interests.

As we age, it's just as important to have the support of family as it is to keep up with regular visits to your doctor. A network of more mobile friends will also help keep you stimulated by visits, sharing books or videos and ensuring that you do not feel lonely or bored.

There is generally no reason why mental faculties should not function as well as they have in the past–and many older women take great pleasure in reading and writing. A local history group may value your memories, and compiling records can be an enjoyable activity.

One inevitable part of growing older is the loss of loved ones. The death of a lifelong partner may seem like an irrecoverable blow. The sadness and depression that follows bereavement is a natural part of the mourning process. But if you can't move on–and many women hide their feelings and find it difficult to talk about their grief–you should seek the advice of your doctor and if necessary take the time to get the appropriate counselling.

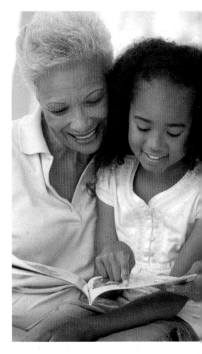

A PURPOSEFUL WOMAN
Opportunities that allow you to pass on knowledge and experience to younger people can contribute to a sense of purpose.

Studies show that women in their 50s are the happiest.

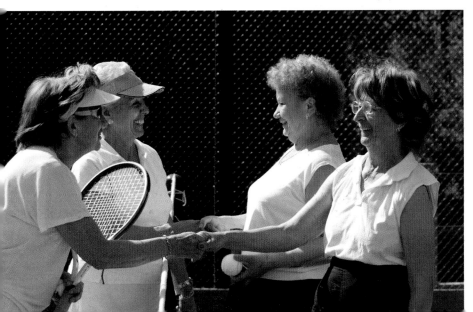

SUPPORT AND FRIENDSHIP
Chatting with your friends is one of the best tonics. In later years, women of the same age can share past experiences and provide a wealth of mutual practical and moral support.

Good Health Basics

Every one of us is entitled to a healthy body. But we have to earn it with good food, sufficient exercise and sleep every night, plus enjoy a range of social relationships and avoid stress. If we do all that, then we may even be able to prevent specific genes that predispose us to illness from being "switched on".

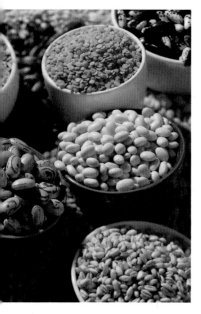

POWER FOOD
Wholegrain foods provide energy and help prevent cancer, heart disease and obesity.

FAT FACTS

Fats have many functions. They help the body absorb fat-soluble vitamins, promote childhood development, help to produce sex hormones and regulate metabolism. Fat is high in calories, having over twice as many as are in carbohydrates or protein, so a diet high in fat can quickly cause a weight problem.

HEALTHY NUTRITION

Providing your body with a healthy balance of nutrients is an art. To get the right balance, you need to ensure that your diet is varied, provides the nutrients your body needs and is both enjoyable and satisfying without placing you at risk of developing illnesses.

To find an approach to nutrition that will be sustainable, you should forget all about diets and dieting that may cause you to feel stressed and will almost always be abandoned. Your own nutritional plan can be established gradually, based on an understanding of why your body needs different types of foods and why too much of some do you no favours. Women often derive a third or more of their calorie intake from fat, and this increases their susceptibility to cancer of the colon and breast, diabetes, high blood pressure, and other disorders. Sugar, salt and alcohol may also adversely affect women's health.

Build your body with protein

From the time a child is conceived, it is protein that ensures the body's growth and good health. It is the body's building material, playing an essential role in making and repairing tissue through wear and tear.

Animal sources of protein are poultry, meat, fish, cheese, milk, yogurt and eggs. Vegetable sources are soya products, pulses (peas and beans), nuts and whole grains. Most people who eat meat consume more protein than the body needs, and the excess is stored in the muscles and liver as glycogen. It can be converted for use as energy when there is not enough sugar circulating in the blood. The aim of healthy eating is to keep the blood sugar level balanced and to have little glycogen or fat stored.

Reach for fibre-rich carbs

The body turns starches and sugars, known as carbohydrates, into glucose, which circulates in the blood to meet your energy needs. Nutritionally, carbohydrates should be the greatest part of a day's eating. There are, however, two categories.

Complex carbohydrates, which provide starch and fibre, are found in whole grains, pulses, vegetables and fruits. These release energy slowly and steadily. Simple carbohydrates are found in sugar and honey and in refined products such as biscuits, desserts, pies, ice creams and some breakfast cereals. They release energy quickly but contain no essential nutrients. In healthy eating, simple carbohydrates should be taken as sparingly as fats.

Ditch extra fat

Most people obtain dietary fat from eating protein foods, in which it is present naturally, through adding it

VITAMINS

Your body can't function without vitamins, which provide the biochemical trigger for nerves, muscles, hormones, energy and waste production. You can make some, but most come from foods. Those transported from the digestive tract in fat (fat-soluble vitamins) can be stored by the body, but an excess of water-soluble vitamins is generally excreted in the urine. Antioxidant vitamins counteract the damaging effect of molecules called free radicals (by-products of energy production thought to trigger the ageing process).

VITAMIN	ACTION	SOURCES
Vitamin A (fat soluble)	A major antioxidant, it keeps eyes and skin healthy and protects linings of respiratory, digestive and urinary tracts	Eggs, full-fat milk, butter, margarine and green, yellow and orange vegetables
Vitamin B$_1$ (thiamine) (water soluble)	Assists in processing carbohydrates, protein and fats for energy	Wholegrain cereals, milk, lean pork, soya beans and other pulses
Vitamin B$_2$ (riboflavin) and B$_3$ (niacin) (water soluble)	Essential for energy and growth	Milk, cheese, cereals, enriched bread and flour, soya beans and green leafy vegetables (especially broccoli)
Vitamin B$_5$ (pantothenic acid) (water soluble)	Required for metabolism, the nervous system and sex hormones	Most vegetables, eggs, wholegrain cereals, salmon, nuts and offal
B$_6$ (pyridoxine) (water soluble)	Necessary for making red blood cells and antibodies	Meat, fish, egg yolks, sweet corn, bananas, avocados, nuts and wholegrain cereals
B$_{12}$ (fat soluble)	Vital for growth, red blood cells and the central nervous system	Fish, eggs and dairy products
Folic acid (folate) (water soluble)	Crucial to the development of fetal nervous system during pregnancy	Liver, kidneys, eggs, wholegrain cereals, peas, beans, nuts and green leafy vegetables
Vitamin C (ascorbic acid) (water soluble)	An antioxidant, it prevents infections, heals wounds, helps absorption of iron and controls blood cholesterol	Fruit (especially citrus), green vegetables, potatoes, tomatoes and peppers
Vitamin D (fat soluble)	Works with calcium to make healthy bones; a small amount is manufactured by the action of daylight on the skin	Milk, oily fish and egg yolks; it is added to flour and some bread
Vitamin E (fat soluble)	Reduces the risk of heart disease and can relieve menstrual cramps and PMS	Most vegetable oils, eggs, nuts, lettuce, seeds, soya beans and seafood
Vitamin K (fat soluble)	Helps in blood clotting, bone formation and kidney function	Green leafy vegetables, beef, liver, green tea, cheese and oats

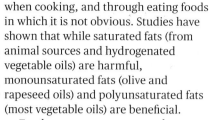

KNOW YOUR FATS
Saturated fats, such as butter or that found on meat, are hard at room temperature. Fats that are polyunsaturated are from vegetable sources, such as sunflower and corn, and oily fish. Olive oil and avocados contain monounsaturated fats. Commercial baked goods and fried foods contain transfatty acids. Saturated fats cause high cholesterol and heart disease. Monounsaturated fats prevent both. Transfatty acids are arguably the most damaging to your health because they create free radicals. These molecules attack the body in myriad ways to set the stage for a variety of diseases.

when cooking, and through eating foods in which it is not obvious. Studies have shown that while saturated fats (from animal sources and hydrogenated vegetable oils) are harmful, monounsaturated fats (olive and rapeseed oils) and polyunsaturated fats (most vegetable oils) are beneficial.

Fat that you can see–on poultry, lamb, pork, beef or ham, for example–should be trimmed before cooking or eating. Hidden fats are the biggest problem–they are included in processed foods such as pies, cakes and biscuits, in fast foods, and in many chilled and frozen ready meals. Always read the labels on prepared foods; note the fat content and remember what it means.

You need to be careful in making choices. Foods that contain good fats–essential fatty acids that help reduce inflammation and lower cholesterol, particularly triglycerides–are oily fish, olive oil and low-fat spreads and dressings based on polyunsaturated vegetable oils. All contain linoleic acid, which works with vitamin E to protect the heart. To reduce intake of bad fats, avoid eating margarine, lard, chips, doughnuts and croissants.

By restricting your intake of saturated fats and transfats you will help to keep your blood level of LDL cholesterol (low density lipoprotein, also known as bad cholesterol) to within normal limits. High blood cholesterol, or hyperlipidaemia, is a key risk factor for heart disease, which is a major health problem for women as well as for men.

Some products may not necessarily be low in fat–the fat content could simply be "reduced" compared to the regular version of the product. Check the calorie values of a normal serving and a lower fat one. Foods can be labelled "reduced" or "low" fat and still have a high calorie count because of added sugar.

Vitamins and minerals

Together, vitamins and minerals are called micronutrients and unlike the macronutrients–protein, carbohydrates and fats–they are only needed in trace amounts. With few exceptions, the body

does not manufacture micronutrients; you must get them from a varied and balanced diet that includes dairy foods, fruits, vegetables, nuts and seeds. Vitamins (p. 17) work in tandem with minerals to keep you mentally and physically healthy.

The antioxidants–vitamins A, C and E–are partnered by selenium, a mineral thought to be important in preventing heart disease and cancer. All minerals have a role, but calcium and iron are especially pertinent for women. Calcium builds bones and teeth, assists in normal blood clotting and in transmitting nerve impulses. Along with magnesium and phosphorus, also essential to bone building and muscle activity, calcium is found in milk, cheese, yogurt, tofu, green leafy vegetables and canned fish, such as sardines and salmon.

To make use of calcium, the body needs vitamin D, which may come from the diet or supplements or through sunlight on the skin. Bone and teeth formation continues through your teens and 20s and, since calcium deficiency can lead to osteoporosis later in life, calcium should be part of your daily diet.

Iron is needed to make haemoglobin, which gives the blood its red colour and carries oxygen to all the cells. If you are deficient in iron you may feel tired, depressed and lack energy. This may happen if you suffer from heavy menstrual periods or if you are not obtaining enough vitamin C for your body to use the mineral efficiently. Iron is found in red meat (beef, lamb, liver), seafood, eggs, broccoli, brussels sprouts, peas, spinach and wholemeal bread.

Stay hydrated

About 70 per cent of your body is water; it is in the bones, blood and every cell. Every day about 2½ l (4¾ pints) leaves the body in sweat, breath, urine and faeces– and you need to drink plain water to make up for this loss. On a cold day, 6 to 8 average glasses (225 ml; 8 ounces) are recommended; in hot weather you may need twice that. If you drink too much, you will simply urinate the excess. If you drink too little, your skin will dry out and you will become constipated. Tea and coffee should not be substitutes for plain water; more than three or four cups a day of caffeinated beverages can inhibit the absorption of iron and keep you from sleeping well. In moderation, alcohol can be part of a nutritious diet.

Try the 80/20 approach

The 80/20 plan is a good way to start. Overconsumption of fats–any type–is the major problem in bad nutrition, and fat is often accompanied by sugar. If you ensure that 80 per cent of what you eat is healthy, low-fat food based on the wider bands of the pyramids and rainbow (right), then you can allow yourself to eat sensible amounts of favourite foods containing fat/sugar for the 20 per cent. The 80 per cent should include proteins (skinless chicken, lean meats, pulses, soya products), carbohydrates (fresh fruits, vegetables, grains, breads, cereals, potatoes and pasta) and little fat (low-fat dairy foods). The changeover can be tackled gradually by substituting lower-fat foods for high-fat foods.

The Food Pyramids

All food pyramids have the same purpose: to help you eat well and healthily. Choose foods from the wider, lower bands and eat less of the foods in higher bands. With all pyramid plans regular daily exercise is a recommended accompaniment.

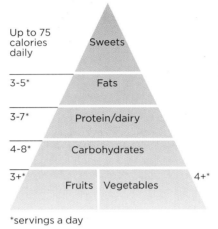

Up to 75 calories daily — Sweets
3-5* — Fats
3-7* — Protein/dairy
4-8* — Carbohydrates
3+* — Fruits | Vegetables — 4+*

*servings a day

Sparingly — Meats, sweets
Small portions, daily to weekly — Poultry, eggs, cheese, yogurt
Often (2+ times a week) — Fish, seafood
Every meal — Fruits, vegetables, grains (mostly whole), olive oil, beans, nuts, pulses and seeds, herbs and spices

*servings a day

Grain products
Vegetables and fruit
Milk and alternatives
Meat and alternatives

5-12*   5-10*   2-4*   2-3*

OPTIMAL WESTERN DAILY DIET

The food pyramid was devised by nutritional scientists to encourage an increased intake of complex carbohydrates and a reduced intake of saturated fats and simple sugars in the daily diet. Recommended servings balance vitamins and minerals needed for health and provide fibre. Exercise is a vital component of a healthy lifestyle.

TRADITIONAL MEDITERRANEAN DIET

The Mediterranean diet is high in plant foods, particularly tomatoes, onions and garlic, and cheese, yogurt and olive oil every day. Fish, poultry, eggs and sweets can be eaten a few times a week. Red meat is optional once every 10 days and alcohol intake, typically red wine, is moderate (2 glasses a day). Exercise and healthy eating is the ideal to aim for.

CANADIAN RAINBOW

The Canadian food guide recommends how many servings people should aim to eat from each of the four different food groups each day. Most servings should be chosen from the groups comprising grain products, and vegetables and fruit. Much smaller sevings should be selected from the milk products group, and choices from meat and their alternatives should be kept to a minimum.

- Sleep more. Studies show that getting less than 7 hours sleep a night turns on appetite genes that make you hungry. Sleeping more can turn them off.
- Avoid alcohol. It's loaded with calories.
- Keep a food diary. Studies have found that just writing down what you eat forces you to eat less.
- Never eat while driving. You'll eat more than you intend.
- Exercise. Exercise. Exercise. In study after study, it's the one thing that helps you lose weight and keep it off.

DIETING AND YOUR WEIGHT

Women are bombarded with images of waif-like models–in magazines, films and on television–presented as the ideal of beauty. These images can be a powerful force, especially for the young, who may come to accept that losing weight and "being on a diet" are a fact of life. The word "diet" in this context does not mean medically advised weight loss programmes designed for severely obese patients. The doubtful "diets" in this case are those that promise miraculous transformation in the short term.

A hundred or more years ago women would not have had time to be as preoccupied with weight as we seem to be today. The everyday preparation of food took energy, and there was little opportunity to overeat. Their daily lives required constant energy, for almost non-stop work in the house and looking after a family. Their metabolism was attuned to burning up calories, with little to spare. Women today have more sedentary lifestyles and endless options for saving, rather than using, energy. But two important points remain true for women who lived then or now: food is good for you, and if you eat more than your body can use, the excess will be stored as fat. For your metabolism to work at an optimal speed, there needs to be a combination of chemical and physical processes.

Diets make you fat

Diet plans favouring grapefruits, cabbage soup, food combinations or even low-fat regimens are not the answer to losing weight. If you have been considering dieting because you think you ought to, give some thought to this fact: the vast majority of dieters eventually go back to their pre-diet weight or become heavier than they were before. Most people who start dieting will continue to do so, on and off, for the rest of their lives. If a range of foods is designated as forbidden, dieters feel guilty if they transgress, which makes them feel worse about themselves.

Dieting makes food an enemy, not a source of sustenance and well-being. So-called yo-yo dieting–losing weight, putting it back on, losing it again and so on–is bad for your health. If you suddenly reduce your food intake, your body, because it is designed for survival, will slow down your metabolic rate in order to store energy more efficiently. This is why people on a diet crave snacks such as chocolate, which gives a quick boost to their energy levels, and why weight loss slows down dramatically after the first couple of weeks.

Weight loss in the early weeks of crash dieting is not, as many women believe, made up mostly of unwanted fat. First you lose those carbohydrates stored in the muscles and liver as glycogen. This is why you feel tired on such a diet and have less strength for lifting and running–because you are losing muscle

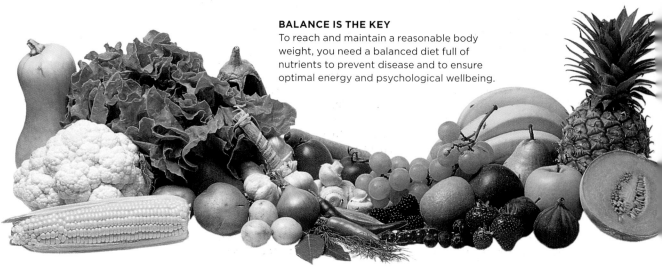

BALANCE IS THE KEY
To reach and maintain a reasonable body weight, you need a balanced diet full of nutrients to prevent disease and to ensure optimal energy and psychological wellbeing.

power. You will also lose a lot of water, which may make you feel less bloated and appear slimmer, when in fact you are still carrying the same amount of fat on your body.

Why do you gain weight?

The way you feel about yourself, and your life, plays a part in weight build-up. It is quite common for people to report that when they are happy, they stop overeating and their body weight stabilizes. Others say they gain weight when they are miserable. But both of these may be too simplistic. There are various factors that are known to play a part in being overweight. Keeping a daily diary of thoughts, feelings and events may help you understand which of the factors relate to you.

An unbalanced diet   Good nutrition is all about balance and variety. You may not be aware of how frequently you opt for certain types of foods, particularly those that are high in fat or sugar. In your diary make a note of everything you put in your mouth over a period of two weeks, then look at your notes carefully. How many days did you have pizza, a burger or other fast food? How many days did you not have milk or fruit or vegetables? How many days did you have sweet snacks or drink alcohol? How many days did you not eat wholegrain cereals or breads?

Not enough exercise   Many people genuinely feel that they do not eat more than friends and family but they put weight on more easily. Perhaps your body is just not expending enough energy. From the mid-30s on, about 225 g (8 ounces) of muscle can be lost each year in women, usually replaced by fat. What is known as your "fat-free mass" determines your resting metabolic rate (RMR), which gets on with the job of converting about 75 per cent of your daily calories for the body to use. The larger your frame and the more toned your muscles, the greater your RMR. The most effective way of improving your RMR is to exercise regularly.

Boredom and depression   Note the time you ate, along with what you ate, and how hungry you felt, in your food diary. Note the reason you ate, too, such as because you were offered food, it was a mealtime, you were putting off doing something else you didn't want to do or you were upset. Eating for comfort may be satisfying in the short term, but if you are really depressed or unhappy with your circumstances, eating will aggravate your problem. It would be better to seek help from your doctor.

Poor self-image   If you have low self-confidence, for whatever reason, you may subconsciously believe your body is not worth respecting, that you deserve to feel fat and unattractive because no one, including yourself, thinks that you're worth anything. This state then becomes self-perpetuating. If you let yourself put on excess weight, you are less likely to feel at your best and you will despise yourself more for not being able to control what you eat.

Poor eating habits   How and when you eat may be part of your problem, especially if you do not have established mealtimes. Do you feel pressured to eat and drink more than you should when out with friends? Do you grab a chocolate bar or fast food when you don't have time for a meal? Do you eat when you have nothing to do or are feeling stressed? Do you finish up food left on your child's plate? Your food diary will help you to identify these habits.

Genetic links   If your parents were overweight, you may have inherited this tendency (although this is the least common cause). It can be difficult to differentiate whether you have inherited poor eating habits or possess a real disposition to store fat. Either way, there is no need to accept being overweight as a way of life. Cutting calories, avoiding saturated fats and exercising can help every woman achieve a healthy weight.

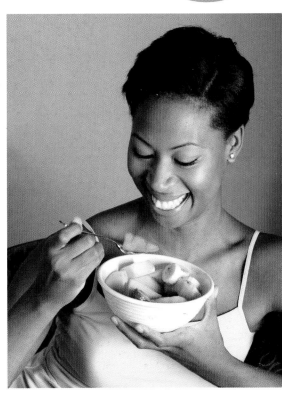

DEVELOPING A HEALTHY FOOD ATTITUDE
Eating a varied, balanced diet and enjoying what you eat can contribute to a non-obsessive attitude to food. You can reinforce this regime by having regular mealtimes and always sitting down to eat.

21

AN EXERCISE PLAN

Today most people do not get as much exercise in their daily lives as they used to—increasingly, jobs and shops are some distance from home, making it impractical to walk to and from them. Also, labour-saving devices have taken much of the exertion out of housework; we spend too much of our working lives sitting in front of computers and too much of our leisure time watching television.

It remains a fact, however, that the route to good health is a combination of regular exercise, nutritious eating, maintaining an ideal weight and enjoying plenty of restful sleep. Lifelong adherence to this may prevent some of the disorders that primarily affect women, including premenstrual syndrome (PMS), constipation and osteoporosis, as well as, in recent years, diabetes and coronary artery disease, which were once mainly male problems.

Regular exercise provides other benefits, such as relieving stress, helping to slow the effects of ageing and reducing the symptoms of debilitating diseases such as osteoarthritis.

Before deciding on an exercise plan, consider your reasons for getting fit. You may want to be fitter to play a sport, to fulfill an ambition, such as running a marathon, or to lose weight and keep it off. You may simply want to feel better, have energy left at the end of the day, be emotionally stable and enjoy activities that entertain and reward you. Exercise should never be seen as a punishment or boring.

To change your shape, you need a programme that combines aerobic and strength training. Fitness training can make you a better sports player, tone your muscles and cut down your body fat. There are three components to an overall fitness programme: aerobic endurance, muscle strength and flexibility. Aerobic exercise is vital for a strong heart and efficient lungs. Muscle strength and endurance mean good support for your skeleton and better posture. Flexibility keeps you mobile as you age, minimizing any risk of straining or pulling muscles in daily life.

One caveat

Varying your exercise and how much you do challenges your body. But it should never be overdone. Excessive exercise can alter a woman's body fat to lean muscle mass ratio. This can lead to menstrual irregularities and can be a problem for athletes and performers, such as gymnasts and skaters, and women with eating disorders who use exercise as a method of burning calories. What is called exercise-induced amenorrhoea may be reversed, but during the time the body does not ovulate, it lacks oestrogen, which can cause calcium to leach out of bones, and bone thinning, leading to osteoporosis later in life.

It is not the exercise that is at fault, but the strenuousness of it. At and after menopause women can reduce their risk of osteoporosis with weight-bearing exercises that help the bones. Walking, hiking, jogging, dancing, step aerobics, tennis and cross-country skiing all improve bone mass, agility and balance. Add training with weights to this and you increase bone density and muscular strength as well.

Set a goal

Take into account the amount of time you have and plan accordingly. Flexibility exercises should be done daily—stretching helps to lengthen the muscles and tendons. You should warm up first with slow, smooth and rhythmic movements, and cool down with the same movements after your session is over. To increase fitness levels, at least three times a week you should do 20 minutes of aerobic exercise to the point of being nearly breathless—sustained running and swimming, for example. This causes you to breathe harder, and the heart to beat faster to supply the muscles with extra oxygen. At this level of activity you should be able—just—to keep up a conversation.

Exercise specialists suggest an activity formula of 70 to 80 per cent aerobic to

TAKE ACTION NOW!

How you choose to exercise is up to you, but you should start without further delay. You may walk, swim, stretch, lift, dance or do sports.

Exercise reduces stress, lifts mood, helps maintain a healthy weight, prevents osteoporosis, helps with sleep and slows the effects of ageing.

20 to 30 per cent anaerobic (not requiring extra oxygen). The combination increases the ratio of muscle to fat more effectively than either approach on its own. If you wish to lose weight, you can work up to the aerobic level, having first of all checked with a doctor that the programme you are beginning will be right for you and your health. Remember that pain is a sign that you should stop. If your joints start to hurt after walking or running, change to swimming, in which the water cushions the joints, so that you can maintain aerobic fitness without placing further strain on your body.

Choose your routine

There is a variety of ways in which to motivate yourself to exercise regularly.

Exercise on your own If you plan to work out with a fitness video or to buy home exercise equipment, before spending too much make sure that you have the self-discipline to go it alone. Goal: at least three days a week.

Go for structure At a gym you will receive the benefits of a tailor-made programme and guidance from experts, but you can go at times that suit you and exercise at your own pace. Investigate weight training using specialized equipment such as Nautilus, or free weights. You must use a trainer to help learn the right techniques and to prevent injury. Do not do more than an hour at a time and don't exercise the same muscle group on two consecutive days. Goal: three times a week, for 45 minutes each time (building up to 60 minutes).

Be sociable Aerobics, aqua aerobics or spin classes are a good choice if you're sociable. In a class you will feel motivated by other members. The instructors are trained to ensure you don't do more harm than good. Goal: two 60-minute classes a week. If possible, fit in a weekly swim or yoga session as well.

Take up a sport Badminton can be enjoyed at all levels; squash can too, but it is faster and more competitive. Tennis and basketball are routes to aerobic fitness and bone strength. Golf has the advantages of walking and fresh air. Country and ballroom dancing are good for bones and for training the memory. Goal: two or more sessions a week.

Be flexible Even if you are resolutely against gyms, classes or playing a sport, you can improve your fitness by incorporating more walking into your daily routine and increasing the pace gradually. Goal: a brisk 30-minute walk five times a week, but build up to this.

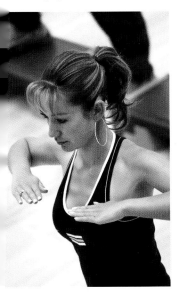

CLASSES CAN BE FUN
Aerobics classes provide social contact, motivation and all-round exercise.

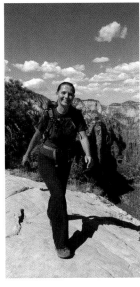

KEEP ON THE MOVE
Brisk walking in beautiful surroundings benefits your mind as well as your body.

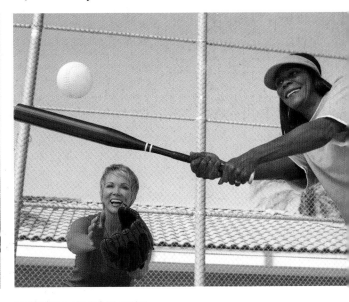

BECOME A TEAM PLAYER
Engaging in a team sport, such as softball, gives your exercise regime a sense of purpose beyond a healthy lifestyle.

THE REWARDING PATTERN OF SLEEP

Sleep is a basic need, as essential for mental and physical health as are nutrition and exercise. It allows your body to repair and restore itself so you can function efficiently and energetically during the waking hours.

On average you spend one-third of your life asleep, although this varies through the years, and less is needed in later life. A one-year-old baby will sleep for about fourteen out of twenty-four hours, but most adults need just seven or eight hours a night. Some say they manage on as few as four hours; others need eleven or twelve to be at their best.

The occasional sleepless night will do no harm, although it may make you feel awful the next day. Continuous sleep deprivation, however, may affect the way you work, your moods and your physical wellbeing because without sleep the body is unable to repair itself. Going without sleep for as little as three days can lead to confusion, serious mental problems and even hallucinations.

Through research on volunteers in sleep laboratories, scientists now know what happens to the body while you sleep. A normal sleep pattern consists of two parts: REM (rapid eye-movement sleep, when your brain is most active and you dream) and NREM (non-rapid eye-movement sleep, when you don't dream).

Volunteers, linked to an electroencephalogram (EEG) that measures brain waves, are woken when electrical activity indicates REM and confirm that they were dreaming. People tend not to remember a dream unless they wake up during it or straight after.

During sleep your brain remains active, analyzing the past day's events and storing and processing information. Sleep may also be a time of mental healing, because dreaming is thought to help you come to terms with any emotional problems.

How sleep happens

Once you are comfortable in bed, your eyes close and you begin to doze; your body twitches as nerves and muscles relax. During this phase, called shallow sleep, you can be wakened easily by the slightest disturbance because you are still aware of your surroundings. After half an hour or so, sleep becomes deeper: you relax, your heart beats more slowly and you become oblivious to your surroundings. Truly deep sleep follows, during which you are completely relaxed. You remain in one position, your heart rate slows down and your breathing is slow and regular.

It was once thought that deep sleep continues until you wake, but scientists have discovered that each of the three stages lasts about half an hour, and that the 90-minute sleep cycle repeats itself through the night. On average, four cycles are needed for a good night's sleep. Toward morning, sleep is more shallow as brain waves speed up again, the heart rate increases, breathing is more rapid and you become more restless. You can seem about to wake and may even open your eyes, but in fact you are asleep.

Your biological clock

The natural sleep pattern is regulated by your biological clock, synchronized by the 24-hour, or circadian, cycle of light and dark. It oversees all body functions, from digestion and waste disposal to sleeping and cell repair.

One of the clock's influences is the so-called third eye, the pineal gland at the front of the brain. As daylight fades, the gland secretes the hormone melatonin into the bloodstream, which makes you sleepy. Melatonin works with another hormone, cortisol. The cortisol level falls

SLEEPING AND DREAMING

Scientists in sleep laboratories, use an electroencephalogram (EEG) to record the brain's electrical activity in volunteers. During dreaming, characterized by rapid eye movements (REM), the brain's activity is similar to that of when a person is awake.

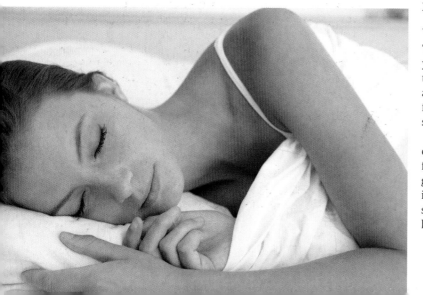

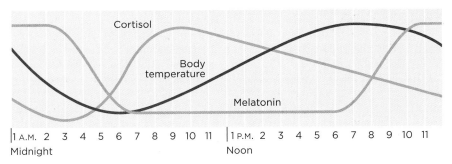

1 A.M. 2 3 4 5 6 7 8 9 10 11   1 P.M. 2 3 4 5 6 7 8 9 10 11
Midnight   Noon

CIRCADIAN RHYTHM
During a 24-hour period, the rise and fall of the hormones cortisol and melatonin tell you when to wake up and when you are tired and need sleep.

gradually and is at its lowest point after you've been asleep for several hours, when your body temperature is also low. At this stage the hypothalamus in the brain prompts the pituitary to direct the other endocrine glands into action to stimulate your metabolism. Your body temperature rises along with the cortisol level and eventually this wakes you up.

When rest is disturbed

If you suffer from sleep disturbance, the balance of these biological processes is upset. In many instances the effects are short term. Periods of sleeplessness occur during pregnancy, and parents may end up feeling exhausted after weeks or months of nighttime feedings after a child is born. Long-distance air travel across several time zones can also play havoc with the body's clock so that night and day lose their meaning.

When sleep disturbance is ongoing, it may need attention. Working mothers who don't get enough rest may be stressed from trying to balance the demands of career, home and children. The most common symptoms of lack of sleep are irritability and loss of concentration, which can have serious consequences. It is estimated that one in five car accidents is caused by sleepiness or sleep disorders, and people who work with machinery put themselves at risk. For safety, people who work night shifts have to establish a pattern that forces the body to adapt to sleeping by day.

Causes of insomnia

Most women experience a degree of sleep disturbance at some point in their lives, but you should consult your doctor if you can't remain asleep for an adequate length of time, and you do not wake feeling refreshed. This is known as insomnia and may be treated by drugs that establish good sleeping habits and reduce brain activity. Insomnia is not unusual at menopause and may also be a symptom of migraine, stress, anxiety or depression. For all of these, medical help should be sought.

Some people suffer from chronic insomnia–they are either unable to fall asleep or they fall asleep immediately after they put their heads on their pillows but wake not long after and stay that way for much of the night. This may have an effect on their metabolism, which relies on being stimulated in the hours before waking by deep breathing.

If your body is showing signs of oxygen starvation–rapid shallow breathing, interspersed with frequent sighing, yawning and erratic breathing rates–deep breathing exercises, to take in more oxygen, may help. Over time this type of shallow breathing results in exhaustion and emotional distress.

TIPS FOR A GOOD NIGHT'S SLEEP

- Try to keep to a regular bedtime routine, even on weekends. Aim to go to bed and get up at roughly the same time every day.
- Avoid stimulants such as coffee or tea several hours before bedtime. Have a warm, caffeine-free drink instead.
- Have your last meal several hours before retiring and avoid too much alcohol—this may help you fall asleep but causes restlessness later.
- Try some relaxation techniques. Have a warm bath, listen to restful music, or do gentle relaxation exercises, such as yoga or meditation.
- Make your bedroom conducive to rest and relaxation. The ideal temperature for sleep is 15–18°C (60–65°F). Make the room as dark as possible. This is important for shiftworkers who need to simulate night.
- Check that your bed is comfortable. Ideally, you should buy a new bed every 10 years. If you sleep with a partner, the bed should be big enough for you both to move easily without disturbing each other.
- If you can't get to sleep, don't lie there worrying about it. Get up and do something else until you feel tired enough to try again.

25

THE LOOK OF HEALTH

Too often women can be affected by negative thought structures. They might have picked up these thought patterns from their families as children, from the society they live in or from the media. Unfortunately, issues such as low self-

The healthiest people seem to be those who love, seek and create pleasure.

esteem and poor body image are common. Negative thought structures can spill over into behaviour patterns involved in parenting, relationships and work. Often women feel pressure to "be perfect". They may overextend themselves and cram too much into their daily lives, fearing failure if they can't do it all. Living up to the demands and expectations of being a girlfriend, wife, mother and working woman may force a woman to set impossibly high goals that are counterproductive to mental and physical health.

Be good to yourself

Researchers have found that being good to yourself has physical health benefits that show on the outside. The healthiest people seem to be those who love, seek and create pleasure. Positive moods and emotions delight the senses and directly affect the immune, cardiovascular and nervous systems. Taking time for yourself, seeking beautiful sights, delicious smells, melodious sounds, delectable tastes and

HOW DO YOU FEEL ABOUT YOUR BODY?
As we grow into women, too often the message seems to be that our worth depends on our looks. Self-acceptance provides better balance.

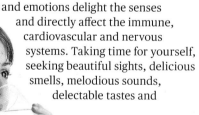

warm touch, enhances wellbeing and is self-nurturing.

This may be the first move you need to take if you feel you are being compromised mentally and physically by the way you are living. When you make the decision to embark on changes you have been considering for a while and discover how cheerful and well you feel, the benefits will start to show in many different ways. You will find you are thinking more clearly and are more optimistic. Self-nurturing is a positive step to reduce risks for illness.

You may not experience an overnight change to glowing skin and shining hair after starting a healthy eating and exercise programme. You can, however, be heartened by the fact that what you put into your body in terms of nutritious food and how actively you engage in strength- and stamina-promoting exercise will show up eventually. All changes take time.

Your determination to succeed will be helped by setting realistic and achievable goals. There are no miracle shortcuts. You need to work at losing weight or maintaining an ideal weight and the support of a personal trainer or group with similar interests will encourage you to get the best perspective and boost you if you are not progressing as well as you had hoped. Concentrate on what you have achieved, and not on your failures. Always try to make sure you get a good night's sleep and sensible rest periods between activities.

Invest in self-esteem

Self-confidence is undoubtedly an attractive quality to foster. It is possible to achieve confidence by committing yourself to a lifestyle in which you take time for your own pleasure (it doesn't have to be expensive or complicated, but should bring you joy). Don't base your sense of worth on other people's approval or gratitude. Don't feel you have to give in order to get praise. Remember not to think of yourself only as a caretaker of others. Finding time to care for yourself and to build your self-esteem also has a good effect on your physical health and wellbeing.

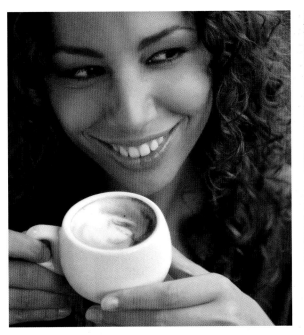

EXUBERANCE OF YOUTH

At this stage of your life, the world is your oyster—there are so many opportunities to seize and you have a positive view of your future development. Being surrounded by family and friends helps you to have a sense of your own individuality and worth.

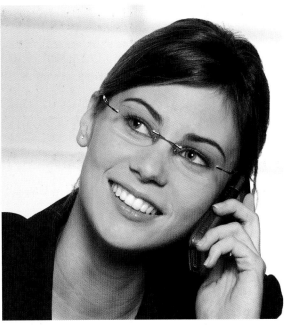

STRENGTH OF PURPOSE

Concentrating on career and burgeoning relationships can bring a sense of contentment with self. You are aware that things do not always turn out the way you had anticipated, but with this realization comes the ability to deal with unforeseen events.

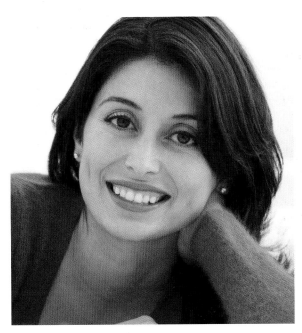

THE SURETY OF MATURITY

Growing confidence comes from knowing yourself and what you want to achieve, and the best ways to do it. If you find you are unable to choose or have difficulty in making decisions, it may be that you need to reassess your priorities.

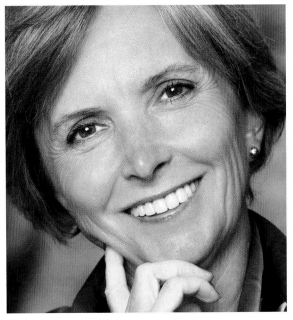

SUCCESSFUL CERTAINTY

Being happy with the age you are shows for all to see. It's not a matter of looking back or forwards but enjoying all the present offers. Accepting that changes can and do occur can help you cope with twinges of anxiety such changes can cause.

A SAFE PLACE TO WORK

People can suffer ill health or injury as a direct result of their jobs. Employers have a duty to ensure that the working conditions of all employees are compatible with their safety, health and wellbeing.

As women make up such a large part of the workforce and work in a wide variety of jobs, it is important that they

KNOW THE DANGERS
Wherever you work, you should be aware of anything that might be a hazard to your health. Substances that are dangerous should be labelled and well displayed for all to see.

know what the minimum requirements are. Workplaces are not all the same, and you should know what you should expect from yours, and what can be done if conditions are not satisfactory.

All parts of the working areas should be cleaned regularly, have good ventilation and be well lit. You should be provided with the correct equipment or furniture to carry out your work properly. There should be separate and easily accessible toilets for men and women (that should not lead directly from a workspace), with hand washing and drying facilities. Women should be provided with an efficient and hygienic way to dispose of sanitary protection. There should be a safe place for staff to keep personal belongings where they are secure against theft.

Buildings need not be old and run-down for working conditions to be poor. Sometimes the most modern and attractive working environment can have an inefficient ventilation system, and the lack of fresh air can cause headaches, respiratory conditions, sleep disturbance and other health problems.

Some types of work involve hazards that need specific rules. Many workplace accidents occur because employees have not been given proper training. Where there are dangerous substances involved, for example, labels should be large and clear–easily recognizable by the words "irritant", "corrosive", "toxic" or "poisonous". You should receive proper instructions about these substances, including immediate action that should be taken if you come into contact with one or if fumes are escaping into the work area.

An employer should routinely carry out an assessment of such substances, making sure they are not putting anyone at risk. People working in laboratories or as cleaners or caretakers are particularly vulnerable, but any member of staff can accidentally touch or inhale a substance that has not been stored securely or labelled correctly.

Some potentially harmful substances are not so obvious, and protective clothing and/or masks may be needed. In a garment factory, the large amount of fluff and dust in the air may get into your lungs; or working with paper and inks can result in cuts and irritated skin. People working with flowers can get rashes from pesticides and from the plants themselves.

Take a break

Regular breaks are necessary for those whose work involves repetitive hand and arm movements in order to prevent the development of serious upper limb disorders. These disorders commonly occur in a wide range of occupations (food and clothing production, assembly-line manufacturing, hairdressing, cleaning and using computers) and account for a large percentage of occupational poor health in women, who are mostly employed in these jobs. Constant pressure to meet tight deadlines, lack of regular breaks and badly designed seating and equipment can all adversely affect the body.

Short, frequent breaks–5 to 10 minutes every hour or so–are better than longer, occasional breaks. These breaks are most effective if you can walk away from your immediate workspace to refresh yourself. Getting some fresh air into your lungs during the course of the day–a brisk walk during the lunch break, for example–is the best antidote to workplace air.

If you experience any pain, swelling, pins and needles or numbness in the arms or legs, you should report it immediately to your supervisor or employer so that action can be taken to find out what is wrong.

Speak out

Whether it is about pregnancy or another issue, you may not be aware of your rights and may feel daunted about approaching your employer to discuss it. Talking problems over with colleagues and then speaking to your manager could be the best solution. If this worries you, you could ask a human resources or union representative to speak to the employer on your behalf. Another option might be to investigate assertiveness training in order to learn how to more effectively articulate your point of view.

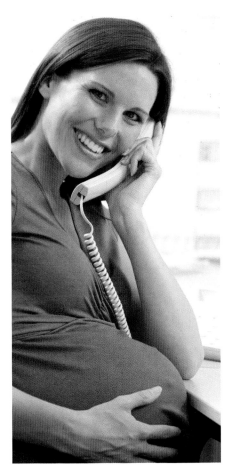

WORK WHILE YOU WAIT
In some types of employment, work that is normally safe may become hazardous if you are pregnant. You should express your concerns and see if you can move to a safer job within the company for the duration of the pregnancy.

Safe working at a screen

- Make sure your desk is at the correct and comfortable height for you.
- You should have an adjustable and stable chair, preferably with a footrest.
- You need sufficient space in front of the keyboard to provide support for hands.
- There should be enough space for you to change position and vary your movements.
- Your desk should be large enough to accommodate all the documents you are working from.
- The screen should not have light shining on it directly. It should be adjustable so you can move it. Your neck and shoulders should not be under stress.
- The screen should be fitted with an anti-glare surface.
- Blink as often as possible to prevent your eyes from becoming dry; alternatively, use eyedrops to moisten them.

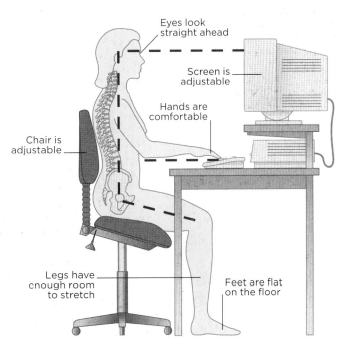

Eyes look straight ahead

Screen is adjustable

Hands are comfortable

Chair is adjustable

Legs have enough room to stretch

Feet are flat on the floor

TYPES OF BONES

There are five types of bones in the human body:

Long bones, such as the femur, are much greater in length than width.

Short bones, such as the wrist bones, are cuboid and sited where extra strength is required.

Flat bones, such as those in the skull, are thin and slightly curved.

Irregular bones, such as the vertebrae, do not fit into any of the above categories. Their shape is non-uniform and complicated.

Sesamoid bones, such as the patella (kneecap), are embedded in tendons to increase the force of the attached muscle.

Bodyworks

Understanding the basics of the mechanisms that keep your body functioning and on the move can help you to be alert to changes that may signal the need for help.

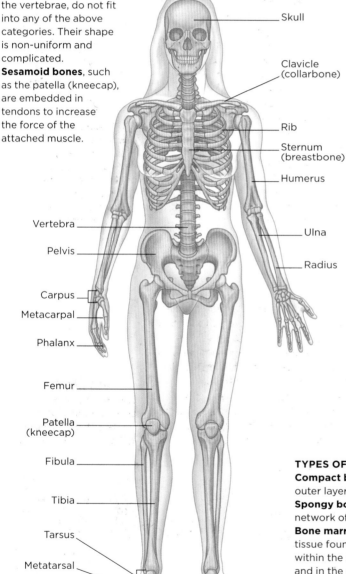

- Skull
- Clavicle (collarbone)
- Rib
- Sternum (breastbone)
- Humerus
- Ulna
- Radius
- Vertebra
- Pelvis
- Carpus
- Metacarpal
- Phalanx
- Femur
- Patella (kneecap)
- Fibula
- Tibia
- Tarsus
- Metatarsal
- Phalanx

THE SKELETAL SYSTEM

There are more than 200 bones in the body's skeletal system, which supports and shapes the body, protects organs and provides mobility.

The bones are connected to about 600 muscles and meet in joints that are held together by ligaments. Exercise is important to maintain healthy bones and strengthen ligaments. Women experience unique skeletal changes at certain times, such as during pregnancy when hormonal fluctuations result in ligaments and joints softening in preparation for childbirth.

How bones form

Bones form the framework of the skeleton. The other important function of our bones is to store minerals such as calcium, phosphate and sodium and to release them into the body as needed. This constant activity within bones results in bone breakdown and

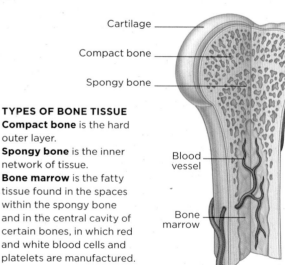

- Cartilage
- Compact bone
- Spongy bone
- Blood vessel
- Bone marrow

TYPES OF BONE TISSUE

Compact bone is the hard outer layer.

Spongy bone is the inner network of tissue.

Bone marrow is the fatty tissue found in the spaces within the spongy bone and in the central cavity of certain bones, in which red and white blood cells and platelets are manufactured.

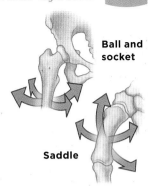

rebuilding, which is called bone turnover. It's a continuous process and is particularly important around puberty, when hormones stimulate the mix of protein (collagen) and minerals to strengthen and thicken the bones.

By the age of 25, bone has reached its maximum length. Cartilage makes up the ends of long bones and occurs at the ends of weight-bearing bones in joints and between vertebrae in the spine, where it acts as a shock absorber. Cartilage is also responsible for nose shape, the ears and the trachea.

Bone turnover continues to increase until you are in your 30s, after which it declines gradually. The fastest decline is in the five years after menopause, because of oestrogen loss, and continues into advanced age. By 70, bone turnover leads to gradual progressive bone loss known as decreased bone density.

Bones are hard on the outside and covered by a fibrous membrane called periosteum; inside they are soft and spongy. Bone tissue consists of minerals, collagen, blood vessels and nerve endings. The centre of the bone is filled with red or yellow bone marrow. Red

bone marrow manufactures red blood cells. Yellow bone marrow is primarily made of fat. In adults, red blood cell production–about 200 billion cells a day–takes place in the spine, breastbone (sternum), ribs, collarbones, hip bones and skull bones.

What can go wrong

The human skeletal system has to work hard to meet all the demands made upon it. The weight-bearing joints–the spine, hips and knees–are the most vulnerable. Osteoarthritis–long-term damage to the cartilage-covered surface of the joints–is common in older people as a result of wear and tear; it affects twice as many women as men. All bones are susceptible to fractures if they are twisted or have excessive strain placed on them. Frequent fractures may indicate bones are more fragile than normal.

Osteoporosis, in which the total bone mass is reduced and the bones become brittle making them susceptible to fracture, is the most common bone disorder affecting women. Preventive measures such as regular weight-bearing exercise can minimize bone loss.

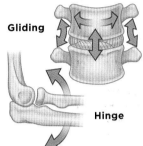

TYPES OF JOINTS
Ball and socket In the shoulders and hips.
Saddle In the thumbs.
Gliding In the spine, wrists and ankles.
Hinge In the elbows, fingers and toes.

Muscle power

Bones depend on attached muscles, which make up 30–40 per cent of the weight of a woman's body. It may take 20 or 30 muscles working together to move you around, yet keep you balanced. The muscles lift and rotate bones, enabling you to carry out actions such as pulling, pushing, squeezing, stretching, walking, running and jumping. They work as opposing pairs, one known as an agonist the other as an antagonist—as one contracts, the other relaxes automatically under the direction of the brain. Only when learning new physical skills or starting a new exercise programme do you become aware of the complex coordination of this partnership. The skeletal muscles—in the legs, arms, neck, chest and face—are joined to bones by tendons, bands of tough,

elastic protein fibres called collagen. Ligaments are also made of collagen and support the joints. Muscles have their own fuel store, which is used to power increased physical effort. The more you exercise, the more the muscles call for oxygen and blood glucose. Actions of skeletal muscles, heart, liver and brain use about 70 per cent of your total energy.

WORKING IN PAIRS
To raise your arm, the biceps contracts and the triceps relaxes; to lower it, the process is reversed.

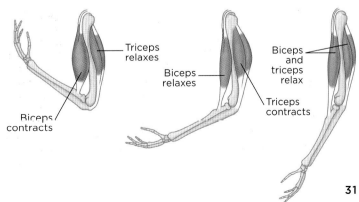

Triceps relaxes
Biceps relaxes
Biceps contracts
Biceps and triceps relax
Triceps contracts

YOUR COMMUNICATIONS NETWORK

The brain and spinal cord are the main parts of the central nervous system. Pairs of nerves branch from both cord and brain leading to every crevice of the body. The cerebrum is the largest part of the brain and has connections with all parts of the body. Beneath it, the cerebellum facilitates precise muscle movement and balance.

THE NERVOUS SYSTEM

There are numerous pathways by which information travels from different parts of the body to the brain. This communication and command network—the nervous system—is essential for the regulation of breathing, digestion, sensations and emotions.

The central nervous system consists of the brain and the spinal cord. Muscular movements, both conscious and unconscious, are controlled from the brain, which sends and receives messages via the spinal cord. The brain is the learning centre in which memory and decision making operate. The central nervous system also mediates your senses of touch, sight, taste, smell and hearing. Through your eyes, ears, nose, tongue and skin sensitivity, it controls your balance, ability to judge distance and to feel pain, pressure and cold. Such sensations are conveyed by sensory nerves to the brain, which instructs the motor nerves by electrical signals to enable the body to react appropriately. The left side of the brain usually controls the right side of the body and vice versa.

The peripheral nervous system consists of 12 pairs of nerves originating in the brain and 31 pairs coming from the spinal cord. These connect the central nervous system with all other parts of the body. The peripheral system includes the autonomic nervous system, which controls the body's unconscious functions, such as the heart and the digestion. This system has two sets of nerves—sympathetic, which works while you are active, and parasympathetic, which takes charge when you are at rest. This system helps the body to respond to emergencies and increased activity.

Each individual nerve consists of a bundle of nerve cells, called neurons, with long branch-like extensions along which impulses or signals travel fast. The impulses travel through sensory neurons, which carry information from the sense organs to the brain and spinal cord. Impulses can also travel through motor neurons, which carry messages from the brain to muscles and glands. Neurotransmitters are chemicals that carry the signal across the synapse—the gap between the sending neuron and the receiving neuron or muscle. Each neuron is protected by a sheath, which, if damaged, disrupts the message network and affects the body's functions.

What can go wrong?

A common neurological disorder is dementia, which largely happens in advanced age, and is a feature of both Parkinson's and Alzheimer's diseases. Stroke occurs when the blood supply to the brain is cut off by a blocked artery, and the body systems controlled by the damaged area are impaired. In multiple sclerosis (MS) the protective sheath of the nerves is damaged, resulting in visual or mobility problems. Women are twice as susceptible to MS as men. Motor neuron disease is a rare disorder in which the motor neurons become damaged. In the spinal cord, nerves can become trapped between vertebrae. In sciatica, acute pain in the buttocks that radiates down the sides of the legs is caused by pressure on the sciatic nerve.

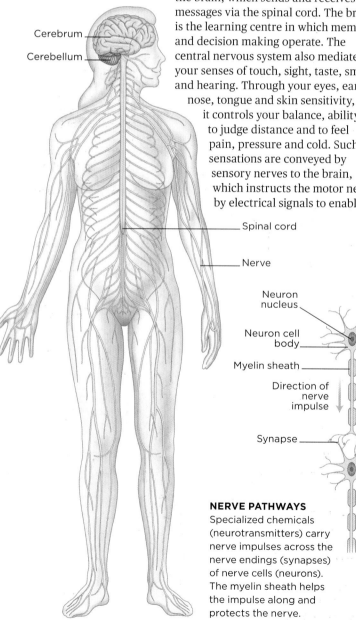

Cerebrum

Cerebellum

Spinal cord

Nerve

Neuron nucleus

Neuron cell body

Myelin sheath

Direction of nerve impulse

Synapse

NERVE PATHWAYS

Specialized chemicals (neurotransmitters) carry nerve impulses across the nerve endings (synapses) of nerve cells (neurons). The myelin sheath helps the impulse along and protects the nerve.

THE ENDOCRINE SYSTEM

In the endocrine system, glands produce the hormones, which are chemical substances that travel through the blood and regulate various functions of your body. Glands are located in various places throughout the body. There are two main kinds of gland: endocrine glands that release secretions into the blood and exocrine glands that discharge secretions into small ducts.

The major endocrine glands are the thyroid, parathyroids, pancreas, adrenals and gonads (sex glands: the ovaries in women, testes in men). The hormones help the body to respond to stress, regulate processes by which the body changes food into energy, and carry messages that maintain the organ's activities. They are crucial for the correct functioning of every body cell and play a central role during growth, development and reproduction.

The major exocrine glands include sweat glands, which secrete fluids that help cool the skin, and sebaceous glands, which secrete sebum to lubricate skin and hair.

The endocrine system is governed by the hypothalamus in the centre of the brain via hormones that it produces, although it is not in itself a gland. The hypothalamus is vital to factors such as sleeping and waking, temperature regulation, stress and excitement.

The pituitary gland is the master gland and measures no larger than the size of a pea. This gland has an anterior and posterior lobe and is also controlled by the hypothalamus. Hormones flow from the hypothalamus to the pituitary, which then stimulates or represses hormone production in the other major glands according to the body's needs.

What can affect it?

Pituitary hormones oversee growth rates, bone growth, sexual development (the ovaries and testes make increased levels of sex hormones at puberty) and fluid levels within the body. The butterfly-shaped thyroid gland is positioned across the voice box in the throat. Thyroxine, which is secreted by this gland, governs energy levels and your metabolic rate. Next to the thyroid are the parathyroid glands. These glands secrete parathyroid hormone, which regulates the correct balance of calcium and phosphorus in the blood to build strong bones.

Lying on top of the kidneys are the adrenal glands, which are responsible for sex hormones and helping the body adjust to stress. They secrete adrenaline (also called epinephrine), which is the hormone that has a direct effect on blood pressure, heart rate, the lungs and digestive system. They also secrete androgens, which are the male hormones that stimulate the development of sexual characteristics. Other important hormones are secreted by cells within the kidney. These include renin, which helps to control blood pressure, and erythropoietin, which stimulates production of red blood cells in bone marrow.

The pancreas, a long, thin gland lying behind the stomach, makes the hormones insulin and glucagon, which work together to keep blood sugar levels balanced. Insulin is produced after you have eaten to help the cells absorb glucose (made from carbohydrates and sometimes fats); it is this function that is impaired in diabetes. Any excess glucose is converted to glycogen for storage in the liver and muscles. When the blood sugar level starts to fall, glucagon stimulates the liver to convert the glycogen back into glucose to bring the levels back to normal.

Some other hormones, such as prostaglandins, are made by tissues and body fluids in response to local trauma to help control inflammation, fever, circulatory disorders and stomach secretions, for example.

KEY PLAYERS
The major endocrine glands—the thyroid, parathyroids, adrenals, pancreas and ovaries—are under the control of the pituitary gland in the brain. The hypothalamus is the link between the nervous and endocrine systems and triggers the pituitary gland.

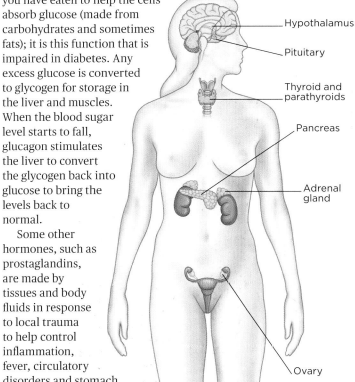

Hypothalamus

Pituitary

Thyroid and parathyroids

Pancreas

Adrenal gland

Ovary

THE CIRCULATORY SYSTEM

Blood delivers oxygen and nutrients to– and removes waste from–all your organs and tissues. The average healthy adult woman has about 4 l (9 pints) constantly circulating throughout the body.

Blood consists of solids and plasma. The plasma is the straw-coloured liquid that is made up primarily of water but contains proteins that enable blood to clot and fight infections. The plasma carries hormones that control growth and bodily functions. The solid component includes three types of cells: red blood cells, white blood cells and platelets.

Red blood cells are responsible for the transport of oxygen to body tissues and the removal of waste matter–carbon dioxide (CO_2), lactic acid–to organs to be excreted. White blood cells help to fight infections and defend the body by producing antibodies against harmful substances that may invade it. Platelets, or thrombocytes, work by plugging leaks in the blood vessels and begin the process leading to the formation of a blood clot.

There are two blood circulation systems. The systemic blood system carries oxygenated blood from the heart to the organs and limbs and deoxygenated blood back to the heart. The pulmonary system is a loop

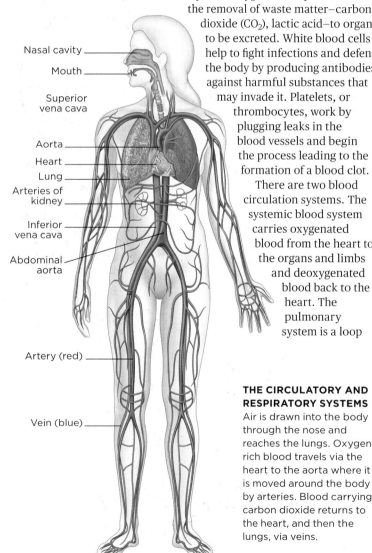

Nasal cavity
Mouth
Superior vena cava
Aorta
Heart
Lung
Arteries of kidney
Inferior vena cava
Abdominal aorta
Artery (red)
Vein (blue)

THE CIRCULATORY AND RESPIRATORY SYSTEMS
Air is drawn into the body through the nose and reaches the lungs. Oxygen-rich blood travels via the heart to the aorta where it is moved around the body by arteries. Blood carrying carbon dioxide returns to the heart, and then the lungs, via veins.

from heart to lungs and back. Bright, scarlet blood is oxygen rich; the darker red it is, the less oxygen it is carrying.

How it works

The power behind the system is the heart, a pump about the size of a clenched fist that sits in the lower chest, left of centre. When the muscular heart wall contracts, deoxygenated blood is sent from the right side into the lungs where its tiny capillaries surround small air sacs called alveoli.

Carbon dioxide moves from the blood to the alveoli. It is then expelled from the body during breathing. Oxygen is picked up by haemoglobin in the red blood cells; it is the oxyhaemoglobin molecule that makes blood bright red. The oxygenated blood returns to the left atrium of the heart, which contracts to pump it into the ventricle; blood is then pumped into the aorta and from there to arteries and smaller vessels supplying organs in the rest of the body.

Arteries have elastic walls, and expand and contract according to changes in the volume of blood. This is the "pulse" you can feel in any artery close to the surface of the body.

Branching off are the smallest blood vessels, the capillaries, which take oxygen to the tissues. Blood laden with waste carbon dioxide enters very small veins, then larger veins as it returns– mostly "uphill"–to the heart. The two main veins are called superior vena cava (brings blood from the head and arms) and inferior vena cava (carries blood from the main part of the body and the legs). Muscles squeeze the thin-walled veins to force the blood on and up, and valves open and shut en route to prevent it flowing back. The entire systemic circuit takes in the region of half a minute to complete.

Blood tests are widely used to diagnose many disorders and infections. A blood sample can be obtained by a needle into a vein on the inner side of the elbow and can provide information about levels of hormones, blood sugar, salts or drugs. Specific blood tests can also provide information about microorganisms such as bacteria and viruses that may be invading the blood.

THE RESPIRATORY SYSTEM

Providing the body with life-giving oxygen to maintain the health and efficient functioning of all organs and cells is the main purpose of the respiratory system. It is also designed to eliminate carbon dioxide, a gas produced when cells use oxygen.

An adult woman at rest needs about 6 l (13 pints) of air a minute. During aerobic exercise, almost six times that amount is needed. The respiratory system is divided into two tracts. The upper tract includes the nose, sinuses, mouth and pharynx (the cavity behind the nose and mouth). The lower tract consists of the larynx (voice box), trachea (windpipe), bronchi (airways) and lungs. The lungs are not identical– the right has three lobes, the left two– but they perform the same function.

The process of breathing consists of inspiration (breathing in) and expiration (breathing out). Inspiration requires taking air from the atmosphere and moving it into the lungs. The diaphragm and chest wall muscles are required to help the process of inspiration by lifting the ribs and widening the chest cavity to expand the lungs. Expiration is the process where the lungs retract, the diaphragm and chest muscles relax and CO_2 is expelled.

Every time you breathe in through your nose or mouth, the upper respiratory tract filters, warms and humidifies the fresh air. From the trachea, the air enters either the right or left bronchus and goes into the corresponding lung. The airways divide into bronchioles (ever-finer branches), the finest of which end in alveoli. These little air sacs within the lungs take oxygen from the inhaled air and convey it into the bloodstream. At the same time, carbon dioxide is transferred from the blood to the alveoli to be exhaled along with some water vapour. There are about 350 million alveoli in each lung, and the total area available for exchange of gases is about 5.4 sq m (600 sq ft).

The lungs are surrounded by a continuous membrane called the visceral pleura and the chest cavity is lined with a similar membrane called the parietal pleura. The narrow space in between is filled with moisture, which, as the lungs move with each breath, provides the necessary lubrication.

The air you breathe is packed with minute particles such as smoke, dust and other environmental toxins that can cause health problems. The respiratory tract has impressive defence mechanisms to combat such invasions–many of the immune system cells are located here. Some of these cells envelop and destroy incoming bacteria or viruses; others manufacture antibodies, which are secreted into the mucous lining of the respiratory tract and provide a continuous wash through it. The mucus also contains other substances that can deactivate or kill bacteria and viruses.

Why you cough

Another protective mechanism is provided by the cilia. These are numerous very fine hairs that line the airways and move in waves to push the mucus, including particles that it may have trapped, up from the bronchioles. The coughing reflex is activated to force secretions and any inhaled particles out of the lungs. Smokers produce more sputum because of inflammation of the airways and therefore cough more.

GAS EXCHANGE

Oxygen passes from the air into the bloodstream through the very thin walls of the alveoli. Carbon dioxide is expelled from the body by means of the same mechanism in reverse.

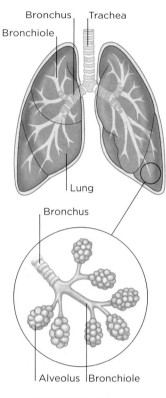

Bronchus · Trachea
Bronchiole
Lung
Bronchus
Alveolus · Bronchiole

THE TREE OF LIFE
The trachea branches into two bronchi, each of which leads to a lung. Each bronchus divides further into bronchioles, which end in air sacs (alveoli).

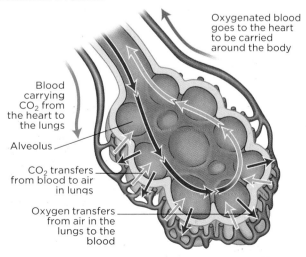

Oxygenated blood goes to the heart to be carried around the body

Blood carrying CO_2 from the heart to the lungs

Alveolus

CO_2 transfers from blood to air in lungs

Oxygen transfers from air in the lungs to the blood

THE DIGESTIVE SYSTEM

All the food and drink you consume is broken down by the digestive system into smaller particles that can be distributed into the bloodstream to nourish all parts of the human body. The process of digestion takes place in a long muscular tube called the alimentary canal, which runs all the way from the mouth to the rectum.

The first stage of the food's journey occurs with chewing, which is very important to good digestion. As the food is chewed, it is mixed with saliva and other digestive juices, which contain enzymes that help to moisten the food and start breaking it down.

The chewed food is swallowed and passes through the oesophagus into the stomach. The process by which the food travels down the oesophagus and stomach is known as peristalsis (contraction of strong muscles in the walls of the oesophagus and stomach). Glands within the lining of the stomach manufacture digestive juices known as gastric juice—a mixture of hydrochloric acid and digestive enzymes—which, combined with churning movements of the muscular stomach, breaks food down to a pulp, much as a food mixer does.

It is at this stage that some medications (for example, aspirin and anti-inflammatory drugs) and water are drawn through the stomach walls. The food that has been churned and partly digested forms a thick liquid called chyme; it passes into the duodenum at intervals when the pyloric valve at the base of the stomach opens. The valve only allows a certain amount through before shutting again.

The duodenum—the first part of the small intestine—contains bile, which is manufactured in the liver and stored in the gall bladder. It also receives enzymes from the pancreas that digest proteins (changing them into amino acids), fats (which are broken down by bile) and carbohydrates. Some nutrients are taken straight into the bloodstream through the duodenum walls, while the rest moves on to the next section, the jejunum, then to the ileum.

The hepatic portal vein brings nutrient-rich, oxygen-poor blood from the intestines to the liver. Here glucose is extracted, converted to glycogen and stored for use as energy. The liver breaks down drugs, toxins, poisons and pollutants and produces pigments from old red blood cells, which give colour to bile, urine and bowel movements. It also stores vitamins A, D, K and B_{12}, makes lipoproteins and cholesterol and helps to make vitamin A from betacarotene. Any amino acids not required are changed into urea to leave the body in urine.

The intestines

The large intestine is primarily for storage of waste food products and absorbing water and minerals. The waste material cannot be digested in the body and accumulates as roughage, which becomes faeces and is eliminated from the body via the anus.

The intestinal bacteria perform a useful function in synthesizing vitamins K and B_{12}, but a side effect of their activity is the production of gas.

THE DIGESTION
The process of digestion begins in the mouth. A ball of chewed food travels down the oesophagus and into the stomach. It passes through the small intestine and into the large intestine, where further breakdown occurs. Eventually waste products reach the rectum. This journey can take as long as 24 hours.

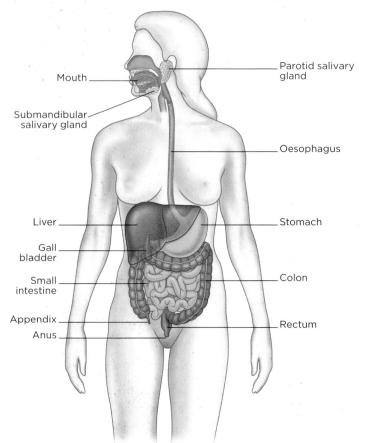

Mouth

Submandibular salivary gland

Parotid salivary gland

Oesophagus

Liver

Gall bladder

Small intestine

Appendix

Anus

Stomach

Colon

Rectum

THE URINARY SYSTEM

About 70 per cent of your body weight is water, and the urinary system plays an important part in keeping the balance right while getting rid of soluble waste.

It is designed to safeguard the health of the blood and to ensure the consistency of the body's water balance, its temperature, acidity and alkalinity. Crucial to this function are the kidneys, two bean-shaped organs behind the lower part of the rib cage. They are like fine sieves through which all the body's blood passes many times a day to remove toxins and maintain the correct volume and chemical composition of the blood.

The kidneys process about 8 l (14 pints) of fluid an hour. Only about 1 per cent becomes urine and the rest–salts, glucose and minerals–returns to the circulation. Urine is almost all water but a little heavier than water. Urine is normally amber coloured and slightly acidic. Only 4 per cent is waste such as urea–a product of the breakdown of protein–that gives urine its colour.

Urine travels through the ureters, which descend from each kidney, to the bladder for temporary storage. The bladder's wall stretches to hold about 700 ml (1¼ pints) of urine until it is expelled through the urethra. Up to 2 l (3½ pints) of urine are passed in 24 hours, but this amount can vary.

The condition of the urine can be a marker or sign of good health. For example, sugar in the urine can alert your doctor to diabetes. Concentrated or less urine production can be a sign of dehydration. Dehydration can occur as a result of insufficient fluid intake, exercising, heat, sweating, caffeinated drinks, alcoholic beverages or drugs.

Thirst is a late warning sign that the body, and the blood in particular, is lacking water for its needs. The body has only to be 10 per cent dehydrated for the pulse rate to increase and blood pressure to fall. To maintain blood pressure, the kidneys respond to an instruction from a pituitary hormone (known as anti-diuretic hormone, which controls the amount of water held by the nephrons–tiny kidney tubes) and reabsorb water rather than releasing it as urine.

THIRST IS A WARNING
When you find yourself needing to drink water, it is a very late response to the body's needs. When the body senses a lack of water, it rations what is available for essential parts (such as the blood and brain), so skin, hair and the urinary system suffer.

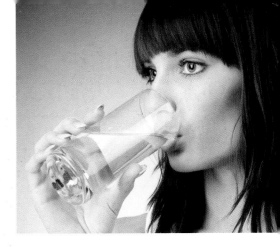

Urinary problems

The shortness of the female urethra and its position close to the anus cause several urogenital conditions, such as infection of the urethra (urethritis) or of the bladder (cystitis).

When a woman is pregnant, she has more fluid in her body and urinates more often. The hormone relaxin, which prepares the body for birth, relaxes the bladder and pelvic muscles. As the uterus enlarges, it presses on the bladder, and frequency of urination increases.

Later in life, urinary incontinence affects at least 15 per cent of women living independently. Incontinence is much more common in females than males. Reasons for this include infection, smaller bladder capacity, early bladder muscle contractions or decreased ability to suppress bladder muscle contractions.

THE URINARY SYSTEM
The kidneys are the body's filters and remove excess fluid and waste materials from the blood. This passes, as urine, into the ureter and then into the bladder, where it can be stored. From the bladder, urine passes into the urethra and out of the body during urination. The process is not under conscious control until the urine reaches the external urethral sphincter—a ring of muscle that can contract to hold back urine.

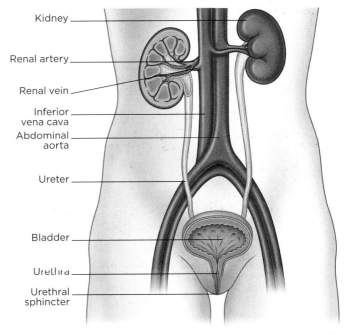

Kidney

Renal artery

Renal vein

Inferior vena cava

Abdominal aorta

Ureter

Bladder

Urethra

Urethral sphincter

THE REPRODUCTIVE SYSTEM

A woman's reproductive system consists of organs located within the pelvis, mainly internally. Male and female reproductive systems differ in shape and structure. Together the systems are designed to produce, nourish and transport the eggs and sperm.

In women, the reproductive system is made up of external and internal organs. The external organs include the vulva and clitoris. The internal organs include

Each month a healthy woman has a 25 per cent chance of conceiving.

the vagina, the uterus (womb) and two ovaries that are connected by fallopian tubes on either side of the uterus. They lie in the abdominal cavity, partly covered by the peritoneum–the lining of the abdomen–and are held in place by the pelvic floor muscles.

The uterus is a hollow, thick-walled muscular sac with a specialized lining (endometrium), which is able to receive and nurture a fertilized egg. Before a woman becomes pregnant for the first time, the uterus is about the size and shape of a pear. Usually, it tilts slightly forwards, but in some women it may tilt slightly backwards (known as

retroverted). The ligaments attached to the uterus allow it to shift a little as the rectum and bladder empty and fill.

On each side of the uterus is a walnut-sized ovary. From the beginning of her life, a woman carries a store of many thousands of immature eggs (oocytes) in the ovaries. During the reproductive years, only about 400 of them will be released and ripen under the influence of luteinizing hormone and follicle-stimulating hormone.

Eggs are produced as part of the monthly process called the menstrual cycle, which begins during puberty. Each month changes occur that prepare the reproductive system for fertilization and pregnancy. The process of ovulation involves at least one egg (ovum) that will grow and begin to mature each month. The fully developed mature egg is released from the ovary at about the midpoint of the menstrual cycle. The egg travels down the 10-cm- (4-inch-) long fallopian tube by means of wave-like contractions of the muscles and hair-like structures called cilia to the uterus where the lining has been prepared to nurture it. If the egg isn't fertilized by a sperm in the fallopian tube–thus becoming an embryo–the lining is shed 14 days after ovulation in the form of menstrual blood.

The first period at puberty is the menarche (pronounced menarkey). The menopause is the end of reproductive years and is usually defined as 12 consecutive months without

A WOMAN'S LIFE CYCLES
The monthly menstrual cycle begins at age 12, on average. It lasts about 28 days and ovulation—release of an egg—occurs on day 14. On average the monthly cycle for women continues for 38 years until the age of 52 (excluding the months of pregnancy). Changes in the levels and activity of the female hormones vary according to the menstrual cycle, pregnancy and breastfeeding.

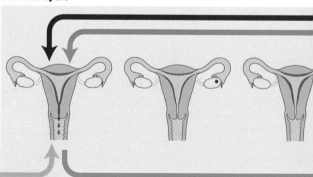

Pre-puberty

Eggs are present, but will only be released when the hormones start the monthly cycle at puberty.

Normal cycle

Menstruation is the monthly shedding of the uterus lining, the endometrium.

Each month at least one egg develops in an ovary, a process called ripening.

Ovulation occur when an egg is released and tra to the uterus.

menstruation. The average age of menopause is 52 years. Perimenopause is defined as the time when the menstrual cycles starts to become increasingly irregular and the onset of symptoms such as hot flushes.

The neck of the uterus (the cervix), is narrow and leads to the vagina, a thin-walled, muscular tube about 7.5-10 cm (3-4 inches) long, between the bladder and the rectum. It provides the entrance for sperm and is the passageway through which a baby is born and through which menstrual blood leaves.

The vagina stretches considerably during sexual intercourse and childbirth. In a virgin it is covered by the hymen, a membrane that may bleed when ruptured during first sexual intercourse.

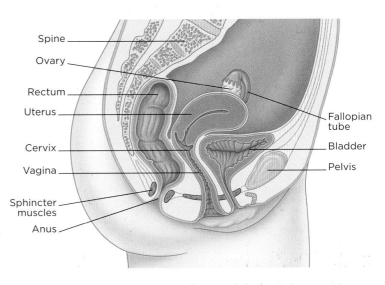

A woman's genitals

The external genitalia (the vulva) covers the opening to the narrow canal called the vagina. The vulva is made up of the labia majora, which are two large folds of skin, shaped like lips and primarily made up of fatty tissue. The vulva is covered with pubic hair. Protecting the entrance to the vagina are the labia minora: delicate, less fatty folds of skin, which become more prominent as a woman ages and fatty tissue decreases. Glands around the vaginal opening release mucus to keep the vagina moist and lubricated so that it can easily accommodate the penis.

The clitoris is a small protruding structure–the female equivalent of the penis–which mainly consists of erectile tissue (as do the nipples). It is highly sensitive to the touch and becomes swollen with blood when a woman is sexually aroused.

A woman is usually at her most fertile in her late 20s. For fertilization to take place, sperm travelling upwards from the cervix must make contact with the egg in the fallopian tube within 24 hours of its release from the ovary. Each month, a healthy woman has a 25 per cent chance of conceiving a child. Most women who want to do so will conceive naturally within a year of trying. If they do not, they can be referred to an infertility specialist by their doctor to investigate potential causes for infertility.

A WOMAN'S BODY

The reproductive system is almost entirely inside the body, where it is protected. Two ovaries, which store and alternately release eggs for fertilization, are situated at the ends of the fallopian tubes. The tubes lead to the uterus (womb). The neck of the womb, or cervix, connects the uterus to the vagina, which is where semen (carrying sperm) enters the body. If an egg has been released and conditions are right, fertilization takes place in a fallopian tube.

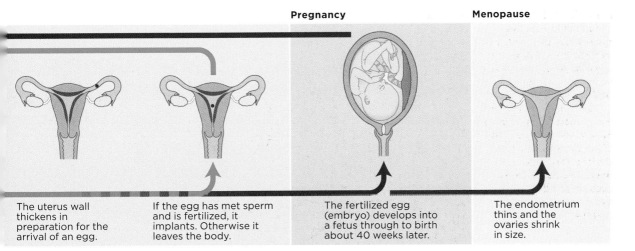

Pregnancy   **Menopause**

The uterus wall thickens in preparation for the arrival of an egg.

If the egg has met sperm and is fertilized, it implants. Otherwise it leaves the body.

The fertilized egg (embryo) develops into a fetus through to birth about 40 weeks later.

The endometrium thins and the ovaries shrink in size.

THE IMMUNE SYSTEM

The immune system defends the body against diseases, infections and harmful organisms that are potentially damaging to the body. The system is an intricate network of cells, molecules and tissues that work together to resist these harmful invaders.

Immunity is the body's ability to resist infection while protecting healthy tissues. The many components of the immune system include physical barriers, such as the skin and mucus in the throat, and chemical barriers, such as enzymes in saliva and acid in the stomach. Phagocytes, a type of white blood cell, also defend the body by engulfing and digesting infectious microorganisms. Immunity is also provided by the lymphatic system, a network of vessels (lymphatics) and filters (lymph nodes) that transports lymph–a watery liquid that begins as fluid flowing between cells.

Lymph fluid is similar to blood but it has no red cells. All body tissue, except the brain and heart, is bathed by lymph. It is not pumped, but circulates when lymph vessels are squeezed by surrounding muscles during movement.

Along the lymphatics are small bean-shaped nodes that contain leucocytes (white cells). One sort, the lymphocytes, recognize foreign matter (antigens) and produce antibodies (immunoglobulins), which in turn stimulate another sort, the phagocytes, to engulf and destroy the invaders. The nodes are concentrated in certain areas–the neck, armpits and groin, and in the deeper tissue around the lungs and liver.

When the body is fighting a bacterial infection, the lymph nodes swell. Swollen glands in the neck, under the arms and in the groin are the most telling sign that your body is fighting an infection. The antibodies are also passed into the blood to be transported around the body to provide future immunity.

LYMPHATIC SYSTEM

Part of the body's defences, the lymphatic system comprises a network of vessels, which transport 1–2 l (2–4 pints) of lymph around the body, and lymph glands, which filter the fluid. Lymphoid organs include the thymus gland and the spleen.

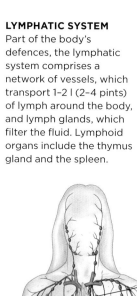

Thymus gland—helps immunity from birth

Minor lymphatic vessel

Major lymphatic vessel

Spleen—filters foreign bodies from blood

Lymph node

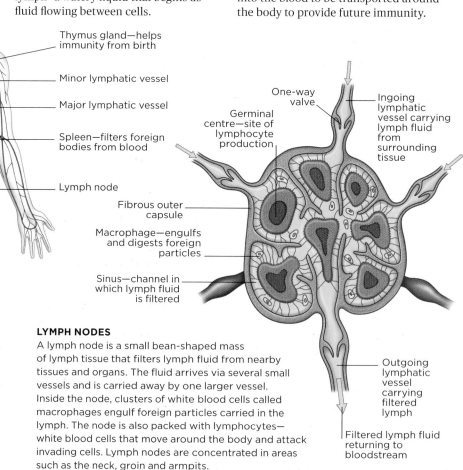

One-way valve

Germinal centre—site of lymphocyte production

Ingoing lymphatic vessel carrying lymph fluid from surrounding tissue

Fibrous outer capsule

Macrophage—engulfs and digests foreign particles

Sinus—channel in which lymph fluid is filtered

Outgoing lymphatic vessel carrying filtered lymph

Filtered lymph fluid returning to bloodstream

LYMPH NODES

A lymph node is a small bean-shaped mass of lymph tissue that filters lymph fluid from nearby tissues and organs. The fluid arrives via several small vessels and is carried away by one larger vessel. Inside the node, clusters of white blood cells called macrophages engulf foreign particles carried in the lymph. The node is also packed with lymphocytes— white blood cells that move around the body and attack invading cells. Lymph nodes are concentrated in areas such as the neck, groin and armpits.

IMMUNE RESPONSES

Certain lymphocytes called T-cells are the fighting force of the immune system—their actions are known as cellular immunity. They do not produce antibodies but stimulate B-cells and macrophages. Some T-cells are killers; others are helpers, suppressors or memory aids. Memory T-cells act as a regulatory mechanism by "remembering" invaders and ensuring that the body's own cells are not threatened. T-cells come from the bone marrow and proliferate in response to antigens in the lymph nodes.

B-cells produce the primary immune response, in which antibodies are produced against an invading microorganism—the antibody immune response. The antibodies produced are carried around the body in the blood and lymph to sites of infection, where they attach to and destroy the antigens with the help of T-cells. The body can make a huge number of different antibodies, each of which targets a different antigen.

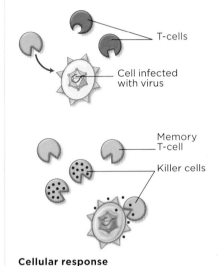

Cellular response

Antibody immune response

Babies have some natural immunity. This can be increased by the antibodies and other substances in breast milk, which is why health professionals advocate breastfeeding. Throughout childhood, you come into contact with a host of infections which, by provoking your body's immune system, provide you with immunity to those diseases later in life.

With some infections, the immunity lasts a lifetime; with others, resistance is only for the short term. This is why children and adults sometimes receive boosts to the immune system through inoculation, also called vaccination or immunization, when they are given a modified strain of the organism causing the disease. Vaccines help to boost the body's ability to defend itself against certain viruses and bacteria.

The type of immunization depends on what is thought necessary and safe at the time; measles, whooping cough, tetanus, polio, rubella, mumps, diphtheria and now varicella, meningococcus C and haemophilus are the ones most routinely offered, particularly in early life. People travelling to places where contagious illnesses are a risk are immunized so the body is stimulated to produce antibodies.

Viruses and bacteria can enter the body in various ways. At obvious entry points—such as the mouth and nose—lymphoid tissue is present to fight invaders. The same illness can be caused by a different strain of the virus so you cannot have immunity to all infections. The common cold is a prime example.

Our immune systems can be seriously affected by stress and exhaustion. Disorders can occur when cells of the immune system are attacked by a virus, as in HIV/AIDS, or when the immune system turns on itself to attack body tissues, as in rheumatoid arthritis (an autoimmune disorder).

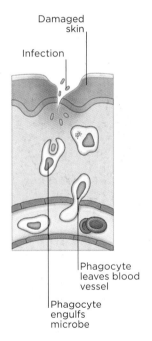

SKIN RESPONSE
The skin is the immune system's first line of defence. Infective agents breaching the surface of the skin are met and "eaten" by phagocytes, a type of white cell in the blood that activates T- and B-cells in lymph to recognize the invader.

THE SKIN AND THE SENSES

The five external senses–sight, hearing, smell, taste and touch, each with its own specific function–are important for giving information about the position and movement of the body and the body's needs. If you lose one sense, your body attempts to compensate by heightening all or some of the others.

The skin–the organ of touch–is the largest organ of the body and has four layers: outer dead cells, the living epidermis, the dermis, and the subcutaneous fat layer that provides warmth and insulation. Fine networks of nerves and blood vessels permeate the layers so that the brain registers temperature, pressure, pleasure and pain experienced on any part of the skin.

The epidermis provides the body with a protective suit that prevents moisture loss from the skin (while allowing waste, such as sweat, to escape), is virtually impervious to harmful substances and has antibacterial properties. In the basal epidermal layer, cells grow, mature, age

and die, moving up to the outer skin, where they are sloughed off by clothing, rubbing or washing.

The next layer down, the dermis, contains the support structure of the skin, including collagen, the elastic tissue that keeps the skin springy. Collagen is a protein and responds to the hormone oestrogen to give skin a supple, youthful appearance. After the menopause, and with age, skin becomes thin and wrinkled through the loss of collagen, moisture and fat, and as a result of long-term exposure to environmental pollution including the sun's rays.

Sight keeps you aware of your surroundings. Behind the iris, the coloured part of the eye, is a lens controlled by a set of muscles and an array of nerves linked to the brain. The lens bends rays of light entering through the cornea so that an image of an object is focused on the retina, at the back of the eye. The two–slightly different–images from the eyes are sent to the brain, which interprets them as one three-dimensional object. A person who

THE SKIN

Millions of specialized cells, including blood vessels, nerves, hair follicles, sweat glands and sebaceous glands lie under the skin's surface. Skin protects and contains the body's organs, releases excess heat and fluid and warns against dangers, such as burning.

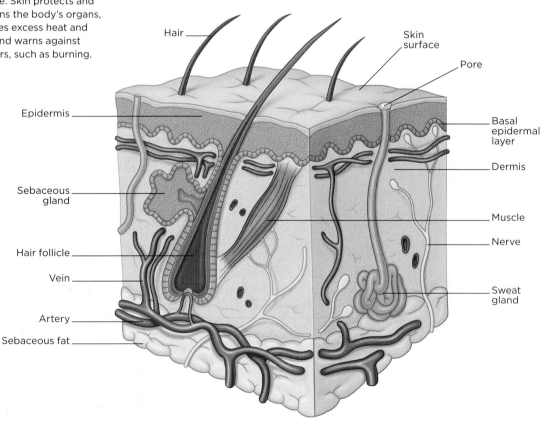

Hair

Skin surface

Pore

Epidermis

Basal epidermal layer

Dermis

Sebaceous gland

Muscle

Nerve

Hair follicle

Vein

Sweat gland

Artery

Sebaceous fat

is colourblind (more common in men than women) is born with a faulty retina.

Bright lights and foreign bodies are kept out of the eyes by the eyelids and lashes. Lachrymal glands constantly secrete tears that bathe the eye with every blink and wash away any irritant that enters. Tears are also an emotional response to both happiness and sadness.

Hearing is the second of your vital senses, allowing you to tune into the world and sounds of danger. The outer ear contains the eardrum, which passes sound waves to three tiny bones (ossicles) in the middle ear, and then to the cochlea in the inner ear, which translates the sound wave into a nerve message that goes to the auditory part of the brain. Also in the inner ear are the semicircular canals, which detect your position in space and maintain your sense of balance.

The sense of smell probably evolved to warn us about bad food and dangers such as smoke from fire. It is also used less consciously to detect pheromones (natural body scents), which are given off in response to sexual arousal or fear.

Taste allows the enjoyment of food; it also warns about potential poisons. The many thousands of "taste buds" in the mouth distinguish different flavours.

SIGHT

Light enters through the pupil and is focused by the lens onto the retina at the back of the eye, where the rod and cone cells are sensitive to light and colour.

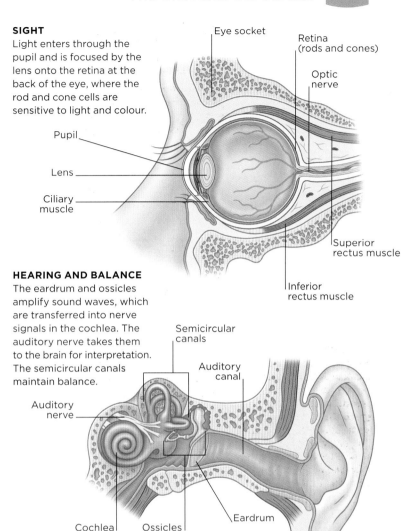

Eye socket
Retina (rods and cones)
Optic nerve
Pupil
Lens
Ciliary muscle
Superior rectus muscle
Inferior rectus muscle

HEARING AND BALANCE

The eardrum and ossicles amplify sound waves, which are transferred into nerve signals in the cochlea. The auditory nerve takes them to the brain for interpretation. The semicircular canals maintain balance.

Semicircular canals
Auditory canal
Auditory nerve
Eardrum
Cochlea
Ossicles
Outer ear

TASTE

The tongue has over 10,000 receptors called taste buds, with different sections in which the tissue is sensitive to sweet, sour, salt and bitter flavours and responds to sensations such as excess heat.

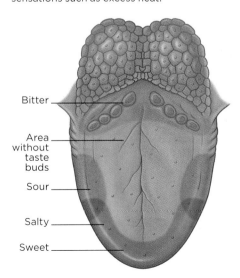

Bitter
Area without taste buds
Sour
Salty
Sweet

SMELL

In humans, smell is more sensitive than taste. There are around 25 million olfactory receptor cells high in the nasal cavity that allow detection of over 10,000 odours.

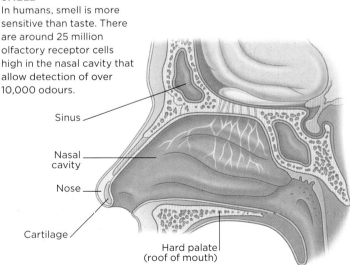

Sinus
Nasal cavity
Nose
Cartilage
Hard palate (roof of mouth)

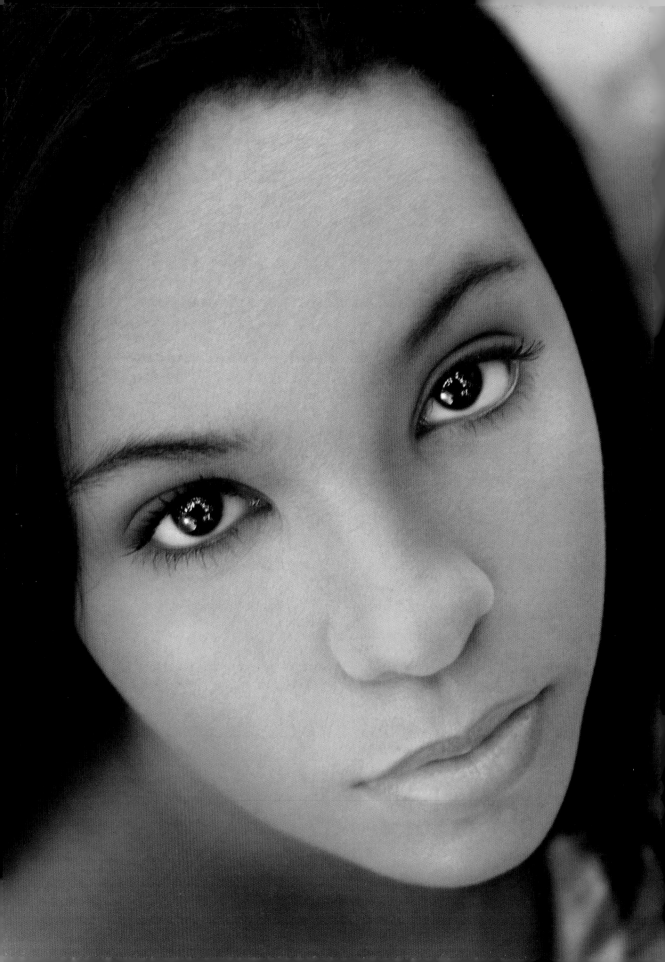

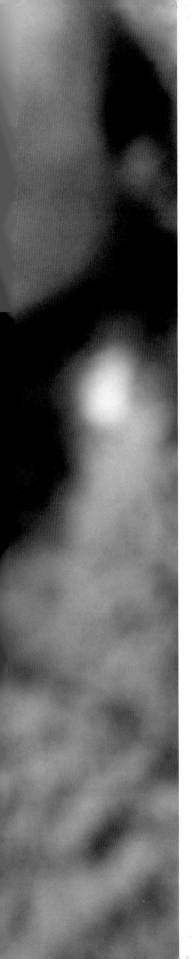

CHALLENGES TO YOUR HEALTH

This chapter discusses a variety of conditions and diseases that can leave you sick and hurting. Learning what they are, how they work and how to reduce your risk can help prevent both the onset and the progression of these diseases. Here's what you need to know.

Skeletal System Problems

Your body's frame and its network of muscles, tendons and ligaments are designed to support your weight through a range of activities. There are over 206 separate bones in the human skeleton. The bones are joined to one another by ligaments, which are strong bands of flexible tissue. When mechanical strain, illness or injury cause problems, they must be recognized and treated to prevent long-term consequences.

TYPES OF JOINTS
Ball-and-socket joints in the shoulder and hip are the most mobile type and give the widest range of movement. Hinge joints allow the elbows, fingers and knees to move. In the wrists, ankles and spine the joints glide. The head, on a pivot joint at the top of the spine, can swivel and bend.

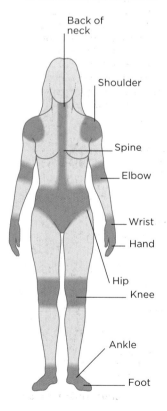

Back of neck

Shoulder

Spine

Elbow

Wrist

Hand

Hip

Knee

Ankle

Foot

VULNERABLE JOINTS

Your body is capable of a range of movements that can occur without your conscious effort. You learned to move as a baby, reaching out to touch, then to grasp. When your bones became stronger you were able to sit up, crawl and then walk. All of these actions are made possible by an array of joints, each one designed to meet the needs of the particular limb involved.

The brain sends out messages and your fingers, toes, arms and legs move, enabling you to write or type, walk or climb stairs, roll your shoulders or ankles, bend to touch your toes, lift a child or shopping bags. But a woman's lifestyle can put her at risk of joint pain. Too much time spent sitting at a desk or computer, without proper care and attention given to correct posture, can cause chronic problems in the back, neck, wrists and elbows. Carrying heavy loads such as a baby or toddler, suitcases or over-full briefcases can strain muscles and place undue stress on your spine, just as wearing high heels can shift your body forwards and compromise the spine's alignment.

In pregnancy your body has a changing centre of gravity because of the weight of the growing baby. Your back muscles have to work harder to maintain an upright stance, and this puts more stress on the strong collagen fibres called ligaments, which have already been relaxed in preparation for the delivery. This can predispose you to backache.

Keep muscles flexible

Muscles, which make up about 23 per cent of a woman's body weight, work with the largest joints (called load- or weight-bearing) to allow everyday movement. Muscles need a constant supply of oxygen to work well. If the skeletal muscles, which give the body its form and are anchored to bones, become slack through lack of exercise or stretching, your movement may be limited resulting in pain or stiffness. Carrying extra weight can also make you prone to musculoskeletal problems.

Build strength

Muscles work better the more they are used, which is why preventive medicine recommends regular, steady exercise. Unaccustomed effort, such as running for a bus, not warming up before an aerobics class or playing a weekend sport, can cause damage such as a pulled muscle or a strained ligament.

The knee is particularly vulnerable. It is supported by four ligaments and 13 muscles, with cartilage protecting the bones. The cartilage can wear down after a sports injury, or from wear and tear over time. Sometimes the ligaments, the supporting tissues of the knee, can tear or become damaged and need physiotherapy or even surgery.

Guard joints

Joints are guarded against friction by bursae, small fluid-filled sacs in the fibrous tissue where tendons and muscles move over bony prominences. But injury, trauma or overuse of joints can result in inflammation and this is known as bursitis.

The most common symptom of these challenges is pain in a knee, elbow or shoulder. Certain repetitive actions also cause joint pain. In tennis elbow, which is not restricted to tennis players, the repeated rotation of the forearm results in inflammation in the tendons of the forearm near the elbow joint. The use of a manual screwdriver over a long period of time will produce the same effect. Treatment involves multiple components including rest, ice compresses, NSAIDs (nonsteroidal anti-inflammatory drugs), cortisone injection and occasionally physiotherapy. You should seek prompt medical attention if there are signs of infection such as fever and inflammation involving a joint.

Watch for inflammation

Women are susceptible to some disabling disorders that can cause joint and muscle pain. Polymyalgia rheumatica (PMR), which can appear after the age of 50, has no known cause. Symptoms tend to occur in the morning and include weakness, stiffness and aches primarily involving shoulders and hips, and there may be pain and swelling in the hands. Other symptoms include a low-grade fever, weight loss and fatigue. In most cases of PMR, blood tests will reveal a raised erythrocyte sedimentation rate (ESR), which indicates the presence of inflammation.

It is treated with a low dose of corticosteroid drugs, generally in the range 5–20 mg of prednisone daily.

The condition may last for months or years, although most people may be weaned from treatment within two years. However, the symptoms can reappear and in some people an associated condition called giant cell arteritis (also known as temporal arteritis) may occur. The symptoms are headaches, a jaw ache and visual problems. Immediate medical attention is needed to prevent sight damage.

Women in their 20s, 50s and 60s are twice as likely as men of the same age to succumb to two autoimmune disorders affecting the joints or muscles. Dermatomyositis and polymyositis target the muscles in the arms and thighs causing inflammation and general weakness. Symptoms include difficulty reaching overhead, combing your hair or climbing stairs. Diagnosis is made by blood tests, electromyography (EMG), which records electrical activity in muscles, and muscle biopsy (removal of a small sample for laboratory analysis). Magnetic resonance imaging (MRI) may be used to pinpoint the affected area for muscle testing and biopsy. Treatment consists of high dose corticosteroid drugs and immunosuppressive drugs such as methotrexate.

TAKE ACTION NOW!

To keep joints strong and healthy:
- Always try to wear low heels
- Take a stretch break now and then when at work or doing the chores
- Avoid carrying very heavy bags
- Keep your muscles flexible
- Avoid repetitive actions
- Move gently when stiff
- Build strength

WHAT GOES WRONG?
The sleeve-like capsule of cartilage surrounding the joint prevents dislocation, and cartilage discs act as shock absorbers. In osteoarthritis, wear and tear over time causes the cartilage to break down, the bones rub together and bony outgrowths called osteophytes are produced to try to repair the damage. In rheumatoid arthritis, the synovial membrane becomes inflamed and thickens, excess synovial fluid accumulates and cartilage damage occurs.

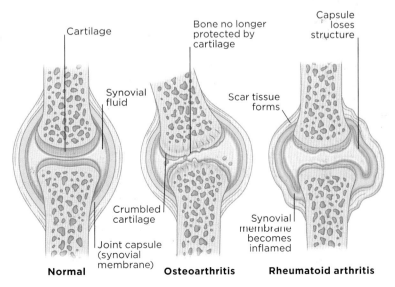

Normal — Cartilage, Synovial fluid, Joint capsule (synovial membrane)
Osteoarthritis — Bone no longer protected by cartilage, Crumbled cartilage
Rheumatoid arthritis — Capsule loses structure, Scar tissue forms, Synovial membrane becomes inflamed

SIGNS AND SYMPTOMS

- The gradual onset of pain in the joints, especially with exertion, that wears off with rest.
- Gradually increasing restriction of movement in the affected joint or joints.
- A "grating" feeling when the joint is moved.

ARTHRITIS

When the tissues surrounding a joint get inflammed, this is called arthritis– a condition with symptoms of swelling, stiffness, redness and dysfunction that can afflict women of all ages. The term rheumatism is sometimes used but it is not a medically recognized condition.

There are several direct causes of arthritis: infection by bacteria or viruses, the degenerative changes associated with age and disorders of the metabolism or immune system. All joints of the body are vulnerable, from the large joints, such as hips, knees and shoulders, to the small joints, such as hands and feet.

The two most common forms of arthritis are osteoarthritis and rheumatoid arthritis. Some forms of arthritis can be inherited, but the genes responsible for this are not yet fully understood. Rheumatoid arthritis, for example, runs in families, and there is a strong hereditary link in both gout and psoriatic arthritis. However, if a family member has one of these forms of arthritis, it does not mean that you are destined to get it. In osteoarthritis, inactivity and overweight are factors that predispose people to the disease.

Painful hands

The hands are a common site for arthritis in many older women. In the condition called erosive osteoarthritis, painful bony growths form in the joints closest to the fingernails (Heberden's nodes) and middle joints (Bouchard's nodes). Pain and stiffness may be present for a few months to a few years, but in general the hands can continue to function. It is not known why the bones change in this way, and there is no proven preventive measure. Degenerative arthritis can also occur at the joints of the bones at the base of the thumb.

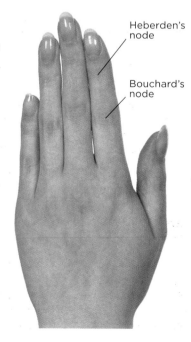

Heberden's node

Bouchard's node

Osteoarthritis

Also known as degenerative joint disease (DJD), osteoarthritis occurs when joints wear out. It's often associated with ageing, although the condition can develop at any age and may be hastened by recurrent joint injuries. The symptoms usually start during middle age and are more common in women than in men. The joints mostly involved are the hips, knees and hands. Most people over the age of 70 suffer from the condition to some degree.

Its main cause is wear and tear on a joint, when bones have lost the protective layer (cartilage) or lubricant (synovial fluid) that prevents them from rubbing against each other. A number of factors can increase the rate at which wear and tear takes its toll. These include previous damage to a joint (especially when the condition develops in a young person) or even misalignment of a joint. The two most important risk factors, however, are a sedentary lifestyle and being overweight.

The progress of osteoarthritis is slow but steady. The cartilage between the bones wears away until, eventually, these bones come into direct contact with each other. At the same time, bony spurs called osteophytes develop around the edges of the joint and the capsule surrounding it becomes thicker and coarser. The cumulative effect is that the joint becomes painful and stiff and its normal movement is restricted. In extreme cases of osteoarthritis the joint may become deformed.

How is it treated?

If osteoarthritis is in its early stages, your doctor is likely to suggest that you do exercises to keep the joints mobile and, if appropriate, try to lose weight–this may be all that is needed to slow down the progression of the condition.

In moderately severe cases, however, painkillers and a range of nonsteroidal anti-inflammatory drugs (NSAIDs), such as ibuprofen, are likely to be prescribed. Losing weight becomes a priority in such cases, although be careful that any exercise taken is not too demanding, in order to avoid further wear and tear. Physiotherapy may be suggested to

Is surgery an option?

Surgery is only an option when there is severe disability and the normal range of treatments has proved ineffective. Various techniques are used, depending on the extent of degeneration and the joint in which it occurs:

Arthroplasty: Part or all of an affected joint is replaced by an artificial one. Arthroplasty is usually the treatment of choice in cases where the affected joint is a hip, knee, shoulder or elbow.

Arthrodesis: The bones of the joint are fused. Arthrodesis is generally performed if the spinal vertebrae are affected.

Other surgical treatments: These include osteotomy, in which the bones in a joint are realigned to relieve pressure, and osteoplasty, in which damaged material is removed from the affected joint.

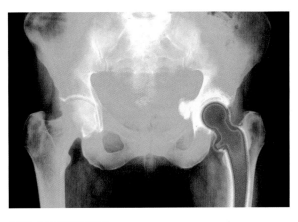

REPLACEMENT HIP
Standard hip replacement joints consist of a metal cup with a long spike attached to one end and a socket made of high density polyethylene. During surgery, the bone ball at the top of the femur is removed and a shaft driven into the femur to take the spike. The metal cup rotates in the plastic replacement socket.

ensure that appropriate exercises are used–some in water–and walking aids, such as a cane, may also be provided to take weight off affected joints. The physiotherapist may also show you how to use hot and cold compresses and other non-drug pain-relieving and anti-inflammatory techniques. Your doctor may, in addition, recommend that you join an arthritis support group to learn more about ways in which to cope with the everyday problems of the condition.

When symptoms become so severe that they interfere with your ability to function, you may be referred to an orthopaedic surgeon for possible joint replacement surgery.

Gout and pseudogout

These are arthritic conditions in which crystals collect in the joint and result in inflammation and pain.

With gout, the crystal is monosodium urate and people with this condition may underexcrete uric acid from their bodies or overproduce uric acid.

In the case of pseudogout, the crystals are formed of calcium pyrophosphate. Pseudogout is often associated with endocrine disorders such as thyroid and parathyroid disease.

Gout is more common in men and rare before the menopause in women. In gout, the usual sites are the joints in the lower extremity and include the toes, feet and knees. Pseudogout tends to occur after the menopause, and most commonly affects the knees but may involve the wrists and elbows. Factors that predispose one to gout or pseudogout include trauma, surgery (3 days after), major medical illness, fasting, alcohol use or infection. The joint symptoms include rapid joint swelling, extreme tenderness and usually involve a single joint.

The conditions are diagnosed by examining a sample of fluid from the affected joint and for gout by checking blood levels of uric acid. Treatment for the initial attack of a painful joint is NSAIDs, steroid injections into the area or oral steroids. Your doctor will discuss treatments to prevent recurrences.

DO SUPPLEMENTS WORK?

Recent research into tissue injury and painful joints suffered by athletes and other sports people has encouraged the development of dietary supplements that may aid repair and recovery of movement. Collagen, glucosamine and chondroitin are essential elements of vulnerable cartilage, tendons and ligaments; when they're under strain, the body is unable to provide sufficient new material to repair any tissue damage as it occurs.

Some studies of patients with osteoarthritis have shown that they benefit from supplements. Others have not. When the pain is eased, sufferers are less likely to remain immobilized, which is one of the major side effects of arthritis and a leading cause of other complications, such as diabetes and heart disease.

If you intend to try dietary supplements, discuss the situation with your doctor first.

After performing a physical examination, your doctor will arrange for blood tests to look for the "rheumatoid factor" common in immune-linked arthritis and markers of inflammation and chronic disease. If there is a suspicion that joints may be damaged, X-rays will be taken to look for evidence of cartilage destruction and bony erosions.

TAKE UP SWIMMING!

If you find your joints are beginning to swell and pain prevents you from pursuing everyday activities, start to go swimming. This activity is gentle on the joints but can also strengthen muscles. Contact your local leisure centre or YMCA for a course specifically designed for those with arthritis.

WHO'S AT RISK?
Different age groups are at risk for different types of immune-related arthritis. The main groups affected are children and young women. Symptoms may fluctuate, or may improve temporarily. The challenge at any age is to find a balance between rest and exercise without allowing the disorder to disrupt everyday life.

Rheumatoid arthritis

Rheumatoid arthritis is an arthritic condition that occurs more commonly in women than men. Although the exact cause of the condition remains unknown, it is thought that the disease may be either immune-related - the result of the body's cells attacking its own tissues - or the result of infection. Rheumatoid arthritis peaks between the ages of 35 and 45, but women over 65 may also be at risk.

Another possible cause of rheumatoid arthritis is genetic susceptibility. Some women are more vulnerable than others to a trigger that initiates the inflammation causing joint destruction.

The first signs appear when the delicate synovial membranes lining the joints become inflamed and start to thicken. Over time, the cartilage and then some of the bone in the joints wears away, while the sheaths of the muscle tendons around them also become thickened and inflamed. The result is pain, stiffness and swelling in the joints, and a reduction in mobility. About 10 per cent of sufferers may become disabled. The joints commonly involved include the wrists, knuckles and spine but may involve any joint. Rheumatoid arthritis can also affect other organs, such as the heart and lungs, and connective tissue in the body.

Rheumatoid arthritis cannot yet be cured, though treatment can reduce its symptoms and delay its progression.

It can go into remission under certain conditions, for example during the months of pregnancy.

Treatment goals are to relieve inflammation and pain and maintain joint function. Initial treatment includes NSAIDs and low dose corticosteroids until the newer disease modifying therapies are initiated. Physiotherapy and strengthening and conditioning exercises help to improve range of motion but need to be included gradually depending on the severity of the disease. New drugs work to slow disease progression and maintain joint function and include methotrexate, sulfasalazine, azathioprine, penicillamine, leflunomide and hydroxychloroquine. Sometimes corticosteroid drugs are prescribed, but they must be closely monitored since they can lead to the onset of Cushing's syndrome (excess of steroid hormones). Obesity, high blood pressure, diabetes and osteoporosis are other side effects of steroids. Surgery may be considered for joint deformities.

Juvenile rheumatoid arthritis

This more commonly affects girls than boys and may strike between the ages of two and four or at puberty. In most cases, the arthritis will disappear after several years, although some children may be left with joint abnormalities. Juvenile rheumatoid arthritis can range from classic rheumatoid arthritis to Still's disease (which occurs between ages 16

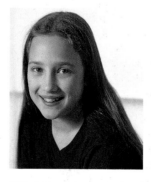

CHILDREN
Children with juvenile rheumatoid arthritis should receive treatment including physiotherapy, which will help to keep growing bodies active.

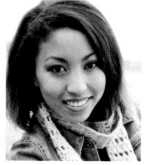

TWENTIES
The twenties are the most common age for systemic lupus erythematosus, but symptoms wax and wane. Care of the skin is needed for sun photosensitivity.

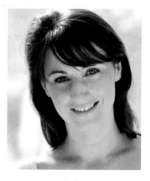

CHILDBEARING YEARS
For some women, being pregnant leads to a temporary remission of arthritis, but the symptoms will return soon after the baby is born.

and 35), in which the fever, swollen lymph nodes and skin rash last for several weeks. The arthritis symptoms–pain and swelling in the joints–may not appear until months later.

Lupus erythematosus

Systemic lupus erythematosus, also known as SLE (*see also* p. 106), is an autoimmune disorder producing inflammation in any of the organ systems or the tissues of the body. The skin, the face, the brain, the kidneys and the joints are especially vulnerable. The cause is unknown but genetic, environmental and hormonal factors seem to play a role in this disease. It affects about eight times more women than men, and symptoms usually appear between the ages of 15 and 40. Treatment of the joint symptoms is similar to that for rheumatoid arthritis although there is no risk of deformity. NSAIDs, hydroxychloroquine, steroids, immunosuppressives and occasionally chemotherapeutic agents are used for all symptoms that manifest as part of this disease (including arthritis, rash, kidney disease and nervous system disease).

Psoriatic arthritis

Psoriasis is primarily a skin disorder that affects women and men equally and has a strong genetic basis. In about 1 in 20 cases, psoriasis sufferers also develop psoriatic arthritis, but the reason for this is not known. Psoriatic arthritis (*see also* p. 132) can be severe and disabling. Pitting of the nails is also associated with the joint disease. It is thought that those with more severe skin disease are at higher risk of developing arthritis. Treatment of this condition includes methotrexate, NSAIDs and recently available tumour necrosis factor inhibitors.

Reactive arthritis

Although more common in men than women, this can occur in either sex after a bacterial infection. The usual sites of the infection are the genital tract (the cervix or urethra) and the intestines. The infection triggers an abnormal immune response. It is sometimes linked with conjunctivitis (inflammation of the membrane lining the eyelids and covering the eyeball) and arthritis in the knee or ankle joints; with this mix of symptoms, the condition is called Reiter's disease. This syndrome is linked to people who carry the blood antigen HLA-B27. About 80 per cent of those with Reiter's are HLA-B27 positive, which means it is inherited.

The first symptoms may be diarrhoea or pain when passing urine, although some sufferers have neither. Swollen, painful, red and tender joints are common. Blood and stool tests can determine the source of the infection. Antibiotics may be prescribed to deal with the infection and NSAIDs for pain. The illness can last for about six months. When the genital tract is involved, it is advised that you practise safe sex until symptoms clear up.

WHEN THE BODY ATTACKS ITSELF

Normally, the immune system recognizes foreign antigens that are harmful to the body and manufactures antibodies to fight them. In an autoimmune disorder, the body loses the ability to distinguish between foreign material and some of its own cells. The body then produces antibodies that act against its own tissue, which in turn can cause inflammation and disease.

Little is known at present about the mechanism of autoimmune diseases, although genetic factors are certainly involved in some conditions. People who suffer from one autoimmune disorder may also be at risk for developing other autoimmune conditions.

Research continues to identify more and more autoimmune conditions. It is known, for example, that SLE (*see left*) is an autoimmune disorder. Antiphospholipid antibody syndrome (APS) is another. This is a disorder that can arise in conjunction with SLE and other rheumatic diseases or by itself. In APS, antibodies are directed against phospholipids, substances found throughout the body. These antibodies promote clotting; patients may experience blood clots, heart attacks, strokes and recurrent miscarriages.

The purpose of treatment of autoimmune diseases is to suppress the immune system's response. Unfortunately, the drugs that do this, which are known as immunosuppressives, tend to reduce the activity of the whole immune system, instead of just the part of it responsible for the disorder. They often have side effects that include an increased risk of infection.

Signs and symptoms

- Tenderness and stiffness in joints, usually the same ones on both sides of the body—the hands, wrists, elbows, shoulders, knees, ankles and feet—often occurs in the early morning and lasts several hours.
- Increasing pain, stiffness and swelling after periods of inactivity (sleep, a car journey, a plane flight). Stiffness lasts more than 30 minutes. There can be joint deformity.
- Painless nodules under the skin over joints.
- Tiredness, fever and weight change.

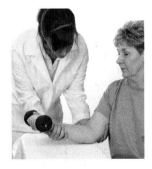

GENTLE THERAPY
Physiotherapists offer treatments ranging from heat and electrical therapy to exercises to help restore movement. Exercise with relaxation techniques can reduce the stiffness and pain of arthritis.

SPINAL CURVES

The spine has four natural curves, which absorb shock and strain during movement. The curves are classified as either primary (present at birth) or secondary (developing duirng infancy). The convex curves of the thoracic and sacral vertebrae are primary. The concave curves of cervical and lumbar vertebrae are secondary.

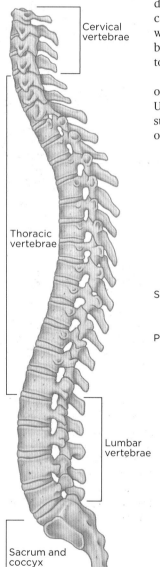

Cervical vertebrae

Thoracic vertebrae

Lumbar vertebrae

Sacrum and coccyx

BACK CONDITIONS

The back's intricate system of checks and balances–in the spine, joints and supporting muscles and ligaments–is vulnerable to damage. That's why you should never move anyone after an accident if you suspect the spine has been hurt.

The bones that make up the column of the spine are called vertebrae. Over time, the cartilage that separates the vertebrae, known as intervertebral discs, can get thinner and lose its ability to act as a shock absorber. Occasionally, the discs can slip or protrude into the spinal canal, putting pressure on a nerve root, which can cause pain. The facet joints between the vertebrae can also become too tight, affecting nerve roots.

There is no doubt that being overweight adversely affects the spine. Unlike muscle, which protects and supports the joints and relieves them of pressure, stored body fat merely

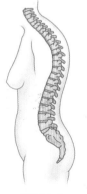

Secondary curve

Primary curve

Secondary curve

Primary curve

ABNORMAL CURVES

Kyphosis, or hunched upper back, may result from bad posture or osteoporosis. Lordosis is too much curve of the lumbar spine and may result from poor posture, pregnancy or obesity. Scoliosis is a lateral curve and may be caused by one leg being significantly shorter than the other.

increases the load that the joints–particularly in the lower back and hips–have to bear. It can increase general wear and tear, leading to osteoarthritis, and can also lead to ailments such as strained ligaments and disc problems.

Overweight people tend to carry much of their extra fat around the stomach, which can weaken the stomach muscles. They are then unable to do the important job of supporting the spine. Anyone suffering from lower back pain will be encouraged to strengthen the stomach muscles with gentle exercises as a first move towards solving the problem.

How problems arise

Crouching, bending, lifting and carrying can cause a great deal of stress on the back. In activities that call for one type of work for several hours at a time–such as pruning, digging, mowing or weeding–stress on the back is made even worse if it is done in irregular spurts.

People who have a sedentary lifestyle spend a lot of time sitting or lying down and if this is combined with lack of exercise and poor posture, a chronic back problem may be the result.

Curves of the spine

The spine has four natural curves and these allow it to absorb the shock waves experienced from the impact of walking and the stresses and strains caused by the body's weight and its movements. Everyone has a naturally slightly different degree of curve but various conditions or postural habits can produce distorted or exaggerated curves. These then fail to absorb shock

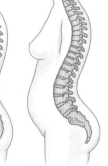

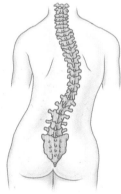

Kyphosis   **Lordosis**   **Scoliosis**

effectively and can lead to nerves not functioning properly.

Why you have back pain

The sciatic nerve is the longest in the body–it is, in fact, six spinal nerves that leave the base of the spine and join up to form one large nerve that runs down the leg. If any part is trapped its effects can be felt a long way from the back.

The sciatic nerve gets "trapped" when a disc presses on it, or it is being pressed against the spine (as can happen in pregnancy). The symptoms are acute and include shooting and unrelenting pain in the area of the body served by the part of the trapped nerve, usually the buttock or the back of the leg.

Another cause of back pain can be when a vertebra collapses on itself and this will cause sciatica-type pain. Mostly this results from severe osteoporosis or bone thinning.

Back pain is not always caused by a back problem. Pain can be "referred" to the spinal region where it is perceived, perhaps because two areas of the body share the same pain pathways. Medical causes of such referred pain can come from a wide range of gynecological, abdominal and chest problems.

THE SPINAL JOINTS

The 33 bones called vertebrae are stacked on top of each other with pads of cartilage known as discs between. The column is held together by strong ligaments and facet joints between the vertebrae.

Normal disc In a healthy spine the discs are plump and resilient. They are compressed during everyday activity and return to normal during rest or sleep.

Slipped disc Under extreme pressure the centre of the disc may break out of its covering and put pressure on a nerve, a painful condition known as a disc protrusion or slipped disc.

Shrunken disc The water content of the discs may diminish with age, leading to a reduction in springiness and painful complications.

TAKE ACTION NOW!

To keep your back healthy:
- Exercise to strengthen abdominal muscles
- Lift with bended knees
- Keep within a healthy weight range
- Stay active

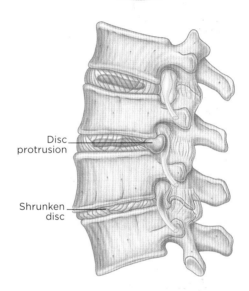

Disc protrusion

Shrunken disc

When back pain strikes ...

It is most important to stop what you are doing and lie down on a bed or the floor. This will have the immediate effect of taking the stress off your spine. Help yourself by making a positive effort to relax both your mind and body.

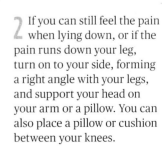

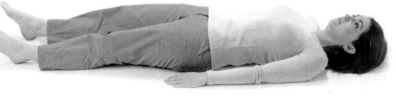

1 Lying flat on your back is an effective way of reducing pressure. You can also bend your knees up but keep your feet flat on the floor and your arms by your side.

2 If you can still feel the pain when lying down, or if the pain runs down your leg, turn on to your side, forming a right angle with your legs, and support your head on your arm or a pillow. You can also place a pillow or cushion between your knees.

PAIN IN UPPER BODY

The neck, shoulders and arms come under considerable strain. Childrearing and domestic activities make women susceptible to problems in these areas.

Neck problems

The neck plays an important role in supporting your head, helping maintain good posture and protecting the vulnerable upper part of the spine that connects to the brain. Its wide range of movement is made possible by strong ligaments and many muscles.

The neck can be the site of problems that may be acute and temporary or chronic. Muscular tension is the most common cause of chronic neck pain and results from stress or poor posture. Some muscles become taut and knotted, putting pressure on nerves in the area, while their opposing muscles become over-relaxed, making the problem worse.

Generally, acute neck pain comes from muscles that go into spasm to protect the joint and prevent movement.

The neck feels "locked", there is often a deep ache and sometimes pins and needles down a limb if a nerve has been trapped. This may result from ageing, trauma or chronic muscular tension.

The postural changes that occur in pregnancy can also cause neck pain. Immobilization in a neck collar, muscle relaxants, NSAIDs and massage therapy may help. If there is no evidence of neurological involvement, chiropractic or osteopathic manipulation and acupuncture can be used. If severe, the doctor may give trigger point or steroid injections into the joints and ligaments.

Women who have osteoarthritis may also develop cervical spondylosis, sometimes called degenerative joint disease. In this condition the discs in the cervical vertebrae wear out, causing stiffness and chronic neck pain.

Shoulder injuries

The shoulder has weaknesses due to its anatomical structure. The socket in which the arm bone sits is small and shallow, its rim of cartilage is weak, and the three short ligaments that protect the joint are unstable. Joint stability and free movement depend on the short, protective rotator cuff muscles around it.

Any damage to the rotator cuff muscles is likely to lead to inflammation of the joint capsule or tendon. Rotator cuff impingement, or painful arc syndrome, is the result of tendons that support the shoulder impinging on the under-surface of the collarbone. If the capsule thickens (adhesive capsulitis) severe pain often shoots down the arm when movement is attempted.

This condition has been found in people with type 1 diabetes, but is also associated with lack of use due to pain, osteoarthritis or wearing a sling. The loss of flexibility occurs more often in the over-50s and some researchers attribute this to ageing. However, the damage may be the direct result of an acute injury such as a fall or from a gradual buildup of frequent strains to the muscles—for example carrying heavy items. It is also associated with various occupations—musicians, for example, are prone to this disorder.

Stay balanced

If you put a heavy bag over one shoulder, your body lurches sideways to keep balanced, forcing your spine into an unnatural position (left) which can, over time, cause injury. That's why it's much better to carry equal weights in both hands. Or use a backpack that is hooked over both shoulders.

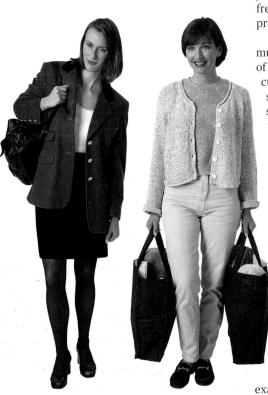

Those with the condition can make only small movements of the joint. To compensate they tend to hunch their shoulders and use the muscles attached to the shoulder blade instead.

Treatment options include a progressive stretching programme with heat and NSAIDs to improve comfort. Corticosteroid injections into the shoulder may be beneficial, as well as physiotherapy, gentle traction and graduated stretching exercises. In severe cases, a specialist may decide to manipulate the muscles and tendons under a general anaesthetic to increase mobility and remove tissue adhesions. This is often reserved for post-operative joint stiffness that does not respond to conservative measures. In extreme cases, it may be necessary to try to repair the cuff surgically, but this in itself may cause further problems.

Rotator cuff injuries tend to clear up over time (about two years) so your doctor may postpone invasive treatment. You will be encouraged to do exercises daily to loosen the joint while taking NSAIDs as needed. As the joint begins to regain normal movement, swimming may be recommended.

Wrist and arm problems

When the hands and wrists are held in an unnatural position for long periods– during repetitive work– inflammation, tendon damage and pain can result. Typing and fine manual work are risk jobs. This is called overuse syndrome or repetitive strain injury (RSI).

Two frequently occurring problems are tenosynovitis and carpal tunnel syndrome. In tenosynovitis the forearm tendons or their protective sheaths become swollen and are unable to slide easily past each other. Carpal tunnel syndrome affects the nerves as they pass through the wrists (*see* box below).

The usual treatment is immobilization of the joint (in a splint for several weeks) and steroid injections followed by physiotherapy to encourage gradual movement and ensure blood flow to the area. The condition may take a long time to correct, and in some cases surgery may be necessary.

Repetitive strain conditions tend to recur. It is important to recognize the signs. Make sure your workplace environment complies with health and safety practice and take frequent breaks–five minutes or so, every hour.

Carpal tunnel syndrome

The carpal tunnel is formed by the first row of carpal bones in the wrist and a ligament (the flexor retinaculum) that runs across and over them. The median nerve, which supplies the thumb, first two fingers and the thumb side of the third finger, passes through this tunnel, with various muscle tendons. In carpal tunnel syndrome (CTS), the median nerve becomes compressed, causing a numbing pain in the hand (often at night or on waking), clumsiness when using the hand (holding a needle or pen is difficult), pins and needles or tingling in the fingers (except the little finger) and, sometimes, pain in the arm and when trying to push the thumb against the little finger. You can find some relief by massaging or shaking the hand.

Carpal tunnel syndrome often has no identifiable cause, although it may be associated with trauma of the wrist and chronic inflammation of the tendon sheaths as a result of RSI (*see* above). CTS is seen during pregnancy and in

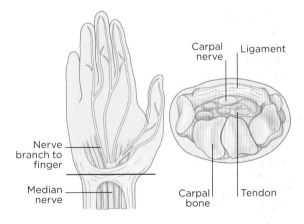

patients with an inflammatory autoimmune disorder such as rheumatoid arthritis. It can also be associated with diabetes and hypothyroidism.

Treatment may involve a wrist splint, exercises to stretch the wrist muscles, steroid injections, and, as a last resort, surgery to release the trapped nerve. Usually, before surgery is attempted, a test called a nerve conduction study is performed.

MUSCLE AND TENDON PROBLEMS

Pain or aching in the muscles or the tendons (the fibrous cord of connective tissue that attach muscles to bones) is a common problem.

Cramps

The cause of a cramp in the leg is not completely understood. It is thought that a chemical imbalance within the muscle may be responsible, resulting in excessive contraction and pain. Other possible causes include a loss of salt, potassium and magnesium, which can occur through excessive exercise, a bout of diarrhoea or alcohol or drug use. During pregnancy muscle cramps are more common.

In the feet, cramping is usually the result of over-stretching your foot; in your calf muscles it may be over-exertion; in your hands and wrists it may stem from a constant repetitive movement. The problem may be avoided by warming up your muscles before exercise and cooling down afterwards. Hydration with adequate fluid intake is helpful in preventing cramps.

Once a cramp strikes, massage the muscles until the pain subsides, usually in a few minutes. Regular night cramps may be treated by a prescribed drug containing quinine or an over-the-counter remedy. Recurrent cramps in the legs, especially when walking and relieved with rest, should be investigated by a doctor. They may be a sign of inadequate blood supply to calf muscles, known as intermittent claudication.

Strains

The usual cause of a strain in a muscle or a tendon–often called a "pull"–is an excessive demand on the tissues as a result of unusual movement, often after periods of inactivity or a result of an injury or trauma.

The degree of damage caused varies from a simple over-stretching of the fibres to a tear in them. In response, the muscle contracts or even goes into spasm to protect the damaged tissues. This disrupts the blood supply and alters the muscle's internal chemistry, which results in pain.

Immediate treatment is by RICE (*see* box opposite). If muscles and tendons are damaged, physiotherapy involving massage, friction techniques and ultrasound may be necessary. When exercising, gentle warm-up and cool-down routines before and after help prevent the problem, as does correct posture and a conscious effort to make movements flow.

Sprains

Ligaments are bands of fibrous tissue that support and stabilize joints by

Pressures on your feet

Many foot problems are the direct result of the feet being subjected to pressures for which they were not designed.

The foot contains 26 bones, linked in a series of joints and supported by numerous ligaments. The whole weight of the body must be carried by these bones and by the arches that they form in the instep. Being overweight and wearing unsuitable footwear can contribute to pain.

High-heeled or narrow shoes, from a medical standpoint, can put strain on the muscles of the lower leg. High heels shift body weight forwards, straining the tissues of the arches. Tight shoes of any type increase the risk of bunions and corns as well as nail or toe deformities.

Pain in the feet can also occur in pregnancy. Choose shoes with low heels, in natural materials such as leather or canvas to allow your feet to breathe. You may need a wider fitting shoe or a different size in the later stages of pregnancy.

Wearing correct footwear will help with your posture and may prevent backache during these months.

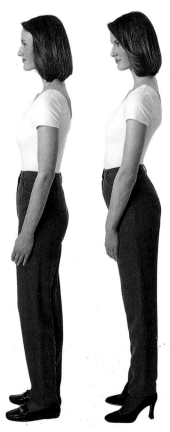

Flat shoes   **High heels**

binding together the bones that they link. In the ankle, where the fibula (the outer bone of the leg) meets the talus (an inner bone of the foot), there are three ligaments. Many common accidents in which you trip or miss a step can cause the joint to lose its stability and twist inwards, resulting in a sprained ankle. The torn fibres bleed and become inflamed, and the muscles in the area go into spasm to prevent any further damage. If you suffer a serious sprain, treatment usually involves application of ice, support from elastic bandages and ultrasound. In some cases, ligaments that have been badly torn may require surgical repair.

Weakness

Women are particularly susceptible to an autoimmune disorder called myasthenia gravis, which involves the muscles used in chewing, swallowing and speaking, and also causes weakness in the limbs. It may become apparent in early adulthood beginning with signs of weakness of the eyelid and double vision. The condition is usually progressive, with some periods of remission.

Treatment of the condition involves drugs to restore nerve transmission to the muscles, immunosuppressive drugs and steroids. Surgery to remove the thymus gland may also be considered in young women.

FIRST AID FOR SPRAINS

R—Rest (stop physical activity).

I—Apply an ice-pack to the injured area for 15-20 minutes each hour while awake (wrap ice in a wet towel to prevent skin damage).

C—Compression using an elastic bandage or air-filled splint to apply pressure to affected area to control swelling.

E—Elevate the injured area for 20 minutes to drain fluid from the injury site and to reduce swelling.

Repeat **RICE** twice a day.

MEDICAL TERMINOLOGY

There are many ways in which your muscles and the associated tissues can cause pain. Here are some of the terms your doctor may use to describe muscular and skeletal problems.

DISEASE	DESCRIPTION
Fibromyalgia	A modern term for what used to be called "muscular rheumatism", fibromyalgia has no known cause, although it has been suggested that it is connected with stress. It mostly affects middle-aged people and may disturb sleep. Symptoms include pain and tenderness in muscles all over the body. There are specific "trigger points" within the muscles that set off sharp, shooting pains—hence the condition's other name "trigger point syndrome". It may also be referred to as fibrositis. Fibromyalgia is treated by deep massage and regular stretching exercises. Antidepressants and muscle relaxant drugs are sometimes prescribed. Some medical centres have fibromyalgia treatment programmes that encompass a multidisciplinary approach to the management of fibromyalgia.
Fibrositis	Another name for fibromyalgia
Myalgia	Muscular pain
Paraesthesia	The medical term meaning "pins and needles", paraesthesia usually occurs in a limb that has been in the same position for a long time. The tingling and numbness indicates temporary disruption to the nerve or blood supply. It can also be a symptom of disc protrusion on a nerve in the lumbar or cervical spine or disorders such as Raynaud's disease, carpal tunnel syndrome, diabetes and hypothyroidism.
Rhueumatism	This is not a word ordinarily used by doctors, but rheumatism is a common description by non-medical people for general pain and stiffness in muscles and joints. So-called rheumatic pain may derive from osteoarthritis, rheumatoid arthritis or polymyalgia rheumatica.
Sciatica	Sciatica is caused by pressure on the sciatic nerve as it leaves the spine. It is the result of inflammation of the facet joints of the vertebrae between which the nerve emerges, or may be due to a disc protrusion between these vertebrae caused by poor posture, lifting heavy objects or unaccustomed activity. Irritation of the nerve by the bony pelvis can occur during menstruation and pregnancy. The nerve compression gives severe pain along its length from the lower back to the foot, often with pins and needles and numbness. Treatment is by anti-inflammatory injection, NSAIDs, rest, manipulation and exercises.

OSTEOPOROSIS

Literally meaning porous bones, osteoporosis is a skeletal and hormone-related disorder that generally afflicts the wrists, spine and hips of post-menopausal women.

Bone thinning leads to fragile bones and increased risk of fracture–often it is only after a fracture that osteoporosis is diagnosed. The condition comes about gradually, causing the thinning of the honeycombed inner layer of the ends of lower arm bones, the hip ends of the thigh bones and the spinal vertebrae.

These bones become extremely susceptible to breaks and the fractures are likely to take longer than normal to heal, increasing the risk of infection and deformity, which may lead to disability or death. It is estimated that about 20 per cent of elderly women who fracture a hip die from complications and half of those who survive are disabled.

In osteoporosis, the gradual collapse of the spinal vertebrae, as a result of the loss of bone density and the load that they bear, causes a reduction in height and a forward bend and hunching of the upper spine. Medically termed a thoracic kyphosis, this is traditionally known as a "dowager's hump".

Who's at risk?

Osteoporosis is the result of bone loss through bone remodelling or bone turnover in post-menopausal women, women who have had a premature menopause, a hysterectomy with removal of both ovaries or reduced oestrogen levels for a prolonged length of time. Other factors that may increase a woman's vulnerability include:

Inadequate bone mass formation This is the most important risk factor. If there is insufficient bone mass before it starts to decrease, the effects of osteoporosis become apparent much earlier. Reasons for the inadequacy may involve any of the other risk factors.

Family history Genetic factors can cause some people to form less bone than average. Osteoporosis is more prevalent among white and Asian women than African and Caribbean women.

Hormonal deficiencies Any condition that lowers oestrogen levels (for instance, anorexia nervosa or exercise-induced amenorrhoea) accelerates loss of bone mass. A lack of calcium or vitamin D through poor nutrition means that less bone is renewed and more calcium leaches out of bone into the blood to make up for the deficiency.

Sedentary lifestyle A sedentary lifestyle and lack of exercise can accelerate bone loss. Regular weight-bearing, repetitive exercise promotes an increase in bone mass.

How bones become osteoporotic

Everyone's skeleton starts out as cartilage and soon after conception begins to be strengthened by calcium, which is supplied by the pregnant woman's diet. In this ongoing process, more cartilage is laid down as the bones—and the fetus—grow. Bone, like any other living tissue, is broken down and replaced throughout life, an activity in women that is influenced by the hormones oestrogen and progesterone. Bone strength is established in young adulthood through a healthy lifestyle, a diet made up of a wide variety of foods rich in calcium and vitamin D (which helps the calcium to be absorbed) and regular weight-bearing exercise, which stimulates bone growth.

Bones reach their peak mass between the ages of 20 and 30, and your bone mass level will depend on hormonal levels, how healthy you are, your genes and if you drink and smoke. Many women with osteoporosis never reached their optimal mass, for reasons mostly related to lack of oestrogen and calcium. This essential mineral is used by the heart, nerves and muscles as well, and if those vital parts do not have enough of it, the bones release it into the bloodstream so affecting the bone-building process.

Bone mineral starts to be lost from the skeleton from the age of about 35 and is part of natural ageing. The greatest loss occurs in the first five years after the menopause. Later the rate of bone mass loss may be as much as 5 per cent a year.

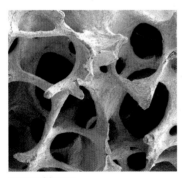

Normal bone

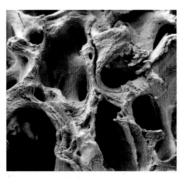

Osteoporotic bone

BONE BUILDERS

If you are at risk of developing osteoporosis, your doctor may suggest ways in which you can increase bone mass and reduce the effect of mineral loss. Your doctor may do some tests to determine if osteoporosis is due to primary (no known cause) or secondary causes (hormonal disorders, genetic disorders or nutritional disorders). If you have been diagnosed with osteoporosis, the following strategies can also play an important part in the medical treatment of the condition.

TREATMENT	ACTION
More calcium	Increase your intake of calcium-rich foods, such as milk, eggs, cheese, bread, leafy green vegetables, canned fish with bones (sardines, salmon), almonds and peanuts. Calcium supplements up to 1,500 mg daily may be taken if you are not able to consume adequate calcium-rich foods in your diet.
Vitamin D	Found in red meat, liver, oily fish, full-fat or semi-skimmed milk, margarine, butter and egg yolks and is also made in the body through the action of sunlight on the skin. Vitamin D supplements up to 800 IU per day are also recommended to maintain adequate levels.
Increase weight-bearing exercise	Regular physical activity of a repetitive nature that allows the bones to bear the body's weight helps the bone-making process. A brisk 20–30 minute walk, two or three times a week, may be enough. In some cases vigorous exercise may not be appropriate.
Stop smoking and reduce alcohol consumption	Smokers and heavy drinkers are at greater risk of developing osteoporosis as well as many other diseases.
Selective oestrogen receptor modulators (SERMs)	Drugs that compete with oestrogen in the body and act by mimicking the effect of oestrogen selectively at the bone. Raloxifene is approved in the UK and Australia for prevention and treatment of osteoporosis in some postmenopausal women.
Bisphosphonates	Bisphosphonates are drugs that affect bone by inhibiting its breakdown, preventing bone loss and increasing bone density and reducing fracture risk. They are prescribed oral tablets taken daily, once weekly, once monthly or once a year as an injection.

Small build Slight women have less bone mass to start with, so the effects of loss of bone mass may become evident more quickly. They are more likely to be predisposed to fractures.

Smoking Tobacco increases the risk of osteoporosis. Smokers on average have menopausal symptoms up to two years earlier than non-smokers.

Excessive alcohol intake Consistently consuming more than two drinks a day is associated with a higher risk of osteoporosis, because alcohol attacks the cells that form bone and inhibits the absorption of calcium.

Excessive caffeine Consistently drinking more than three cups of caffeine-containing drinks a day, such as coffee, tea and cola, can increase the risk of developing osteoporosis. Adequate calcium intake can counteract this.

Prescription drugs Long-term use of a number of drugs can cause osteoporosis. They include thyroid hormone, anticonvulsants, antacids that contain aluminium, methotrexate (used to treat cancer, immune disorders and arthritis), heparin (used to prevent blood clotting), cholestyramine (used to reduce levels of cholesterol in the blood) and some glucocorticoids, such as cortisone and prednisone, which are given to treat osteoarthritis, rheumatoid arthritis, asthma, allergic reactions, multiple sclerosis and chronic skin disorders.

Certain medical conditions Bone loss may be caused by two conditions: Cushing's syndrome, in which the adrenal glands are over-active and produce excess glucocorticoids; and hyperparathyroidism, an over-activity of the parathyroid glands. The hormone from these glands controls blood calcium levels, and if there is not enough, it removes calcium from bone tissue. Thyroid disease and malabsorption (from digestive disorders) may also affect bone mass.

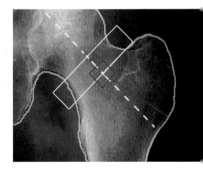

FRACTURE POINT
An X-ray of the hip obtained by dual-energy X-ray absorptiometry (DEXA). The hip is one of the most vulnerable areas and likely to fracture in anyone susceptible to osteoporosis.

Diagnosing osteoporosis

Bone mineral density (BMD) can be measured by dual-energy X-ray absorptiometry (DEXA). In this test you lie fully dressed on a table for about 15 minutes while a low-powered X-ray scanner is moved above your spine, hips and wrists. A bone densitometer

It is estimated that about 20 per cent of elderly women who fracture a hip die from complications, and half of those who survive are disabled.

A DEXA BONE SCAN
The density of your bones can be measured by this type of X-ray scanner. The scan takes only a few minutes, and the results are recorded on a computer for analysis by a doctor.

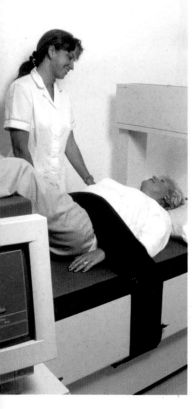

calculates the density of the bone by analyzing how much radiation is absorbed by it and how much passes through. The information is processed by a nearby computer.

The results are graded according to a World Health Organization classification, comparing your BMD with the average bone mass of a young female adult. Under this system, osteopenia is defined as a BMD between minus 1 and minus 2.5 and osteoporosis has a BMD of less than minus 2.5. The measurements are particularly relevant for menopausal women, women who experienced premature menopause due to ovarian failure or conditions that lower oestrogen levels because these result in oestrogen-deficiency states.

DEXA is recommended for women over 65 and before that age in women with risk factors. Your consultant will use the results of the DEXA to determine if you need additional treatment and whether you need to increase calcium intake or exercise.

How osteoporosis is treated

Calcium and vitamin D supplementation does not increase bone mass, but it may be prescribed to prevent bone loss. Generally, the typical daily requirements for a postmenopausal woman not using hormone therapy (HRT) are 1,500 mg of calcium (carbonate or citrate), with 400-800 IU of vitamin D. Women on HRT and premenopausal women should take 1,000-1,500 mg per day. An excess of vitamin D–more than 2,000 IU a day–can lead to kidney damage and the formation of calcium deposits in the skin.

Bisphosphonates are the first-line therapy in the treatment of osteoporosis for postmenopausal women. They can be used when there is a contraindication to HRT–in conditions such as liver disease, breast cancer, blood-clotting disorders and unexplained vaginal bleeding–or when a woman chooses not to have HRT. The other medications are the SERMs (selective oestrogen receptor modulators), the most prescribed being raloxifene. Bisphosphonates inhibit breakdown of bone; raloxifene mimics the effect of oestrogen on bones, but does not appear to reduce the risk of hip fractures.

Oestrogen therapy can prevent osteoporosis from developing in those at risk if given early enough. Many doctors suggest it should be taken from the start of menopausal symptoms, when hormone levels begin to fluctuate (measured by blood testing). It can halt bone loss in those with osteoporosis and, in some cases, restore some bone mass.

Progestogen is also given to reduce the risk of developing uterine cancer, which is possible when oestrogen is given on its own. This is not necessary in a woman who does not have a uterus. Various HRT regimes are available, depending on individual circumstances and preferences and include oral or transdermal (skin patch) preparations.

Whether or not to have HRT is a decision a woman should make with her doctor after careful study of the facts and discussion of the risks and benefits. Women are advised to use HRT at the lowest dose possible to manage symptoms and for no more than 3-5 years during the early postmenopausal years. HRT for osteoporosis is not recommended in the over-60s; they should be offered bone-building drugs. Combination HRT (oestrogen and synthetic progesterone) increases the risk of heart disease, blood clots and breast cancer.

Calcitonin may sometimes be prescribed as a nasal spray to prevent bone loss. It has been found to help relieve painful spine fractures.

Osteomalacia

The adult form of rickets, osteomalacia is a condition in which a deficiency of vitamin D leads to insufficient calcium being laid down in bone. As a result, the bones become soft and weak and are prone to fracture. In severe cases, the bones of the legs may bow under the weight of the body. Other symptoms are diffuse bone tenderness and pain, muscle weakness and a waddling gait.

Lack of exposure to sunlight, which helps the body make vitamin D, is the main cause in women who rarely go out of doors or are housebound. In recent years, the condition has been diagnosed in people who diet excessively over a long period, and women with eating disorders such as anorexia nervosa.

Vitamin D and calcium deficiency can sometimes be attributable to a failure of the intestines to absorb them properly, or to liver disease. Osteomalacia responds quickly to treatment with vitamin D supplements and a diet rich in calcium. Milk (not fat free) is a main source of vitamin D and should be consumed daily.

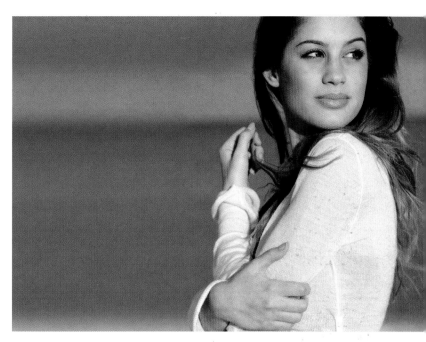

SEE THE LIGHT
Vitamin D can be obtained from sunlight on skin, from certain foods or taken as a supplement. The strength of bones depends on the way in which the mineral calcium works with vitamin D.

Colles' fracture

More frequent in women than men, Colles' fracture is the most common fracture in adults over 50. It is instinctive to put a hand out to break a fall making the bones of the wrist susceptible to damage. Such a fracture is often the first sign of a disease that has weakened the bones and made them brittle. It affects the wrist, which suffers from the impact when the palm hits the ground. The scaphoid bone at the base of the thumb may be fractured, too. The radius and ulna in the forearm are forced out of position, which forces the wrist into an unnatural upward position.

The bones may need to be surgically realigned under a general anaesthetic, and then the whole joint immobilized in plaster for about six weeks. There is a danger of the joint remaining stiff after this and physiotherapy may be required to restore the full range of movement. Anyone who has had a Colles' fracture would be advised to discuss the implications with her doctor.

An older woman might not be able to put out her hand quickly enough, and it is more likely that she will fall on her hip and fracture it.

WRIST DAMAGE
The many bones that make up the wrist can be damaged by a fall and take time to repair themselves. The situation is made worse if the break is a symptom of bone disease or another medical condition.

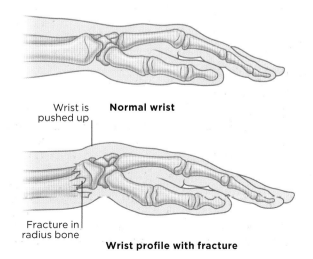

Wrist is pushed up

Normal wrist

Fracture in radius bone

Wrist profile with fracture

Blood and Circulation

Every cell in your body depends on a constant supply of blood for nourishment, oxygen and protection. Unfortunately, there are many problems that can disrupt the flow—including anaemia, atherosclerosis, stroke, varicose veins, scleroderma, and cancers of the blood and lymph nodes.

ANAEMIA

People with anaemia either have too few red blood cells or the cells are not able to carry enough oxygen for the body's needs. A blood test to measure the level of haemoglobin–the protein that transports oxygen–will determine if you have the condition and whether further investigation is needed–there are several reasons why it may develop in women.

The symptoms of anaemia include tiredness and breathlessness, especially after any kind of physical effort, very pale skin, a general feeling of weakness and being unusually cold.

The most common cause of anaemia is that your food intake does not include one of the components needed to manufacture the red cells in blood. Iron is particularly important as it is essential to make haemoglobin–dietitians recommend a daily intake of 14.8 mg. Vitamin B12 activates the making of red cells in bone marrow and the daily intake should be 1.5 mcg. Folic acid, a B vitamin, is important for cell division– 200 mcg per day is recommended, but this should be increased to 400 mcg during pregnancy.

Who's at risk?

Iron and vitamin B12 (which are usually obtained from animal sources) may be missing from the diet of vegetarians who do not have a well-balanced food intake. People who have pernicious anaemia lack the substance that enables B12 to be absorbed from the intestines into the blood and will usually need monthly injections of the vitamin. A number of diseases cause red blood cells to be destroyed, among them sickle cell disease and thalassaemia, in which the red blood cells are abnormal.

Loss of blood can also result in anaemia, which is why it sometimes

Blood constituents

Blood is composed predominantly of red cells. White blood cells are part of the immune system and defend against infection and disease, reacting to the presence of alien substances such as bacteria or viruses by destroying or neutralizing them. Other cells called platelets are part of the mechanism that enables blood to clot so it can seal a wound. Oxygen-rich blood in the arteries is bright red, while blood in the veins is darker.

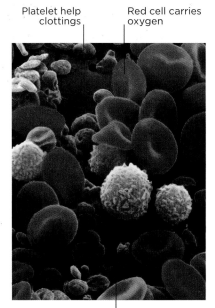

Platelet help clottings

Red cell carries oxygen

White cell for defence

WHAT'S YOUR BLOOD TYPE?

You inherit your blood type or group from your parents. There are four types: A, B, AB and O. In the UK and Australia the most common is O. The compatibility of blood types is crucially important in blood transfusions, since people cannot receive blood from incompatible types:

A can receive A or O;

B can receive B or O;

AB can receive any type;

O can only receive O.

Another element of blood typing is the rhesus (Rh) factor. The Rh system classifies blood according to the absence or presence of certain red blood cell protein molecules (antigens). About 85 per cent of people have the antigens and are Rh positive; the rest are Rh negative. Special care must be taken to match Rh negative blood in transfusions. Problems may arise in pregnancy if the woman is Rh negative and the father is Rh positive; the baby may in turn be Rh positive and the mother's antibodies may attack the baby, causing haemolytic disease.

Any underlying problem such as a stomach ulcer or unusually heavy menstruation will need to be treated. A blood transfusion may be necessary if the anaemia is severe. Iron may also be prescribed–as pills or, in some cases, injections–if you are not getting enough in your diet or are not absorbing it properly. You should not take iron supplements without your doctor advising you to do so.

Build iron into your diet

Adding iron to your diet means eating plenty of fresh green vegetables (such as broccoli, watercress and cabbage), either raw or lightly cooked, plus consuming blood builders such as almonds, eggs, shellfish, beans and lentils. Vitamin C helps the absorption of iron, so eat plenty of fresh citrus fruit, such as oranges, kiwi fruit, green and red peppers, tomatoes and potatoes (with the skin on, if it's organically grown). Avoid too many drinks containing caffeine, such as tea, coffee or cola that can prevent iron from being properly absorbed by the body.

WHEN YOU'RE PREGNANT

During pregnancy, you need a constant supply of iron for the extra red blood cells that make up a part of the increasing volume of blood swirling through you and the baby. The ratio of haemoglobin to blood volume may be slightly lower than normal because of this increase in total volume, but this doesn't necessarily mean that you are iron deficient.

Anaemia usually develops, if at all, in the last trimester of pregnancy, although it may occur earlier if you are carrying more than one baby. You will have regular blood tests as part of your antenatal monitoring and if you are found to be anaemic, you will be given advice on boosting your iron intake. Your doctor may also prescribe supplements.

affects those with peptic (digestive) ulcers. Women who experience heavy menstrual loss over a long time may become anaemic. It can occur in pregnancy when the baby draws on the mother's iron for its developing blood supply, or if the mother was deficient in iron before the beginning of the pregnancy. This deficiency can continue postnatally. Taking aspirin and NSAIDs can irritate the lining of the stomach and over a long period of time can cause microscopic blood loss.

Your options

If you suspect that you're anaemic, you should consult your doctor rather than trying to treat the condition yourself. Some symptoms may have other causes.

A blood test will determine your haemoglobin level–normal is about 12 g per 100 g of blood–and haematocrit (the ratio of blood cells to total volume of blood). If the level is low, your doctor will aim to establish the reason before deciding on treatment.

Anaemia can occur in pregnancy when the baby draws on the mother's iron for its developing blood supply.

IRON-RICH FOODS

The mineral iron is essential for the health of your blood throughout your lifetime. To ensure that you have a regular daily supply, choose from a variety of green vegetables and protein-rich foods. Keep up your intake of fresh foods containing vitamin C, so that the body can absorb the iron.

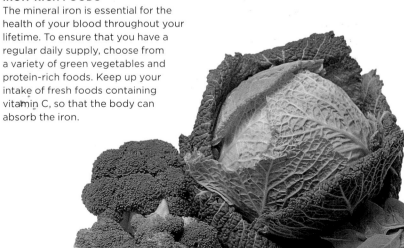

ATHEROSCLEROSIS

Commonly known as hardening of the arteries, atherosclerosis reduces the blood flow and increases the risk of various disorders, such as angina (chest pain), heart attack and stroke.

As part of the process of ageing, small deposits of fat begin to build up on the insides of your arteries causing the walls to become less flexible and more rigid. This natural deterioration can be exacerbated by conditions such as hypertension, diabetes, obesity, high blood cholesterol or lifestyle factors,

Women develop atherosclerosis later than men mainly due to oestrogen.

such as smoking, a high-fat diet and lack of exercise. Over time, the inner surfaces of the arteries become lumpy, narrowing the space for blood to flow through.

If the walls develop small cracks as well, they are sealed by patches called plaques, made up largely of blood fats such as cholesterol, dead cells and calcium. These plaques can eventually block the artery or they may break off and be carried around in the bloodstream until they end up blocking the blood flow completely. The consequences depend on whether the blockage is complete or partial and which artery is affected.

REDUCE YOUR RISK

To reduce your risk of atherosclerosis, take these steps.

- Don't smoke and stay out of smoky rooms. Avoiding tobacco smoke is the most important step you can take to reduce your risk. Smoking is an important risk factor in itself, and also multiplies the effect of any other risks, such as raised cholesterol levels.

- Lower your blood pressure. Elevated blood pressure may be an indication of arterial damage, so regular monitoring is needed. If yours is high, ask your doctor about medication. Since high blood pressure has no symptoms, all women should have their blood pressure checked yearly.

- Improve your diet. Try to have at least five portions of fruit and vegetables each day. Reduce your overall fat intake, choosing monounsaturated fats rather than saturated fats (those from animal sources) and keep intake of sugar and salt to a minimum.

- Exercise. Aim for 30 minutes a day of brisk walking, cycling or swimming, or three 20–30-minute sessions of more vigorous aerobic exercise every week.

- Step on the scales. Try to stay within the normal weight range for your height. Obesity is a risk factor in itself and may also increase your chances of developing type 2 diabetes (adult onset) and high blood pressure, which in turn can make you more susceptible to arterial disease.

BLOOD VESSELS AND WHY THEY NARROW

In normal arteries the walls are muscular and elastic and with the help of the heart push the oxygen-rich blood around the body to all the cells. For a variety of reasons the walls lose this elasticity and as fatty deposits, called atheroma or plaques, build up on them, the space through which the blood flows becomes narrower. The heart has to work harder to circulate the blood.

Mild sclerosis

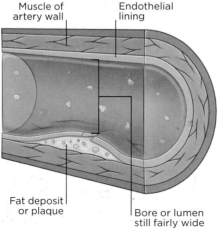

Muscle of artery wall

Endothelial lining

Fat deposit or plaque

Bore or lumen still fairly wide

Severe sclerosis

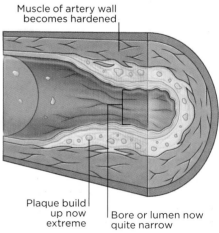

Muscle of artery wall becomes hardened

Plaque build up now extreme

Bore or lumen now quite narrow

RISKS DIFFER WITH AGE

While some women may be genetically predisposed to atherosclerosis and may need close monitoring, other women may develop the condition due to diet or lifestyle. If you eat foods high in saturated fats, cholesterol may collect in your arteries. If you don't exercise, your weight and blood pressure may suffer. If you smoke, toxic gases from the cigarettes can damage the artery linings. Be aware of the risks for each stage of life.

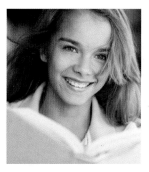

TEENS
Eating high-fat "junk" foods during childhood and the teenage years can be the start of bad eating habits and fatty deposit build-up, although without symptoms at this stage.

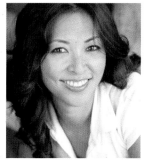

30s
Women have protective oestrogen, although it starts to diminish in the mid-30s. Oestrogen keeps the level of good cholesterol in the body high until the menopause.

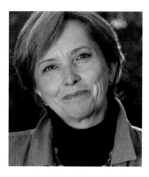

OVER 50
After the menopause, when the secretion of oestrogen stops, a woman's risk of developing atherosclerosis approaches that of men (for whom the condition is more common).

Who's at risk?

A number of interrelated factors determine whether a particular individual will develop atherosclerosis. Some you can do nothing about, while others can be reduced by a change in lifestyle.

A minority of people may have an inherited disposition to develop fatty deposits because they produce abnormally high amounts of a type of cholesterol known as LDL (low-density lipoprotein). People in this category usually have one or more close relatives who have experienced coronary heart disease (CHD) or strokes at a relatively early age (under 50). Atherosclerosis is one of the causes of cerebrovascular disease, in which the arteries of the brain are narrowed.

Women develop atherosclerosis later in life than men mainly due to the female sex hormone oestrogen, which appears to provide a certain amount of protection in premenopausal women. The hormone promotes high-density lipoproteins (HDLs) that protect against the development of CHD. After menopause, HDLs tend to fall and LDLs to rise. Other factors that increase the risk include premature menopause (including removal of the ovaries), hypertension, smoking, diabetes and obesity, and everyone becomes more susceptible in advanced age. Regular monitoring of cholesterol levels and blood pressure is important for all women, but essential for those at high risk.

Atherosclerosis is a common and increasing problem in most Western countries. As well as the five steps outlined (see box left), which should be followed even if you have already developed atherosclerosis, your doctor may suggest other treatments, including drugs. Aspirin can help to dissolve blood clots; statins reduce cholesterol levels; and a range of other drugs are designed to improve blood flow. Angioplasty can be used to open up arteries, and surgery can remove or replace blocked sections of arteries, although this may not be appropriate for every woman suffering from the condition.

ULTRASOUND

Doppler ultrasound is a non-invasive test used to diagnose atherosclerosis. It assesses the state of the blood vessels by measuring the rate of blood flow in the arteries and the heart.

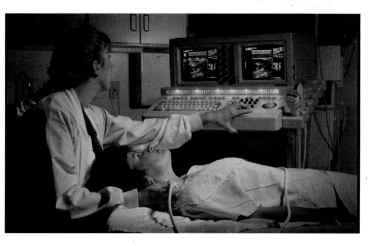

STROKE

Sometimes referred to as cerebro-vascular accidents, strokes are more common in men and older people. A stroke affects the blood supply to the brain, and its consequences will vary greatly depending on the degree of damage and on which part of the brain has been affected.

The most usual cause is a blood clot blocking an artery in the brain, known as an infarct or ischaemic stroke. Until investigations are done, it will not be certain whether the clot was formed elsewhere in the circulatory system and was carried in the bloodstream to the brain (known as an embolism), or whether it formed in the brain artery itself (thrombosis). In most people, the artery has narrowed because of atherosclerosis and a blockage occurs when a piece of plaque breaks off.

A stroke may also be caused by bleeding into the brain (called a cerebral haemorrhage), after a weak part of an arterial wall (aneurysm) has given way. Often the only symptom of cerebral haemorrhage is a severe headache. Brain cells and the surrounding tissue die when their blood supply is cut off.

If the damage is only minor, the person may recover completely, or may have problems with speech or vision or a part of the body may have been weakened or become paralyzed. There may be longer lasting paralysis or loss of sensation down one side of the body or the face, difficulties with comprehension, slurred speech, incontinence and loss of balance. The most dangerous type is bleeding into the brainstem, which directly affects breathing and heartbeat.

New treatments, if given early, can prevent permanent damage. Intensive treatment from rehabilitation specialists can minimize the after effects of brain damage and can often enable the person to regain some movement in paralyzed parts and recover the ability to speak.

"Mini" strokes

Transient ischaemic attacks, also known as TIAs and sometimes referred to as little or mini strokes, are caused when the blood supply to the brain is briefly and temporarily interrupted, usually by a tiny clot that then disperses. Symptoms last for less than 24 hours and include dizziness, weakness or numbness in one arm or leg, loss of vision and/or difficulty in speaking. The condition is more common in older people and it always needs to be investigated fully so that treatment in order to prevent further clots can be given if necessary to avoid a full stroke.

Reduce your risk

Regular blood pressure checks are essential–untreated hypertension is a major risk factor. If you are on medication to reduce your blood pressure, you must continue to take it, even if you have no symptoms. High cholesterol is also linked with stroke and blood cholesterol levels should be regularly tested and controlled with medication if necessary.

SCANNING THE BRAIN
One way to look at the brain is with magnetic resonance imaging (MRI). The body is placed in an enclosed unit with an intense magnetic field. Radio waves emitted by the body's atoms are detected and built up into a picture for analysis.

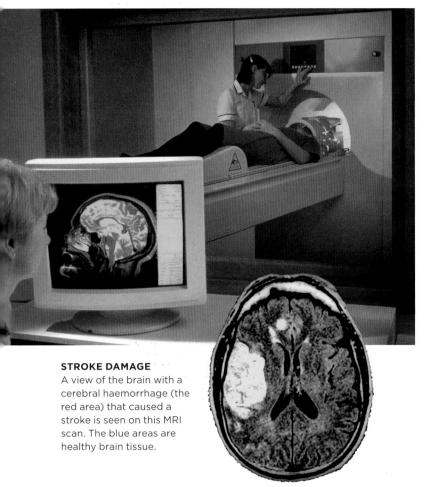

STROKE DAMAGE
A view of the brain with a cerebral haemorrhage (the red area) that caused a stroke is seen on this MRI scan. The blue areas are healthy brain tissue.

As well as following the advice given for preventing atherosclerosis, you should in addition try to limit your intake of alcohol to a maximum of one drink a day and avoid binge drinking or drinking without eating food.

Consuming less salt is also important as this can help to bring down elevated blood pressure–a contributing factor in many strokes. If you have diabetes or are extremely overweight or obese, you run a higher risk of having a stroke. Smokers fall into the same category. In some migraine headaches, accompanying symptoms such as numbness or tingling in the arms or legs may indicate that there are changes in your cerebral blood flow and should be brought to your doctor's attention.

THE SALT CONNECTION

Salt—chemical name sodium chloride or NaCl—plays an important role in maintaining the body's fluid balance and blood pressure. One of the key conclusions of nutritionists is that people in Western countries consume too much of it. Average consumption is 7.5 ml (1½ teaspoons) a day, yet as little as 2.5 ml (½ teaspoon) can lead to high blood pressure in susceptible people, and this in turn can lead to stroke. Cutting down such high levels is recommended.

Most foods—including vegetables, fruit and grains—contain some salt, but over 75 per cent of the salt we eat is hidden in prepared foods, added both for taste and preservation. Always read labels on bought, preprepared or packaged food. If you see salt or sodium or Na among the first few ingredients listed, the amount of salt in the food is high. If salt comes last on the list, the amount included may be low. If sodium bicarbonate (commonly called baking soda) is included on the list, that food should be avoided by anyone with heart or kidney problems.

It is worth knowing that if you prepare all your own meals, you should not add salt when cooking and use only coarse sea salt in a grinder at the table (rather than from a shaker that allows more to come out). If you do this, you will still provide the body with sufficient salt for fluid balance and health.

Making sense of clots

Peripheral vascular disease is the name given to blocked arteries or other conditions of arteries, such as aortic aneurysm. Symptoms include painful cramps in the feet, calves, thighs or hips when walking or exercising, but stop with rest. Smoking is the most common cause.

Phlebitis is a general term meaning inflammation of a vein. Thrombophlebitis describes clotting at the site of the inflammation usually in the superficial leg veins. The skin over the affected areas is tender and feels hard when touched. Although it can be unpleasant, phlebitis is not a risk to a woman's general health. The symptoms can be eased with rest, warm compresses, painkillers or NSAIDs, by propping your feet up to help blood flow or by gentle use of an over-the-counter remedy such as zinc oxide. Wearing support tights or stockings can help.

A blood clot that affects a deep vein—called deep venous thrombosis—is potentially serious. It can be fatal if the clot breaks away and travels through the bloodstream to block an artery in the lungs, called a pulmonary embolism. Thromboembolic disease is treated with blood-thinning drugs such as aspirin, heparin and warfarin, which dissolve the clot and prevent any more forming. In rare cases, people with varicose veins face an increased risk of this disease.

A woman thinking of taking oral contraceptives or hormone replacement therapy should tell her doctor of any personal or family history of thrombosis, as oestrogen medications—even if prescribed in low doses—may increase the risk of clotting.

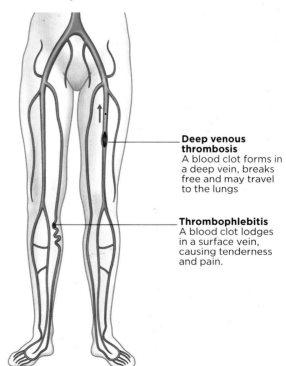

Deep venous thrombosis
A blood clot forms in a deep vein, breaks free and may travel to the lungs

Thrombophlebitis
A blood clot lodges in a surface vein, causing tenderness and pain.

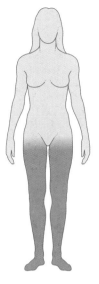

VEINS UNDER PRESSURE
The leg veins are the most hard-working in the body. They need to be strong to go against gravity in order to return deoxygenated blood to the lungs for cleansing, oxygenation and redistribution.

VARICOSE VEINS

From a medical point of view, varicose veins are rarely considered to be a serious problem. However, their appearance can sometimes cause concern, and they may be an indicator of a more serious circulatory disorder such as thrombosis.

Varicose veins occur mainly in the legs and may be disfiguring; they are usually hard, lumpy and blue because the walls of the veins become enlarged or twisted. They may also cause various symptoms such as aching, heaviness, skin damage, ulcers and swollen ankles. As these can also be symptoms of other medical conditions, you should discuss them with your doctor.

Women and men are probably equally susceptible to varicose veins. It is a condition that tends to run in families, which implies an inherited weakness in the blood vessels. They also seem to be more common in people whose job involves standing for long periods of time. Varicose veins can occur during pregnancy. They are also found in people who are overweight or obese.

Which veins are affected?

The veins most likely to have problems are those closest to the skin–known as the superficial veins. In particular, the long saphenous vein, which runs up the inside of the leg from the ankle to the groin, and the short saphenous vein, which is visible on the outside of the leg from the ankle to around knee level, are commonly involved.

WHAT TO EXPECT FROM TREATMENT

Since healthy, deep veins are capable of keeping the blood flowing, superficial veins that are badly affected can be stripped out under a general anaesthetic or epidural block anaesthesia. Before this is done, your veins are assessed using a Doppler ultrasound technique, which measures blood flow and enables the surgeon to identify and mark the veins that are varicosed. After the operation, there will be some bruising that will fade and some pain and discomfort. For a few days postoperatively you will need to wear compression stockings that help blood flow.

Injection treatment, known as sclerotherapy, can work well for small veins, especially those below the knee. It involves injecting the affected veins with a substance that, in effect, causes the walls to become glued together so that blood cannot flow through. The vessel collapses and the blood then reroutes itself to nearby veins.

Tiny spider veins are not considered a medical problem, but they can be sealed with laser surgery or sclerotherapy for cosmetic reasons.

Most of the blood that flows through veins has to travel upwards. Not being pumped in the same way as blood in the arteries, it would flow back under the influence of gravity without the valves that allow only so much blood through before shutting, then reopening. It is thought that varicose veins are caused when these valves stop working properly, possibly because the vein walls become

HOW VEINS BECOME VARICOSED
In a healthy body, veins have valves that work in a similar way to canal locks. They automatically open to let a certain amount of blood through, then shut while the next amount accumulates. If the valves aren't working well or the walls of the vein stretch, blood collects in one area and distorts the system. The medical term for this distortion is "varicosed".

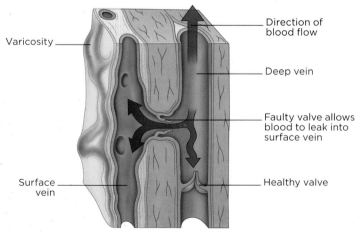

Varicosity

Surface vein

Direction of blood flow

Deep vein

Faulty valve allows blood to leak into surface vein

Healthy valve

weak and distended. The blood collects and distorts the vein, slowing the flow from one valve to the next.

Should they be treated?

Most people want their varicose veins dealt with for cosmetic reasons, but some seek help when skin changes occur–commonly eczema and/or skin darkening or discoloration, which may eventually result in ulcers. If you experience bleeding from varicose veins, which is relatively unusual, this is a sign that they need to be treated, as is a sudden feeling of heaviness in the legs and swelling. See your doctor if any of these occur.

Varicose eczema

The supply of blood to any area affected by varicose veins is reduced and the skin therefore receives less nutrient-enriched blood. It is at these places that eczema may develop. The scaly patches and blisters that characterize the condition may be treated with corticosteroid ointments and you may be advised to wear support compression tights or stockings to help reduce the swelling.

Varicose veins in pregnancy

One of the common complaints of middle to late pregnancy is varicose veins. The head of the fetus presses down on the pelvic veins, causing blood to pool in the legs and placing pressure on the walls of the veins. You will be advised to avoid gaining too much weight and not to be on your feet for long periods. Sleeping with your legs raised will help and daily exercise will improve circulation. The tendency to develop varicose veins increases with each successive pregnancy you have.

Haemorrhoids (commonly known as piles) can also be a problem for pregnant women who are susceptible to constipation. Haemorrhoids are varicose veins of the anal canal, a direct result of straining to pass faeces. When you strain, the blood bears down on the lowest vessels, causing them to stretch. Unlike other veins, the blood vessels in the anal canal have no valves to regulate the flow of blood and the pooled blood becomes a haemorrhoid. It can be internal or, if it extends from the anus, prolapsed. Consult your doctor before using any ointments and suppositories from a pharmacy. A high-fibre diet and drinking plenty of still water may help to ease the problem of constipation.

If haemorrhoids continue to be a problem after your baby is born, they can either be injected with a chemical to shrink them or tied with an elastic band to halt circulation to the area. In serious cases–that is, when the haemorrhoids are large and don't respond to treatment or bleed–anaemia can result.

Pregnant or not, it is important to report all instances of bleeding from the anus or blood in the stools to your doctor. It may need further investigation with a proctoscope or colonoscope to examine the anus, rectum or colon.

Relieving varicose veins

Here's how to ease the effects of varicose veins:

- Take short walks. Just get up and walk around whenever possible—repeatedly lifting your heels off the ground. This activates the "muscle pump", which helps to keep blood moving and prevent the formation of clots. Exercise that stimulates blood circulation is beneficial for women at any age and during pregnancy.

- Keep weight down. Excessive weight is thought to be a contributory factor in varicose veins. They may be less problematic if you keep your weight within the normal range for your height.

- Put your feet up. You can relieve heaviness and aching by raising your legs so that they are supported level with or above the rest of your body. Just keep in mind that sitting immobile in a chair for long periods will make symptoms worse.

- Wear support stockings. Avoid over-the-counter stockings; ask your doctor to prescribe the correct level of compression and get them from a medical supply store. Support stockings compress veins, discourage clots and ease discomfort. However, it is not advisable to wear them at night.

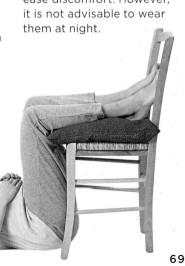

SCLERODERMA

A relatively rare condition that mostly affects women, scleroderma changes the look and feel of skin on the face, arms, hands and feet, and it can also involve some internal organs.

Also known as progressive systemic sclerosis, the disorder is part of a family of disorders characterized by skin thickening, due to disturbance of connective tissue called collagen, and a drastic reduction in the number of blood capillaries that feed the skin. This tissue, which normally gives skin its elasticity and bounce, becomes hardened and has fewer sweat glands and hair follicles. The skin thickens and appears shiny and smooth to the touch. The underlying subcutaneous fatty tissue and muscle may also be affected. If the skin tightens, it can limit the range of motion of joints and limbs.

It is not known what actually causes the collagen to overproduce. Scleroderma tends to be regarded as an autoimmune disorder in which the body produces antibodies against its own tissues. If the sclerosis is progressive, other organs including the kidneys, lungs and heart may be affected.

Scleroderma is a multi-system disease that may be managed by a medical team comprising a rheumatologist, a nephrologist, a chest physician, a gastroenterologist, a dermatologist and a cardiologist. It is a chronic disease that needs to be carefully monitored so any physical changes can receive prompt attention. There is no cure and drugs must be prescribed, which include corticosteroids, anti-hypertensives, antacids and NSAIDs. In severe cases calcium channel blockers may be used.

HOW SCLERODERMA IS DIAGNOSED

Diagnosis of the condition is based on a physical examination and occasionally a skin biopsy may be done. The doctor will look for what is known as CREST syndrome:

C—calcinosis (calcific deposits under the skin).

R—Raynaud's phenomenon (*see* box below).

E—oesophageal dismotility (thickening of the oesophagus, which prevents simple digestion).

S—sclerodactyly (thickening skin on the fingers affecting shape and movement).

T—telangiectasias (collection of tiny blood vessels on the skin's surface, most usually the face).

WHO'S AT RISK?

Scleroderma can occur at any age, but it's most likely to be found in Afro-Caribbean women in their 20s, and in white women between the ages of 20 and 40. Thought to be an autoimmune condition, it can be limited (affecting only the hands and face) or diffuse (skin over the entire body is involved). The condition is rarely life threatening, but it can be disabling and affect quality of life.

The blue finger problem

Raynaud's phenomenon is a circulatory disorder that mostly affects women under 40 and has no known cause. It can be triggered by emotion and appears when the temperature drops. Sufferers are hypersensitive to cold because the small arteries close to the surface of the skin go into spasm, restricting blood flow.

During an attack, usually lasting only a few minutes, the fingers and toes (and sometimes the nose and/or the earlobes) turn white, then blue and feel numb. They may turn red and you may have a tingling or burning sensation.

Prevention is the first line of defence. Dressing in warm layers when going out in cold weather and remembering to protect the head (from which most body heat is lost) and hands and feet will help. Stopping smoking is crucial. Be alert to changes such as ulcers, sores or discoloration on fingers or toes. Report them to your doctor as they may indicate lack of blood to these vulnerable parts.

Fight back
- During a Raynaud's attack, have a warm (not hot) bath.
- If you are prone to attacks at night, keep a hot drink in a flask by your bed.
- Regular, vigorous exercise may help by improving your circulation and toning your muscles. You should be careful not to become chilled following exercise.

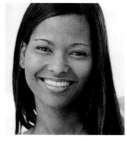

Between 20 and 30

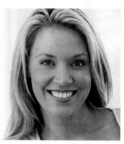

Early 20s to late 30s

BLOOD AND LYMPH CANCERS

There is a close relationship between blood and lymph. Both reach all parts of the body and may be involved in the spread of cancerous cells. Women are at relatively low risk rate for these cancers.

Leukaemia

There are several different types of leukaemia (cancer of the blood) and some are more dangerous than others. All involve excess production of various types of white blood cells and tumours may form in bone marrow, spleen and lymph nodes.

Symptoms differ according to the type of leukaemia, but may include tiredness and generally feeling unwell, aching bones, susceptibility to infections, night sweats and a raised temperature. Diagnosis is by blood test and bone marrow sampling. Sometimes leukaemia that causes few or no symptoms may only be diagnosed when a blood test is done for some other reason. Chronic types mostly affect people over 50.

Leukaemia classified as "acute" and chronic myeloid or lymphocytic are treated with powerful chemotherapy and, in some cases, with a bone marrow transplant. For some chronic forms, a milder form of chemotherapy with fewer side effects may be adequate.

Multiple myeloma

This rare condition, which involves uncontrolled growth of plasma cells in bone marrow, generally appears in middle to old age. It can interfere with the production of normal red and white blood cells and result in anaemia and risk of infection. Diagnosis is by X-rays and bone marrow biopsy; treatment includes anticancer drugs.

Hodgkin's disease

At the earliest stage of this uncommon cancer, the only symptom may be enlarged, painless lymph nodes in the neck or under the arm. However, as malignant cells develop in the lymphatic system, fever, loss of appetite and weight and night sweats add to a general feeling of being unwell. The cause of the disease is not known, but it is more likely to affect women between the ages of 20 and 30, and over 55. Gradually, as the lymphoid tissue spreads, it impairs the immune system, leaving the body vulnerable to infections that would not worry a healthy person.

The progress of the disease is assessed by tissue biopsy (from a lymph node, affected organ or bone marrow), chest X-ray and CAT or MRI scans. If diagnosed in its early stages, Hodgkin's disease can be cured. Chemotherapy is the most likely treatment, in some cases combined with radiotherapy. In other cases, relatively low-dose radiotherapy on its own is likely to be effective.

Non-Hodgkin's lymphoma

A malignancy of the lymph system (not Hodgkin's disease), non-Hodgkin's lymphoma mostly affects people over 50. It may begin with painless swelling of lymph nodes in the neck or groin, but the spread of cells can speedily overwhelm the immune system. Other symptoms include weight loss, fever and fatigue.

Treatment is decided after biopsy. Radiotherapy may be given if the cells are contained in a group of lymph nodes. If the disease affects the spleen, liver or other organs, treatment is anticancer drugs possibly with radiotherapy. A bone marrow transplant may be the only option in serious cases.

CELL CHANGES
Healthy white blood cells are carried in blood and lymph fluid to fend off disease. When something causes certain white cells to grow uncontrolled, the healthy ones are crowded out and the abnormal ones proliferate. As all blood cells are made in bone marrow, a bone marrow transplant may be viewed as the best way of treating blood cancer. Development of drugs that work on affected cells may eventually change this.

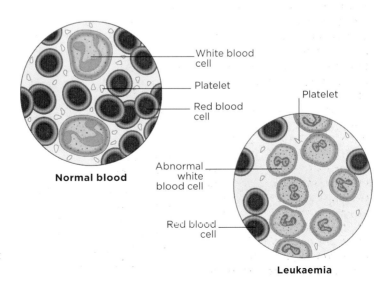

White blood cell

Platelet

Red blood cell

Normal blood

Abnormal white blood cell

Platelet

Red blood cell

Leukaemia

Women and heart disease

The heart is a pump that sends blood to all parts of the body every second you're alive. It's a complex organ made up of four chambers, which are separated by valves and operated by powerful muscles. Cardiac disease affects not only the heart, but your whole body.

REDUCING RISK

Women before the menopause are much less likely to develop coronary heart disease (CHD) than men.

As women age, however, they become more vulnerable to heart disease and by their 70s are nearly on a par with men. The loss of oestrogen may play a role but studies suggest CHD in women is more complex. In fact, postmenopausal hormone replacement therapy or selective oestrogen receptor modulators (SERMs) to reduce the risk of CHD is no longer advised.

Postmenopausal hormone replacement therapy or selective oestrogen receptor modulators (SERMs) to reduce the risk of CHD is no longer advised.

You may not be able to change pre-existing or inherited conditions that predispose you to heart disease, but heart disease itself is less likely to occur if you adopt a healthy lifestyle.

Don't even THINK of smoking There is no doubt that smoking is one of the most important risk factors for heart disease. Smokers are 2–4 times more likely to develop CHD as non-smokers; even second-hand smoke exposure increases the risk of heart disease.

Among other things, the chemicals in smoke can cause temporary narrowing of the blood vessels and an increase in the stickiness of blood platelets, which makes clotting more likely. Chemicals also contribute to plaque build-up on the inner walls of arteries, which can result in angina and heart attacks.

Eat far less fat You should aim to reduce saturated fat and transfatty acid intake (in foods from animal sources), and substitute polyunsaturated or monounsaturated fats. Eat a lot more fresh fruit and vegetables, pulses and wholegrain foods including bread, brown rice and oats.

Exercise Your heart will become stronger and fitter with regular exercise, which will also have a positive impact on

How the heart beats

Your heart rate alters according to what you are doing. When the body is at rest, the nutrients in the blood are transported to the cells for repair. Activities such as eating and walking need energy, so heart rate increases. When the body is in action, when playing tennis for example, the lungs take in more oxygen, and the heart beats faster to produce the energy needed for the movements of the game.

other risk factors such as cholesterol, diabetes, obesity and high blood pressure. Aim to leave yourself feeling slightly breathless but still be able to talk to give your heart a reasonable workout.

Lose extra pounds If you have accumulated excess fat it's especially important to bring your weight down to the normal range for your height.

Monitor blood sugar High blood sugar (glucose) increases your risk of CHD. Keep yours in check with daily exercise and a diet rich in high-fibre vegetables such as beans.

Know your numbers You should have your blood pressure checked at least once every year, and also have your cholesterol measured. Elevated blood pressure and hyperlipidaemia (high cholesterol) are considered important contributing factors to CHD and heart attack.

The blood flow in the heart

The average woman's heart weighs 255 g (9 oz), about 56 g (2 oz) less than that of a man. Protected by the breastbone and the ribs on the left side of the chest, the heart beats around 70 times a minute, the rate increasing when demand for blood goes up, during exercise or at times of stress, for example, when the body systems prepare for "fight or flight".

The heart has four chambers, two on each side, separated by a membrane called the septum, which stops oxygen-rich blood from mixing with blood depleted of oxygen. Valves between upper and lower chambers on both sides open and close to ensure that blood flows in one direction only. The coronary arteries carry blood rich with oxygen and nutrients to the heart muscle or myocardium. This muscle contracts under stimulation from a series of electrical impulses controlled by nerves—the heart's natural pacemaker. These impulses are measured during an electrocardiogram (ECG).

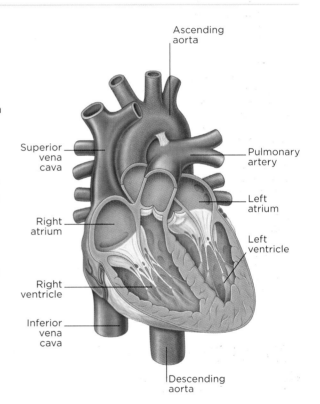

Ascending aorta

Superior vena cava

Right atrium

Right ventricle

Inferior vena cava

Descending aorta

Pulmonary artery

Left atrium

Left ventricle

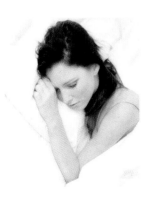

Sleeping 60 beats per minute

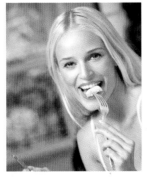

Eating 65 beats per minute

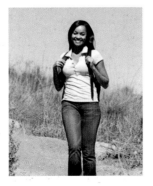

Walking 100 beats per minute

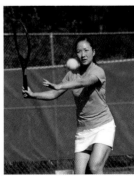

Tennis 110 beats per minute

WHAT CAN GO WRONG WITH THE HEART

One of the problems with heart and blood vessel disease is that it may develop slowly over many years without causing any symptoms. What's more, symptoms that are relatively minor may be attributed to some other cause. Women in particular may be slower in seeking help and in recognizing their symptoms. Women may experience different symptoms compared with men, which may be described as atypical.

Too often they can be thought to be the inevitable consequences of getting older rather than important indicators of disease. A prime example is recurrent indigestion, which may be an atypical symptom of angina in some women.

When you stop what you're doing and rest or go into a warm environment, angina should ease within 10 minutes.

An increased awareness of your health will help you take steps to reduce your risks, if necessary. It also helps to be aware of the forms heart disease can take.

Angina

The condition's full medical name, angina pectoris, simply means pain in the chest, and it occurs because some muscle fibres in the heart are not receiving the oxygen they need.

This happens as a result of narrowing of the arteries, but people don't usually get any symptoms until the problem is quite advanced–when the arteries have narrowed by more than 70 per cent and blood flow to the region of the heart they supply is drastically reduced.

Chest pain caused by angina often comes on when the heart's demand for oxygen increases even slightly and exceeds the blood supply to the heart, so relatively minor exercise, such as walking uphill, going out into cold air or a strong wind, or sexual activity can trigger the pain. When you stop whatever you are doing and rest or go into a warm environment, the pain should gradually ease within 10 minutes.

Once the condition has been diagnosed, you will be prescribed medication to stop it even faster. If it doesn't go away or comes on when you are resting or even asleep, you should go back to your doctor as this might mean the condition has become unstable and could culminate in a heart attack. Fatigue without chest pain may also be a sign of a problem and should be brought to your doctor's attention.

Normally, angina doesn't damage the heart muscle. Once the oxygen supply is restored to the heart muscle, it recovers.

Heart attack

A heart attack occurs when one of the coronary arteries becomes blocked by a thrombosis (or clot), which is why it is referred to as coronary thrombosis. Clots can develop in an artery that has become narrowed from atherosclerosis, and no blood or oxygen can reach the area of the heart supplied by that artery. If the blood supply is not restored, that part of the muscle will die within five to ten minutes–this is called a myocardial infarction (MI). The extent of the damage depends on the size of the blocked artery and whether it is the only blood vessel supplying that part of the myocardium (heart muscle).

It may not be easy to distinguish the pain of a heart attack from that caused by severe indigestion, particularly in the early stages. The pain may be felt in the

WHAT HAPPENS IN A HEART ATTACK

When a coronary artery is narrowed or blocked by fatty deposits on the artery wall, or by a blood clot, blood supply to the heart is restricted or stops and the heart muscle tissue "suffocates" through lack of oxygen. Cardiac muscle fibres begin to die causing chest pain. Clot-busting therapy, using drugs as fast as possible, can reinstate blood flow in 60 to 90 per cent of those who have a heart attack.

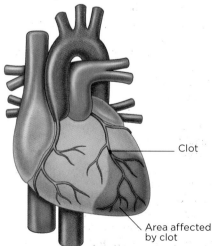

Clot

Area affected by clot

centre of the chest or on the left side, and sometimes spreads into the shoulders and upper arms or into the neck and jaw. A person having a heart attack may look pale and sweaty and may also feel faint and sick. Don't hesitate to call an ambulance as prompt treatment is vital. Sometimes a severe heart attack can disturb the normal rhythm and result in the heart stopping altogether (cardiac arrest).

Abnormal rhythm

Many people have felt at one time or another that their heart is not beating regularly or seems to miss the occasional beat. In fact, this is quite common, although not everyone notices when it happens. Usually, it is not a problem. If you have other symptoms such as chest pain, nausea, lightheadedness, sweating or loss of consciousness, you should seek help to rule out a medical condition.

Abnormal rhythms are most likely to occur when you are under severe stress. They are sometimes brought on by drinking too much alcohol or caffeinated drinks such as coffee, tea or cola.

Abnormal heart rhythms, also called arrhythmias, are a possible complication following a heart attack. If the myocardium has been damaged it can affect the heart's electrical pacemaker, causing it to beat so that blood is not pumped in and out properly. Called fibrillation, it can affect the upper (atrial) or lower (ventricular) chambers of the heart. As it can be fatal, drugs may be prescribed to control it.

Arrhythmia can sometimes cause the heart to stop completely. Immediate use of a device called a defibrillator, which delivers a short, sharp electric shock, can restart it. If there is a persistent risk patients may need a defibrillator surgically placed in the chest, called an implantable defibrillator.

Another condition, Wolff-Parkinson-White syndrome, is characterized by an arrhythmia known as tachycardia (rapid and irregular heartbeats) and may be treated by surgery.

Heart failure

While this term means that the heart is no longer capable of pumping sufficient

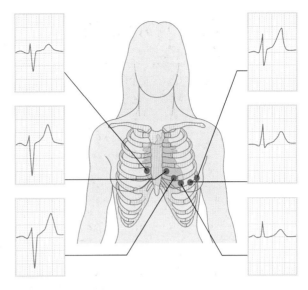

blood around the body to supply its normal requirements it doesn't mean that the heart has given up altogether. A person may live for many years thanks to modern treatment, especially drugs, that can be used for heart disorders.

The problem may arise as a consequence of diabetes, or blood pressure being too high for a long period, which makes the heart thickened and stiff. More often it is a result of coronary heart disease. In an attempt to compensate for damage to large parts of the myocardium, the heart can enlarge but is unable to pump as efficiently as before. This can cause the lungs to fill up with fluid and water, which leaves the person breathless, and causes legs and ankles to swell because of fluid retention.

Valve disorders

The four heart valves play a vital role in ensuring that blood flows in one direction only and in the right amounts. If they become damaged, they may prevent sufficient blood being pumped with each heartbeat, or they may allow blood to flow back in the wrong direction. Some people are born with defective valves, although this does not always cause problems. A bout of rheumatic fever in childhood may affect the valves later in life, as can bacterial infection. Symptoms may include breathlessness and angina, but their nature and seriousness depend on which valves are affected.

MONITORING THE HEART
An electrocardiogram (ECG) picks out rhythm abnormalities, detects old or recent heart attacks, and provides information on whether the heart is under strain because of disease, or is enlarged. An ECG is done in the doctor's surgery or hospital, is painless and takes about 10 minutes. Electrodes are placed on the chest, arms and legs to chart the pattern of electrical energy on a graph. Using many leads means every part of the heart can be evaluated.

LIVING WITH HEART DISEASE

Women with cardiovascular problems need to be as vigilant as men about their health. They have as great a risk of complications and death as their husbands or sons diagnosed with heart disease. Treatment as well as prevention of further risks are both important.

Getting your life back

Recovering from a heart-related illness may involve confronting and dealing with emotions that your physical situation has brought. Apprehension, anxiety, anger and depression are commonplace. You may be aware of similar feelings in family members who may not have thought women were susceptible to problems that for so long have been male related. They too will need guidance about how to improve your chances of returning to health.

With greater understanding of the way women are affected, more help is now provided by national bodies, usually charities, which have a countrywide support network. Cardiac rehabilitation centres and clubs provide a backup service with information and advice. Some may offer counselling and stress management classes to teach coping strategies. Sharing experiences with others can bring reassurance, and following advice can reduce problems.

You will likely have many questions about relationships, resuming sexual activity, returning to work, responses you may have to surgery or drugs, or what you are physically capable of doing. Those involved in rehabilitation understand and should take the time to answer your questions. There may be a programme that encompasses a range of aspects of recovery, from medication and diet to exercise and stress management. Each of these is important. Physical activity, built into everyday life in combination with a low-fat, low-salt diet, can restore the quality of life that heart disorders threaten to take away.

A new start

The purpose of rehabilitation is to get you to identify the most beneficial changes for you, an approach summed up as "heart-smart concepts".

You need to pinpoint the greatest stresses in your life and find ways to deal with them. Reducing their effects may be the most immediate way to improve your health. In turn this may help you conquer other heart-related problems, such as smoking, overeating or an unbalanced diet. Physical activity, even if you are overweight, is health giving.

In a heart rehabilitation programme, physiotherapists and your doctor choose exercises geared to you, so you reach a level that will help you relax, breathe well and stretch muscles, to benefit blood flow and pressure, and lift your spirits, encouraging wellbeing.

WIDENING YOUR ARTERIES

Modern surgery can expand your arteries if they have become narrowed by fatty plaques. A catheter (fine tube) is inserted through your skin into the femoral artery in the leg. The catheter is threaded through the body to the coronary artery.

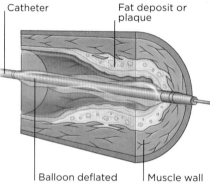

Catheter | Fat deposit or plaque

Balloon deflated | Muscle wall

Inside the catheter is a tiny balloon, which the cardiologist can inflate at the point where the fat deposit is causing the constriction. The blown-up balloon widens the bore or lumen to improve blood flow through the artery.

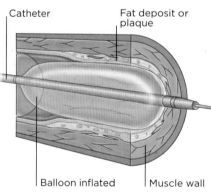

Catheter | Fat deposit or plaque

Balloon inflated | Muscle wall

To prevent the artery collapsing or being blocked again by fat deposits, the balloon is deflated and a coronary stent is left in its place. This is a fine mesh of stainless steel that can be expanded to brace the muscle wall.

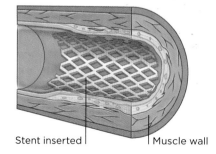

Stent inserted | Muscle wall

HEALING THE HEART

The aim of your medical team will be to alleviate the disorder, return you to health and improve your life expectancy. Treatment for any heart condition will be planned on an individual basis, but the following chart lists some of the most common medical and surgical options for women as well as men.

CONDITION	MEDICINAL TREATMENT	SURGICAL TREATMENT
Angina	Drugs to reduce the amount of oxygen needed by the heart and/or dilate the blood vessels to improve the flow, aspirin or glyceryl trinitrate placed under the tongue to relieve symptoms; also, aspirin and cholesterol-lowering drugs	Angioplasty: inserting an expandable balloon into the narrow artery to stretch it; sometimes a wire mesh (stent) is left inside to hold the walls apart. If severe, coronary artery bypass graft (CABG) may be carried out
Heart attack	Aspirin to make blood platelets less sticky; thrombolytics ("clot-buster" drugs) to dissolve clot within 12 hours; beta-blockers to slow heart; ACE inhibitors to dilate blood vessels; statins and other drugs to lower cholesterol; glyceryl trinitrate to relieve angina attacks	Angioplasty or coronary artery bypass graft (CABG) to bypass the blocked section with either a piece of vein or artery from the chest wall or one from an arm or leg: may be single or multiple bypass
Abnormal rhythm	Drugs such as digoxin, beta-blockers, amiodarone or other antiarrhythmic drugs	Implantable defibrillator or pacemaker for recurrent ventricular fibrillation
Heart failure	Drugs to relieve congestion, such as diuretics (water tablets); ACE inhibitors; glyceryl trinitrate to relieve angina, and other drugs	None
Heart block (upper and lower chambers of the heart out of synchronization)	None	Operation to place electronic pacemaker under the skin of the chest to help heart muscle contract
Valve disease	Drugs to treat symptoms of heart failure; prophylactic antibiotics; drugs to reduce stress	Operation to stretch narrowed valves or replace damaged valves with synthetic or tissue ones
Mitral valve prolapse	Drugs to help with arrhythmia, or murmur and possible anxiety; prophylactic treatment to protect the heart may include oral antibiotics before and after surgery and dental work (routine antibiotics before dental procedures are no longer recommended in cases of mitral valve prolapse alone); prophylaxis is for patients at the highest level of risk for heart-valve infection (bacterial endocarditis), such as patients with a prosthetic cardiac valve, patients who have had bacterial endocarditis before, or patients with specific types of congenital heart disease	None

HIGH BLOOD PRESSURE

The medical name for blood pressure (BP) that is consistently above a recognized norm is hypertension. It is directly associated with increased risk of stroke and heart disease. Hypertension usually affects the middle aged and elderly, with a much higher incidence in those people who have a family history of the condition.

When the heart muscle contracts to pump blood through the body, pressure in the arteries is at its peak. This is called the systolic pressure. The muscle then relaxes before the next contraction and the pressure drops to its minimum, the diastolic pressure. When your blood pressure is measured, it is expressed as two figures, for example, 150/85–the higher systolic and lower diastolic pressures, respectively.

A silent threat

There is usually no way you can know whether your blood pressure is high without having it measured; you can't feel it, because hypertension does not have any symptoms until it gets to a dangerously high level.

However, if it stays high, it causes serious and progressive damage to the blood vessels, making the linings rough and causing narrowing and thickening of the artery walls. Eventually, these changes can lead to coronary heart disease (CHD), stroke and eye damage from bleeding in the retina (particularly in diabetics).

Women who take oral contraceptives, who smoke and those over the age of 40 should have their blood pressure checked annually. Ideally, it should be less than 120/80. Elderly women often have systolic readings above 140, a condition called isolated systolic hypertension, which should be treated.

Do you need medication?

You will need medication if your BP readings are high on two or three separate occasions, in spite of attempts to lower it by lifestyle changes. Modern drugs are effective and can reduce the risk of stroke by 35 to 40 per cent and CHD by 20 to 25 per cent. Diuretics or beta-blockers can be used to slow the heart, and various drugs can open up blood vessels. You must take them as prescribed, even though you may feel well. If you experience any side effects, don't stop taking the medication. Consult your doctor who may prescribe a drug from a different group. Medication will control but not cure hypertension and you will need to continue to take it for the rest of your life.

MONITORING
Having blood pressure measured is quick and painless. It frequently goes up when you visit your doctor—a phenomenon called "white coat hypertension".

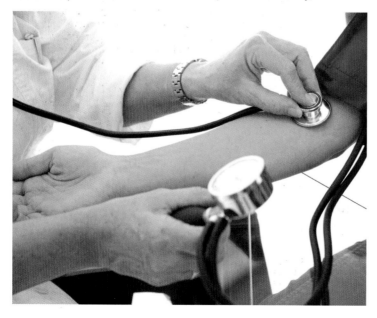

REDUCE YOUR RISK

To reduce your risk of hypertension:
- Exercise every day.
- Avoid tobacco smoke.
- Limit your intake of salty processed foods and snacks, and don't add salt to your food when you are cooking. Consuming a lot of salt significantly raises the risk of hypertension.
- Keep your weight within a healthy range.
- Consider having a glass of wine once a day. It may help keep blood pressure down. More, however, can drive it up.
- Eat fruit, vegetables and low-fat dairy products, since these contain potassium and calcium, which help control blood pressure.
- Analyse your lifestyle and make changes to reduce chronic stress.

HIGH CHOLESTEROL

Many women do not realize that cardiovascular disease (CHD) is their greatest potential health problem. They, as much as men, can benefit from identifying their risk factors and reducing them. That's why all women from the age of 20 should be screened for high cholesterol, a key risk factor for heart disease. The medical term for this condition is "hyperlipidaemia" (excess fat in the blood).

Checking the level of lipids (fats) in the blood, one of which is cholesterol, is one of the foremost indicators of the health of the heart. If high cholesterol is left untreated, it increases a woman's risk of developing CHD, especially after the menopause. Establishing a healthy eating pattern (using the healthy eating diagrams in Chapter 1 as a guide and the accompanying advice on serving sizes and total fat content) is considered the first step for women concerned about living well and living longer.

Who's at risk?

In most cases, high cholesterol is caused by excessive consumption of dietary fat and cholesterol, combined with a lack of physical activity. Women who smoke, are overweight or obese and have high blood pressure and/or diabetes are at particular risk. Other medical problems, including liver and thyroid disease, excessive alcohol intake and diabetes that remains undiagnosed, can also cause increased lipid levels in the blood.

Two further important risk factors are premature menopause (before the age of 45) and a family history of premature CHD in a close relative (especially in a mother under the age of 65 or a father under the age of 55).

Women with these risk factors who have high cholesterol will generally be placed on a restricted diet for a trial period of three to six months. The saturated fats found in butter, lard, cheese, meat and meat products and transfats found in hard margarines and products made from them, such as cookies and pastries, should be reduced and/or replaced by polyunsaturated fats (found in sunflower, soy and fish oils) and monounsaturated (found in olive oil, rapeseed oil and nuts).

The restricted diet will be followed, if necessary, by treatment with lipid-lowering drugs. In addition to diet and medication, women will be given advice

All women from the age of 20 should be screened for high cholesterol.

and instruction on a course of exercise to help them achieve and maintain a desirable body weight for their build and height. It is generally considered that 20 to 30 minutes of exercise every day is adequate.

A CHOLESTEROL PRIMER

One of the essential components of cell walls is cholesterol, a natural waxy substance that is made in the liver and carried around the body in the blood.

High levels of cholesterol in the blood are a risk factor for heart disease. Surplus cholesterol settles on the walls of the arteries, forming plaques that narrow the space through which blood flows. The excess in the blood comes from the way the body processes animal (saturated) fats in the diet. On the other hand, vegetable fats (unsaturated, polyunsaturated and monounsaturated) are chemically different from saturated fat and metabolized in a different way. They may have a beneficial effect on cholesterol.

Transfat comes from adding hydrogen to vegetable oil through a process called hydrogenation. Transfats are more solid than oil, which makes them less likely to spoil. That's why they're used in the manufacturing of foods. Initially, transfats were thought to be a healthy alternative to animal fats because they are unsaturated and come primarily from plant oils. However, scientists discovered that transfats appeared to both increase LDL cholesterol (also known as bad cholesterol) and decrease HDL (good cholesterol). They should be avoided wherever possible.

Cholesterol has three measurements: total, HDL (high-density lipoprotein) and LDL (low-density lipoprotein). Here are the goals set by scientists in two regions:

CONDITION	EUROPE	UNITED STATES
Total cholesterol	<5.2 mmol/L	<200 mg/dL
HDL cholesterol	>1.5 mmol/L	>60 mg/dL
LDL cholesterol	<2.6 mmol/L	<100 mg/dL
Triglycerides	<1.7 mmol/L	<150 mg/dL

Your doctor may use the term "cholesterol ratio", which is the total cholesterol divided by the HDL. The optimal ratio for women is 3.5 to 1; above 5 to 1 is a health risk.

Do you have any of these symptoms?

- Constant thirst and a dry mouth
- Extreme appetite
- Need to empty your bladder frequently
- Tiredness or increased irritability
- Blurred vision
- Unexplained weight loss
- Frequent urinary or vaginal infections

Endocrine System Problems

The endocrine system consists of various glands that secrete hormones into the bloodstream to regulate bodily processes. When those hormones become unbalanced, disorders such as diabetes and thyroid disease are the result.

WHO IS AT RISK?

Diabetes can strike at any age, from birth to old age. If you have parents with diabetes or are overweight, you are more likely to develop the illness (type 2). You are also susceptible if you have elevated blood pressure, you are pregnant or have polycystic ovary syndrome (mostly under the age of 40).

DIABETES

The hormone insulin is produced by your pancreas to enable the cells in your body to make use of the fuel they need, which involves processing the glucose in the blood. When someone has diabetes–type 1 or type 2–either not enough insulin is being produced or it is not being used properly, or both. Any interruption of the insulin supply results in glucose levels in the blood becoming too high. All brain and red blood cells need a constant supply of glucose, but too much is life threatening.

Diabetes mellitus is the fastest growing illness in Western countries, yet it is not understood why some people get it and others don't. Currently, there is no cure for the condition, but depending on the type, it can be controlled effectively by exercise, diet and medication.

If the condition arises quickly, it suggests that the insulin-producing cells in the pancreas have stopped working, an autoimmune problem caused by the

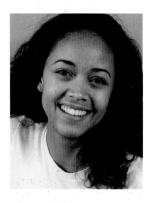

TEENAGERS
The genes inherited from your parents may play a part in whether you get diabetes. In young people the disease may be triggered by a virus.

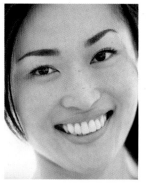

20s AND 30s
During the 20s and 30s either type 1 or 2 diabetes may occur. The sudden onset of symptoms is likely to indicate that insulin production has stopped.

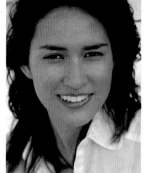

PREGNANT WOMEN
Approximately 3 per cent of pregnant women develop a variation called gestational diabetes. It will be picked up in antenatal tests after the 24th week of pregnancy.

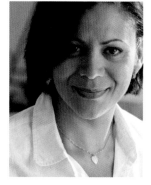

OVER 40
Type 2 diabetes is the most common type of diabetes in women over 40, perhaps because weight gain, a major contributing factor, is common at this time.

body attacking itself. This is type 1 or insulin-dependent diabetes. It is also called juvenile diabetes, although it can begin in adulthood.

If diabetes occurs gradually, "insulin resistance" sets in. Insulin is produced normally but for some reason blood glucose cannot enter cells making the insulin ineffective. Called type 2 diabetes, it usually begins after the age of 40 (hence its former name adult-onset diabetes) and is more common than type 1. Type 2 diabetes is associated with obesity and may be familial.

Type 2 diabetes is prevalent in South Asian and Afro-Caribbean women. In the UK diabetes occurs in 2-3 per cent of the population. Symptoms may not be noticed for up to 9 years. Close to a third of those people who have diabetes may be undiagnosed.

A blood test every three years is advised for women over 45 without risk factors, or over 40 if they are overweight or have a family history of diabetes.

How to handle diabetes

Lifelong regular injections of insulin are currently the main treatment for type 1

diabetes, although a balanced diet and regular exercise is also essential to all diabetes management.

Among the diagnosed type 2 diabetic population over a third manage their diabetes by exercise and diet alone. Sometimes this needs to be combined with medication that can help make better use of the insulin the body produces or slow down the speed at which sugar is absorbed.

Some type 2 diabetics may need insulin. Following a low-fat, high-fibre diet with plenty of vegetables, fruit and wholegrain foods is key. Limiting consumption of refined carbohydrates loaded with sugar, which quickly raise the blood glucose level, benefits everyone who suffers from diabetes.

Those with type 2 diabetes can frequently keep their blood sugar down with 30 minutes of exercise a day.

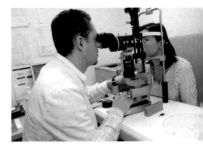

EYE TESTS
Many people who have undiagnosed type 2 diabetes find out during a routine eye examination: the ophthalmologist may notice changes in the retina. Damage to blood vessels at the back of the eye can cause loss of sight and even blindness. Laser treatments can slow down the progression.

30 minutes of exercise a day can often keep type 2 diabetes at bay.

The big picture

The main long-term risk for people with diabetes is high blood pressure and high cholesterol, which leads to blood vessel damage. That can cause coronary heart disease or a stroke, and can affect eyesight and damage the peripheral nerves, especially in the feet. Kidney disease is another common problem.

You should try to maintain blood glucose levels. Monitor your blood sugar level by regularly using a finger-prick blood test and a glucometer so treatment can be adjusted if necessary.

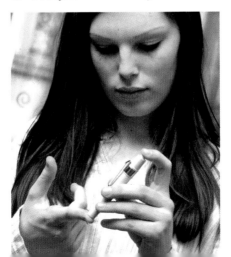

DIABETES IN PREGNANCY

When you are pregnant, your urine is tested for any trace of sugar. This can appear, usually after the 24th week, because hormones from the placenta may affect the body's response to insulin, making it less effective. Glucose in the bloodstream rises and overflows into the urine.

This condition is known medically as gestational diabetes. If nothing is done, the baby may grow too large, resulting in a difficult delivery, and it may develop hypoglycaemia (low blood sugar).

Often a change of diet may be enough to solve the problem, but some women may need to be treated with insulin until giving birth. Once the placenta is delivered, the diabetes usually disappears, but 30 to 50 per cent of women may develop type 2 diabetes later. A woman with gestational diabetes is more at risk of urinary tract infections and preeclampsia. A baby whose mother had gestational diabetes may have a greater risk of developing diabetes in future.

WHEN YOU NEED INSULIN
Insulin as a medication is destroyed by the digestive system if taken orally. That is why it is most often injected into the fatty layer under the skin: a quick-acting form by day to counter the rise in blood sugar from food; at night a longer-acting one. As many as four injections in a 24-hour period may be needed. You can use a syringe, a pen (shown left) with disposable cartridges or a jet injector that uses pressurized air. Those whose blood sugar fluctuates irregularly can use a pump placed in the skin, which injects insulin continuously.

THYROID DISEASES

Women are particularly susceptible to the problems of metabolism caused by autoimmune disease. For example, hyperthyroidism (overactive thyroid) is eight times as common in women as in men. If the thyroid gland doesn't work properly bones, nerves and other body tissues suffer.

The thyroid gland, about the size of a small plum and located in the front of the neck, is under the control of the pituitary gland, which is connected by a stalk to the brain, and responds to signals from a part of the brain called the hypothalamus.

For reasons possibly related to oestrogen, menstrual irregularities are often symptomatic, the thyroid gland may become overactive or underactive– conditions known as hyperthyroidism and hypothyroidism. Both are usually autoimmune disorders.

Who's at risk of an underactive thyroid?

Because iodine in the diet is essential to the manufacture of thyroid hormones, shortage of it is the most common reason worldwide for people to develop hypothyroidism.

In Western countries today, the cause is more usually an autoimmune disorder called Hashimoto's disease: in this, white blood cells take over thyroid tissue, which is then attacked by antibodies. Genetics and environmental factors may have an influence.

Hashimoto's disease progresses reasonably slowly and is not always promptly recognized. Sometimes the condition is mistaken for depression, which is in reality a symptom. Also, an expected side effect of treatment for hyperthyroidism can be hypothyroidism, as not enough tissue remains. The symptoms of hypothyroidism in its severe form, known as myxoedema, might be due to psychological problems or ageing.

Routine screening is sometimes given after the menopause to measure the levels of thyroid-stimulating hormone (TSH): too little TSH indicates that the thyroid is overactive, too much that it is underactive. Another test identifies antithyroid antibodies, which indicates an autoimmune link.

How to handle hypothyroidism

In principle, this condition can be corrected by hormone replacement, using a synthetic form of the thyroid hormone thyroxine to bring levels back to normal. There may, however, be a certain amount of trial and error to find the right dose. Your doctor will normally start you on a low dose that can be increased if necessary (for example, if symptoms recur or if blood tests indicate abnormal levels), and you will have to continue taking the pills for the rest of your life.

Regular testing of TSH levels is needed to ensure that the treatment is not causing hyperthyroidism, which can then affect bone density and result in osteoporosis. Women who are hypothyroid have an increased risk of atherosclerosis and heart disease because they tend to have high levels of blood fats (including cholesterol) that cause deposits in the arteries.

Who's at risk for an overactive thyroid?

The causes of hyperthyroidism can be congenital, or caused by previous thyroid treatment, or drugs such as lithium carbonate (used to treat people with bipolar disorder) and amiodarone (used for an irregular heartbeat).

Through questions and close scrutiny your doctor will pinpoint the symptoms

DO YOU HAVE AN UNDERACTIVE THYROID?

Symptoms of an underactive thyroid are:

- Weight gain
- Dry, brittle and thinning hair
- Dry skin
- Forgetfulness and mental sluggishness
- Lack of energy and constant tiredness
- Depression
- Scanty or irregular periods
- Increased sensitivity to cold
- Constipation

THYROID AND PARATHYROID GLANDS
The thyroid gland consists of two lobes situated on either side of the trachea (windpipe). The four tiny parathyroid glands are found behind the thyroid gland, the superior at the top and the inferior below.

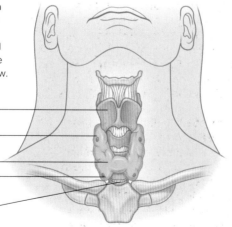

Thyroid cartilage

Superior parathyroid gland

Thyroid gland

Inferior parathyroid gland

Trachea

IT'S A WOMAN'S DISEASE
Women are more much likely than men to have a thyroid disorder. During the reproductive years long menstrual cycles can indicate hypothyroidism, while scanty or lack of bleeding can be a symptom of hyperthyroidism. The disorder may appear after giving birth and may be mistakenly diagnosed as postnatal depression.

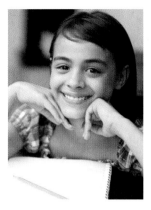

CHILDREN
Girls as young as five can develop Graves' disease. This is a very common disorder that can be diagnosed through a simple blood test.

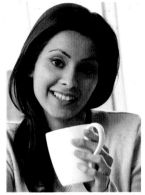

20s TO 40s
Women may not realize that their symptoms perhaps relate to thyroid excess or deficiency. Both can affect the menstrual cycle and fertility.

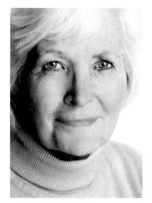

OVER 60
Hashimoto's disease may affect 1 in 10 women over the age of 60. They are 10 times more likely than men to develop a goitre (enlarged thyroid gland).

and confirm the diagnosis with a blood test for TSH. Graves' disease causes the disorder in around 80 per cent of people. This is an autoimmune disease in which the body's own antibodies attack the thyroid gland and stimulate it into releasing excess hormone and thus speeding up the metabolic rate. It is not known why this happens, although there may be a genetic link. In the other 20 per cent of hyperthyroidism, the cause is thyroid malfunction.

How to handle hyperthyroidism

Your doctor may prescribe antithyroid drugs to suppress hormone production, but these don't work for everyone.

Another treatment–although not for pregnant women–is radioiodine, taken as a drink, which destroys thyroid tissue. Assessing the correct dose can be difficult; some people need more than one treatment while in others so much tissue is killed that they then have to take thyroxine pills to compensate for the loss. Alternatively, or if neither of these treatments works, most of the thyroid gland can be removed surgically; some people may need to take thyroid hormone replacement after such surgery.

Other thyroid disorders

Thyroid cancer is a rare disorder and is treated by surgical removal of the thyroid gland. Most types of thyroid cancer have a high cure rate.

Subclinical hyperthyroidism, usually affecting women over 60, develops from toxic nodules that form on the gland. These may have no symptoms but can cause bone density loss, irregular heartbeat and make heart problems such as angina worse. Radioiodine or surgery are the usual treatments.

Check for osteoporosis

Hypo- and hyperthyroidism can affect bone mineralization. The parathyroids (four tiny glands found near the thyroid gland) are responsible for regulating the levels of bone-building minerals–calcium and phosphorus–in the blood. Any treatment that affects the healthy functioning of the thyroid or parathyroid glands and their hormone production can influence the strength of your bones and teeth. Parathyroid overactivity is picked up by blood calcium screening, or if osteoporosis has been diagnosed.

See your ophthalmologist

Graves' disease can cause protrusion of the eyes (known as exophthalmos). Eye problems can occur at any stage in the course of the disease, even after the thyroid is back to normal. The changes are irreversible and require steroid treatment, or in some cases surgery.

DO YOU HAVE AN OVERACTIVE THYROID?

Symptoms include:
- Sweating and feeling too hot all the time
- Anxiety and nervousness
- Restlessness and insomnia
- Weight loss despite increased appetite
- Palpitations, racing heartbeat
- Diarrhoea
- Trembling hands
- Bulging eyes

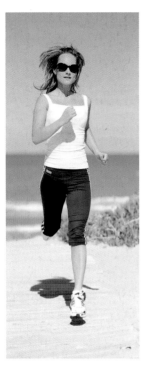

FEEL GOOD!
Exercise releases feel-good hormones in the brain, which can ease depression, improve digestion and reduce bloating.

PREMENSTRUAL SYNDROME

Approximately 80 per cent of women are affected, to a greater or lesser extent, by premenstrual syndrome (PMS) at some time in their lives. The impact may be mild and infrequent, or very frequent and quite disabling.

For PMS to be diagnosed, only one of the following symptoms is required: mild psychological discomfort, bloating and weight gain, breast tenderness, swelling of hands and feet, various aches and pains, poor concentration, sleep disturbance and change in appetite. Symptoms occur in the second half of the menstrual cycle–that is, the 14 days before the beginning of the next period. They peak shortly before menstruation and usually stop when the menstrual flow begins. They may be at their worst in the week immediately before menstruation and may continue for the first couple of days of bleeding.

Symptoms of PMS

Although the physical, behavioural and emotional symptoms ascribed to PMS are plentiful–up to 150–the most common can be classified into four groups:

Mood swings Feelings of anxiety, tension and irritability.

Fluid retention Giving rise to weight gain, swollen ankles and fingers, a bloated feeling in the abdomen and breast discomfort.

Depression Tearfulness, forgetfulness, confusion and insomnia.

Cravings For carbohydrates and especially sweet foods, increase in appetite, palpitations, faintness, dizziness and headaches.

Although the cause is clearly related to cyclical fluctuations in hormones, no one is sure precisely how symptoms are triggered or what determines who gets which ones. It may be that some women are naturally more sensitive to hormonal influences or become so as they get older and changing hormone levels build up over time. The menstrual cycle may also affect food metabolism–some women can control PMS symptoms by regulating their intake of carbohydrates and fats.

Identify the symptoms

Symptoms that come and go without any pattern or that trouble you in the first half of your menstrual cycle are unlikely to be related to PMS and will need medical evaluation to find the cause. Anxiety and depression, for instance, may have nothing to do with PMS. Your doctor will want to rule out an underlying physical disorder or a personal problem such as an abusive home situation or sexual experience. Recurring pelvic pain is not a PMS symptom and needs full medical investigation.

Some women may experience PMS symptoms for the first time as they approach the menopause, when the levels of reproductive hormones decline. However, any problems directly resulting from menopausal changes are likely to respond better to hormone replacement therapy (HRT). Discuss your available options with your doctor.

To see if there is a link between your symptoms and the onset of your period, your doctor will probably suggest that you keep a daily diary for two months. You will be asked to record when symptoms occur, what they are, the level of severity, how long they persist and whether they prevent you from performing normal activities. You may be given a self-rating form called COPE (calendar of premenstrual experiences), which is easy to complete.

Support your body

Try reducing your consumption of salt, which encourages fluid retention, and avoid tea, coffee and most carbonated drinks, which contain caffeine and can exacerbate tension and anxiety.

You should plan to have several small meals a day based on complex carbohydrates such as wholegrain bread,

About 80 per cent of women are affected by premenstrual syndrome (PMS) at some time in their lives.

brown rice and pasta, cereals and pulses, and keep fatty and sugary foods to a minimum. This should prevent large swings in blood glucose levels, which may contribute to both physical and psychological symptoms.

Eat plenty of fresh fruit and vegetables every day to help balance blood glucose and prevent constipation. Foods with the amino acid tryptophan (*see* chart below) increase serotonin, a "feel-good" brain chemical. Higher intake of calcium and vitamin D may have a beneficial effect, although research is not clear how.

Exercise that makes you slightly out of breath will boost your production of endorphins, the body's natural opiates, which ease aches and pains and lift your mood. Gentler forms of exercise such as yoga, Pilates and t'ai chi will help you relax and relieve anxiety. Taking time to care for yourself is essential in helping you manage your PMS symptoms.

PMS or PMDD?

Premenstrual dysphoric disorder (PMDD) is a disabling form of PMS. As well as PMS symptoms, a woman may have mood changes just before her period starts that are severe enough to interfere with her ability to function at home or at work. The effect is similar to that of major depression and needs treatment with drugs.

WAYS TO HELP PMS

Method	Action
AEROBIC EXERCISE	
Increase heart rate for 20 minutes daily	Produces endorphins that relieve symptoms
DIET CHANGES	
Cut down on caffeine, salt, alcohol and chocolate. Eat more complex carbohydrates and foods containing tryptophan (sunflower, pumpkin and evening primrose seeds) and potatoes. Increase calcium and vitamin D intake	Improves mood and assuages cravings
RELAXATION EXERCISES	
Meditation, yoga, prayer	May alleviate tension or depression
MASSAGE	
Whole body or hands/feet (reflexology)	Relaxes
AROMATHERAPY	
A few drops of lavender, chamomile, juniper or geranium oils added to a warm bath	May be relaxing
DRUGS PRESCRIBED FOR PMS	
Combination oral contraceptive pill controls the body's hormones	Provides a more consistent hormonal milieu
ANTIDEPRESSANTS	
Pills to treat depression or tearfulness. This method appears to be the most effective	SSRIs (selective serotonin reuptake inhibitors) raise the level of the feel-good brain chemical, serotonin

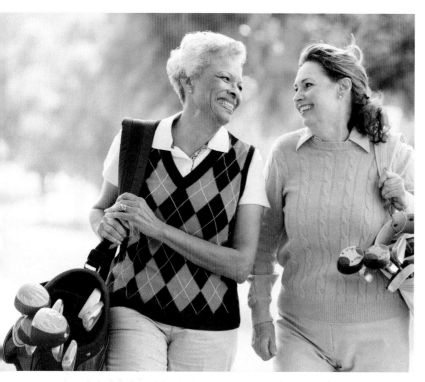

KEEPING ACTIVE
Get into the habit of regular weightbearing exercise before the menopause and continue to enjoy it afterwards. Getting out into the fresh air—playing golf or tennis or walking—helps to slow down bone loss and maintains muscle tone, helps to prevent weight gain and keeps your cardiovascular system healthy.

THE MENOPAUSE

The menopause marks a new phase in life and women react to the absence of menstruation in different ways, both physically and emotionally. Some women gladly welcome the absence of periods and not having to think about contraception any more; others regret the loss of their fertility.

For the vast majority of women, the monthly cycles stop around the age of 50, after years in which bleeding has varied from heavy to scanty, or been irregular. With the decline in the amount of the female hormone oestrogen being secreted by your ovaries you ovulate less frequently, so conception and pregnancy become increasingly unlikely in that time known as perimenopause. After 12 months without bleeding you are postmenopausal.

The time span of perimenopause is usually about four years although it may be longer or in some cases abrupt. Some women experience premature menopause, either naturally or as a result of medical or surgical treatment involving either the removal or destruction of the ovaries.

Women under 40 will be advised on the benefits and risks of hormone replacement therapy (HRT). It can reduce their risk of developing osteoporosis in the future. Menopausal symptoms can appear earlier in women who smoke. Some women will go through the menopause with few or no problems, but the majority experience symptoms that can range from being a minor nuisance to quite troublesome.

A range of symptoms

Hot flushes, which can occur at any time, are the most common problem and one that many women find difficult to cope with because of their unpredictability. Insomnia–often made worse by night sweats–leaves you feeling tired and lethargic. You may lose confidence and get more headaches than you used to. Other common symptoms include mood swings, irritability and depression, although these may have more to do with other changes happening in your life at this time.

You may find you "leak" urine when you cough, laugh, sneeze or run. Lack

PUT YOURSELF FIRST!

For some women, the changes that occur at the menopause may coincide with changes in their personal lives. A relationship may go wrong, working women may be made redundant or reach the peak of their career ambitions, and those who have devoted most of their energy to their families may feel at a loss when their children leave home or need less of their mother's support.

It is not unusual for women to put on weight around this time, and you may feel less attractive as wrinkles and other skin changes become more noticeable because of oestrogen loss. Higher stress can result in weight gain and decline in mood. Learning to put yourself first will help you to be positive about making the necessary changes that will carry you into, through and beyond the postmenopausal years.

If you feel you can't handle what is happening to you, seek support. Talk to your doctor about counselling, psychotherapy or, if you're depressed, possibly antidepressants.

of oestrogen can affect the cells lining the vagina, so that it becomes drier and lacks lubrication, making intercourse uncomfortable or even painful. You may lose interest in sex, perhaps even find it difficult to respond to your partner.

It is important to reassure yourself that what you are going through is a natural life event, that you are healthy and the symptoms can be alleviated. Find someone to talk to. Your doctor may be the one to help you get through this time or you may find a counsellor more useful. Sharing your thoughts with your partner or a friend may help you clarify problems and give you a different perspective on the solutions.

Are you baby-safe?

"Change of life" babies are usually born to women who thought that they could not get pregnant again. If you haven't been sterilized, continue contraception for two years after your last period if you are under 50, or for one year if over 50. HRT treats symptoms of menopause but does not restore fertility.

It can be difficult to know when you have reached menopause if you are taking the combined contraceptive pill or progestogen-only pill, have been using HRT for several years or been fitted with the intrauterine contraceptive system, all of which may prevent you from noticing symptoms. When you reach the age of 50, you should ask your doctor if changes need to be made to your prescription.

Live well

Keep moving. Run up stairs, walk instead of driving or taking the bus. Regular exercise that causes you to breathe more deeply, to take in more oxygen and increase your heart rate, is known to help reduce mood swings and hot flushes and improve concentration and energy levels. You should start slowly–30 minutes at least three times a week–and build up to five or more days a week.

Running, brisk walking, dancing, tennis, golf and badminton are weightbearing activities that benefit bone strength.

If you are very overweight, talk to your doctor and a dietitian about a weight-loss diet combined with physical activity that will gradually help you reach an acceptable weight. Take control of your diet. Include plenty of calcium-rich foods, especially low-fat dairy foods, green leafy vegetables and pulses (*see* box below) and oily fish.

Spend at least 20 minutes a day outdoors so that your skin is able to make the vitamin D needed to absorb calcium efficiently. Remember to use skin protection–it won't hinder the process of vitamin making, but it will protect your skin from the risk of skin cancer and the drying, wrinkling effects of photoageing.

Oestrogens in plant foods

There is a theory, although not yet proven, that Asian women are less likely to report menopausal symptoms. This is thought to be related to their high intake of phytoestrogens, substances found in many plant-based foods. If eaten regularly it seems they may compensate for declining oestrogen levels and decrease cholesterol levels. The two main groups are lignans and isoflavones.

Opt for soya products (beans, milk, tofu, miso), pulses (black beans, mung beans, alfalfa sprouts), wholegrains (rice, wheat, barley), fennel, celery and rhubarb. Do not take any herbal preparations without discussing them with a herbalist, because some preparations may have side effects in people with certain conditions. Take note that the possible long-term effects of phytoestrogens are not yet fully known.

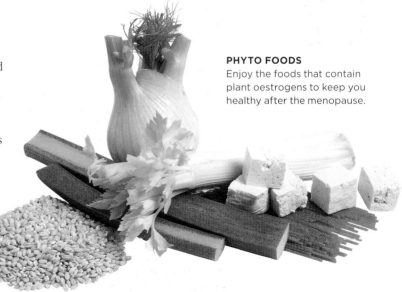

PHYTO FOODS
Enjoy the foods that contain plant oestrogens to keep you healthy after the menopause.

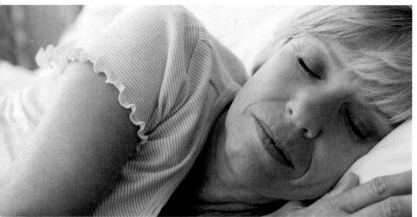

A PEACEFUL NIGHT
Many women going through the menopause find the symptoms of hot flushes and night sweats intolerable, particularly when they interfere with sleep. HRT can help alleviate these problems and allow a full night's rest.

Raloxifene is an oestrogen alternative used in postmenopausal hormone therapy. Its purpose is to confer oestrogen's alleged bone-preserving benefits, without the risks of breast or uterine cancer. Raloxifene is a SERM—selective estrogen-receptor modulator—which mimics oestrogen in some tissues while blocking the hormone in others. Taken as a pill, a SERM may meet the needs of older postmenopausal women who cannot, will not or should not use HRT but may be concerned about osteoporosis. Raloxifene improves bone density of the spine, and stops bone loss without affecting the breast and uterus. It does not, however, treat menopausal symptoms; in fact, you may experience side effects such as mild leg cramps and hot flushes.

Although it is an oestrogen from a plant source, it is not hormone replacement and so will not alleviate a menopausal problem such as vaginal dryness. While oral oestrogen in HRT is known to boost the levels of HDL or "good" cholesterol and to lower LDL, the "bad" form, raloxifene has no effect on HDL and only lowers LDL. Raloxifene is not advised for women with cardiac risk factors or a history of heart disease or with a personal or family history of thrombosis (blood clots). They are at increased risk of blood clots or stroke.

HORMONE REPLACEMENT THERAPY (HRT)

At and after the menopause, which occurs on average around the age of 51, a woman's symptoms, such as hot flushes and night sweats, may become troubling.

Although doctors once thought that HRT both relieved these symptoms and protected the body from a variety of diseases, recent research has forced them to take another look. According to new research in the United States by the North American Menopause Society, a leading group of menopause experts, you may be at greater risk of heart attack or stroke if you start HRT at age 60 or above for the

HRT is the most effective way to treat vaginal symptoms, such as dryness and related discomfort with sex.

first time. However, if you begin HRT earlier, during perimenopause to relieve hot flushes, night sweats or other menopausal symptoms, you may have the same or even a lower risk of heart-related complications as a woman not taking HRT.

Further, HRT is the most effective way to treat vaginal symptoms, such as dryness and related discomfort with sex. You may also wish to talk with your doctor about HRT's role in the prevention of bone loss, mental slowing

(dementia)and colon cancer. A thorough discussion with your doctor about your symptoms and individual risks and understanding about the benefits and risks of the different hormonal formulations available is crucial before you start any HRT.

What to expect

If you have your uterus, you will initially take both oestrogen, for treatment of menopausal symptoms, and progestogen to protect from uterine cancer. You will have period-like bleeds, although not necessarily every month, depending on the HRT formulation. There are HRT formulations designed to minimize bleeding. If you have had a hysterectomy, you can receive oestrogen only. You may need to try delivery systems and dosages to find the one that suits you. If you have vaginal dryness alone, you may want to consider vaginal oestrogen therapies, which come in the form of creams, suppositories or a ring.

If you don't notice a difference, discuss further options with your doctor.

Who should not take HRT?
HRT may not be suitable for anyone who has had breast or uterine cancer, heart disease or deep-vein blood clots.

A gynaecologist will want to ensure that a woman with factors such as being overweight, hypertension, diabetes, gallstones, fibroids, endometriosis, breast problems or osteoporosis caused by long-term use of steroids receives appropriate counselling about HRT. If you are unable to take HRT, there are non-hormonal alternatives that may provide some symptom relief.

THE TYPES OF HRT

It is important to get as much information as you possibly can about the various types of HRT so that you can find out which are most suited to you as an individual and your particular symptoms. Take time to discuss your health and lifestyle before deciding which to try.

TREATMENT	METHOD	POINTS TO CONSIDER
Oral: oestrogen and progestogen	Pills are taken by mouth, absorbed through the stomach, broken down by the liver and distributed in the blood. Can be sequential or continuous combined.	Simple to take. Side effects may include nausea and breast tenderness. Need to take as prescribed, as lapses negate the effect. Must not be taken by women with liver disease. Breakthrough bleeding may occur.
Oral: tibolone	A synthetic steroid that treats menopausal symptoms, prevents bone loss and improves libido and mood. Does not affect breast and uterus.	Only for postmenopausal women.
Transdermal patches	See-through patches contain either oestrogen or both hormones, applied to abdomen or buttocks. Hormones are absorbed through the skin into the blood so are not initially metabolized by the liver.	Can be either sequential (oestrogen for so many days, progestogen for so many days) or continuous combined (for period-free, postmenopausal women, but breakthrough bleeding may occur). Patches are visible, don't always adhere to dry skin, can cause allergies, can leave adhesive marks when changed (either once or twice weekly).
Vaginal therapy	Direct treatment for vaginal and urinary symptoms.	Wide range of methods: creams, pills (via vagina) or silicone ring replaced every three months. Vaginal therapy is not approved for prevention of osteoporosis. Progestogen is generally not needed to protect the uterus.
Intrauterine device	Releases progestogen and provides contraception for perimenopausal women.	Must be inserted by a doctor. May be used with oral oestrogen. Lasts up to five years.
Implant	Pellet inserted under skin in groin or buttock (done under local anaesthetic). Releases oestrogen as body demands. Testosterone may be added for libido.	Must be inserted by a doctor. Used with oral progestogen to prevent thickening of endometrium (for women with uterus). Lasts about six months. You need to avoid excessive levels in the blood.

Digestive System Problems

When the system is working well, every part of your body benefits from the food you eat. In some women, however, for reasons not always known, the system's efficiency is compromised by a range of problems that can potentially cause long-term risks to health.

OBESITY

When your body weight is too high in relation to your age and shape you raise your risk of serious health problems.

Between the start and end of the 20th century, due to changes in diet and lifestyle, the shape and weight of men and women changed a great deal, but not for the better. By the millennium, more people were classed as overweight than of normal weight.

More importantly, 27 per cent of women and 24 per cent of men were classified as clinically obese–their weight was at least 20 per cent more than that regarded as desirable for their frame (bones of the skeleton). A worrying number of children were in this category.

FAT DISTRIBUTION
Near right: A certain amount of fat is natural on a woman's body.

Centre: If throughout her life a woman's weight comes more from muscle or bone than fat, her outline is pear-shaped.

Far right: If a woman aged between 40 and 60 builds up fat around waist and stomach, and she becomes apple-shaped, she runs the risk of heart disease, stroke, diabetes and gallbladder problems.

| General fat distribution | Pear shape | Apple shape |

What causes obesity?
Your natural body weight is influenced by many factors, including your age, sex, shape and genetics. You gain weight when what you eat is not used by the body as energy (calories) and is instead stored in adipose (fatty) tissue. In women, this is usually around the hips, thighs and buttocks, the arms and shoulders. In men, fat builds up around the waist and stomach.

Obesity tends to run in families, not only through genetics but because most people acquire their eating habits from their families. Very rarely, obesity is caused by glandular problems, such as an underactive thyroid or overactive adrenals. Getting older can have an effect, too; older people use less energy, may have joint and mobility problems, lose muscle mass, have slower metabolic rates and store more fat.

Problems caused by obesity
It is important to understand that obesity is not simply a cosmetic problem. Even moderate weight gain as an adult increases your risk of illness later. Many overweight people have high blood pressure and blood fat levels that have been linked to a number of health concerns, including coronary heart disease (CHD), stroke, some cancers (including colorectal and breast cancer), gallstones and adult-onset diabetes.

If you are clinically obese it means your metabolism is putting stress on many organs in your body and the extra load on the bones and joints can make pre-existing medical conditions, such as osteoarthritis, worse. Storing weight around the stomach (apple shape) is associated with greater risk of disease than storing fat on the hips and thighs (pear shape). However, if you lose 5 to 10 per cent of this accumulated extra weight and switch to a healthy eating plan with exercise, you can substantially reduce your risk.

How fat are you?

To calculate your body fat in relation to your frame, doctors use the Body Mass Index (BMI). This figure is reached by dividing your weight (without shoes) in kilograms by your height in metres squared (rounded off to nearest decimal point). A woman who is 1.6 m tall and weighs 60 kg can work out her BMI as: 1.6 multiplied by 1.6 = 2.6; then 60 divided by 2.6 = 23.1.

For women, the desirable BMI is between 19 and 24. If it is under 19, you are underweight; 25-27, you are overweight; 27-30, you are obese; over 30, you are clinically obese.

Doctors may do another assessment: the waist-to-hip ratio where your waist measurement is divided by your hip measurement. If your waist is 75 cm (30 in) and your hips 92.5 cm (37 in), your ratio is 0.8. Women should ideally have a ratio of less than 0.8 (the waist is not greater than 80 per cent of the hips); if 0.9 or higher, they have more than three times the risk of heart disease as women with a ratio of less than 0.7, even if their weight is normal.

A third measurement determines lean body mass (reflecting bones and muscle) and fat mass. Exercise programmes aim to turn body fat to muscle.

Fat and the menopause

Women tend to put on weight between the ages of 40 and 60. Though overall oestrogen levels drop, oestrogen is still produced by body fat, if it is substantial. Some women attribute weight gain to hormone therapy, but reduced activity resulting in loss of muscle mass may be more pertinent. Walking for at least 30 minutes daily reduces the risk of CHD and stroke by 40 per cent. Walking strengthens muscles and bones by placing one and a half times the body weight on them.

YOUR METABOLISM

Your metabolic rate is the speed at which your body turns food into energy. Regular aerobic exercise, which makes you out of breath, tends to raise your metabolic rate, even once the exercise has ceased. This burns fat to produce energy, leads to a healthier circulation and keeps your muscles in better shape. With regular exercise, your body will tend to burn rather than store extra calories. If you crash diet (eat very few calories) rather than exercising, your body responds by decreasing its metabolic rate. When you return to your normal eating pattern, your body can no longer burn extra calories as efficiently, so excess energy is stored as fat and you put on weight.

Acid reflux and hiatal hernia

Doctors call it gastro-esophageal reflux disease, and it occurs when stomach acid comes up the food pipe into the mouth. It affects about 30 per cent of adults and most pregnant women.

The common symptoms are heartburn (burning sensation) and regurgitation of food or acid, both of which happen after meals, when bending over or lying down. Some people may also have chest pain, which can be mistaken for a heart attack, and wheezing and coughing.

The cause usually lies either with the muscular valve or a hiatal hernia, where part of the stomach rises through a hole in the diaphragm (the hiatus) into the chest. Hiatal hernia is common in middle-aged women, in smokers and people who are overweight. Heavy lifting, sneezing or coughing can also cause this type of hernia.

Tests—gastroscopy or barium swallow—may be done to confirm the diagnosis, and you will be advised to change your lifestyle: reduce alcohol, stop smoking, lose weight, exercise daily and raise the head of your bed about 10 cm (4 in). Eat small, frequent meals, chew food well and reduce fat intake.

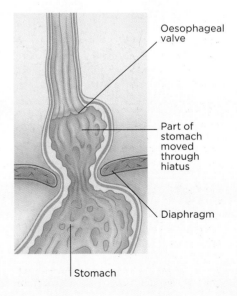

Oesophageal valve

Part of stomach moved through hiatus

Diaphragm

Stomach

HEPATITIS

DID YOU KNOW?

There is no cure for hepatitis. Sometimes drugs such as interferons (that have a nonspecific antiviral action) or antivirals are given. They stop or slow replication of the virus in the body. This may allow the liver to heal itself.

Hepatitis (inflammation of the liver) is usually caused by one of three viruses. It can also stem from lifestyle and overindulgence. In some cases it is life threatening.

The viruses that cause hepatitis are known as A, B and C; D and E also exist, but are much rarer. Non-infectious hepatitis can occur as a result of alcohol abuse, industrial chemicals, some autoimmune disorders (in which your immune system attacks your liver) or drug overdose, for example paracetamol. Other viruses, such as glandular fever or cytomegalovirus, can cause hepatitis.

Hepatitis can be acute or chronic, and will need medical attention. The acute illness lasts for a few months, has no long-term effects and gradually you feel better. The chronic illness is more serious, since it can destroy the liver.

Helping yourself

Noninfectious hepatitis can be prevented by avoiding excesses of alcohol.

Viral hepatitis is spread in contaminated blood, water and food and is most likely to be caught in developing countries. Vaccines are available against hepatitis A and B and are usually recommended for people at high risk, including health care workers and travellers to these countries.

Good hygiene is essential while travelling. Drink only boiled or bottled water, avoid ice in drinks and don't eat food stored or prepared in unhygienic conditions. You should also avoid unprotected sex or sharing needles.

What to expect

Many hepatitis patients recover without treatment; the doctor will recommend rest for a few weeks until the jaundice disappears. Because of the liver's role in digestion, you may be advised not to take certain drugs (such as birth control pills) or alcohol. Jaundice can last many months, leaving you feeling very tired, even after the infection has passed. You should help the liver recover by avoiding alcohol for as long as your doctor says.

If you have hepatitis A you must avoid spreading it to other people in your household. Use separate eating utensils and be extra vigilant about hygiene. People who have contracted hepatitis B or C can be carriers; a mother can pass hepatitis B to her child by breastfeeding.

A HEPATITIS PRIMER

There is more than one type of hepatitis and the symptoms depend on the virus involved. A diagnosis is made by a physical examination, and urine and blood tests. Approximately 10 per cent of patients with hepatitis B later acquire chronic hepatitis; this is extremely rare for people with hepatitis A.

DISEASE	SYMPTOM
Hepatitis A (HAV)	Causes an acute flu-like illness, with headaches and fever, aching joints or muscles, nausea, diarrhoea and vomiting, loss of appetite and abdominal pain. If the condition is severe, within a few days there may be jaundice—yellowing of the skin and whites of the eyes caused by a buildup of bile pigments in the blood. You may also pass pale-coloured stools and dark urine.
Hepatitis B (HBV)	Has similar symptoms to those above, but is a greater problem since it can lead to a chronic illness, with severe, persistent liver inflammation that can result in cirrhosis and liver failure. It may also cause cancer of the liver.
Hepatitis C (HCV)	Mainly chronic, but symptoms may be no worse than generally feeling unwell. It, too, can lead to cirrhosis. It is most usually the result of blood transfusion, which is less likely now that donated blood is screened. Both this type of hepatitis and hepatitis B can be sexually transmitted.

CIRRHOSIS

This life-threatening disease of the liver is characterized by the progressive destruction of cells within an organ that is central to your body's health. Chronic alcoholism over a number of years is the most common cause of cirrhosis, although chronic viral hepatitis and, in some rare cases, inherited diseases can also be the culprits. Even though a woman may drink less than a man, she may be at an equal risk of developing cirrhosis because of her smaller body size and slower metabolism of alcohol.

Primary biliary cirrhosis, which represents about 20 per cent of all types of cirrhosis, mainly affects women aged between 30 and 60. It occurs when the small bile ducts, which deliver bile to the intestines for the digestion of fats, become inflamed and blocked. It is an autoimmune disorder.

A subtle onset

The onset of cirrhosis may be fairly gradual and no specific symptoms may be noticed at first. Signs to be aware of include tiredness and sleep disturbance, generalized itching, swollen feet and legs, menstrual disturbances, nausea, loss of muscle bulk and slight jaundice.

In more advanced cirrhosis, the cells are replaced with fibrous scar tissue and the liver becomes less effective. There may be malabsorption of vitamins, such as vitamin D, leading to loss of bone mass. A build-up of female hormones causes spidery small red marks to appear on the chest and upper body, while an accumulation of waste products can affect the brain, causing confusion and coma.

Once the liver begins to harden, blood pressure in internal organs may increase, leading to sudden internal bleeding. The cell death and scarring can be serious enough to cause liver failure.

A good chance of recovery

The liver has a remarkable ability to repair itself. If the early signs of cirrhosis are recognized, most people have a good chance of recovery. Since the liver cell damage is most commonly caused by heavy alcohol consumption, alcoholics must stop drinking alcohol. They may be helped to stop by drug treatment that disrupts alcohol metabolism in the liver leading to nausea and vomiting if alcohol is ingested.

Steroids or antiviral drugs may be given to treat chronic hepatitis and there are other drugs that can be used to control symptoms such as itching. If no action is taken or the cirrhosis is far advanced, permanent damage may occur and the only chance of a long-term cure will be a liver transplant.

ALCOHOLIC NEUROPATHY

Excess intake of alcohol can cause alcoholic neuropathy, a condition resulting in permanent nerve damage. It is usually associated with vitamin deficiencies, usually of the B vitamins. The symptoms include numbness, abnormal sensations, muscle weakness, incontinence, constipation and diarrhoea. The symptoms may develop gradually and progressively worsen over weeks or even years. However, it is possible to control the condition with medication and replace the missing nutrients with dietary supplements.

KEEP TO YOUR LIMIT

Even light drinkers who consume an unusual amount over a short period may be at risk of developing fatty liver—a condition that produces pain and tenderness, caused when the liver becomes swollen with fat and water that it is unable to process in the normal way.

THE LIVER
The liver has a vital role in the control of chemicals in the body. It absorbs oxygen and nutrients from the blood, regulates levels of glucose and amino acids, manufactures proteins and removes toxic substances.

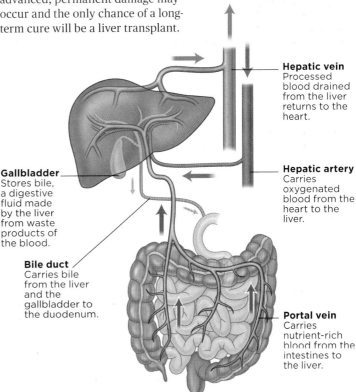

Hepatic vein
Processed blood drained from the liver returns to the heart.

Hepatic artery
Carries oxygenated blood from the heart to the liver.

Gallbladder
Stores bile, a digestive fluid made by the liver from waste products of the blood.

Bile duct
Carries bile from the liver and the gallbladder to the duodenum.

Portal vein
Carries nutrient-rich blood from the intestines to the liver.

GALLBLADDER DISORDERS

The gallbladder is a small pear-shaped sac lying directly beneath, and connected to, your liver. It has a profound effect on digestion.

Every time you eat, the gallbladder responds by releasing bile, a yellow fluid produced in your liver that breaks up fats from food and blood. In addition, the gallbladder is involved in removing waste products to the small intestine through a tube-shaped duct.

Inflammation of the gallbladder–known medically as cholecystitis–is a common condition in women. The most usual cause of the inflammation is gallstones, which develop if the bile becomes too concentrated and hardens.

Are you at risk?

No one knows why some people get gallstones and others don't. However, there is increasing evidence that oestrogen influences the making of cholesterol, which in turn combines with bile pigments to form crystals–gallstones–that vary in size from a tiny bead to a pigeon's egg. Stones may take years to form with no symptoms if they remain in the gallbladder. It is when they leave and get caught in the ducts that pain occurs.

Gallstones affect one in 10 people and are two to three times more common in women than in men. You are at greater risk if you are over 50, overweight or diabetic, have high triglyceride levels in the blood, have had several children or take contraceptives or hormone therapy in pill form (these are metabolized by the liver). Also at risk are women with a history of rapid weight-loss diets with low-calorie intake: not enough bile acids are generated to dissolve the cholesterol allowing crystals to form.

Stuck stones

Although you can have gallstones without being aware of it, if a large stone gets stuck in the common bile duct you will certainly feel it. Typically, it causes intense pain on the right-hand side of the body under the ribs (called biliary colic). The pain may be very brief or may last for up to several hours and can spread towards the shoulder blades. In addition, symptoms may include bloating of the stomach, nausea and vomiting.

If the gallstone prevents bile from reaching the intestines, the stools may turn putty-coloured and, if the liver can't get rid of bile, this can lead to jaundice. Occasionally the gallstone blocks the bile flow in the common bile duct, leading to a serious condition, pancreatitis (an inflammation of the pancreas).

Getting rid of the problem

If you are not in any pain, gallstones can be left to their own devices. If the stones are causing discomfort, however, bile salts may be prescribed to try and dissolve them, although these can take up to two years to work and the stones can often recur.

Lithotripsy (shock-wave therapy), which uses high-frequency sound waves, may be performed in an attempt to break up the stones. Alternatively, as a long-term solution the gallbladder may be removed by simple, same-day surgery. This is called a cholecystectomy.

You can function perfectly well without a gallbladder, because your body is able to create a reservoir of bile within the liver.

GALLSTONES

Gallstones (yellow mass at left) vary in size and can occur singly or in groups. Signs of bile-duct obstruction include jaundice, clay-coloured stools and fever. Surgeons remove the gallbladder laparoscopically, using a flexible endoscope—a fibre-optic viewing instrument.

THE CHOLESTEROL LINK

Gallstones may contain either cholesterol or bile pigments or a mixture of the two. Cholesterol stones can grow very large—big enough to block the common bile duct—whereas pigment stones are generally much smaller. Stones made of cholesterol are formed if bile contains too much cholesterol, which is made from the breakdown of saturated fats. Therefore, eating a diet that contains little saturated fat (from meat and dairy products) is a good preventive measure. If you already have gallstones, fatty foods can make your symptoms worse.

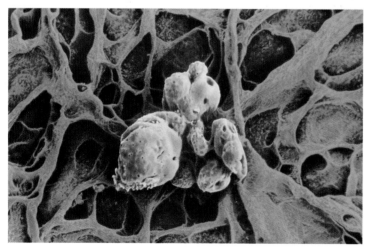

DIGESTIVE TRACT ULCERS

Ulcers are sensitive raw patches that occur in the lining of the digestive tract from the oesophagus to the stomach and duodenum (the first part of the intestines). Collectively, stomach (gastric) and duodenal ulcers are called peptic ulcers.

Digestion is a carefully balanced process. Your stomach produces hydrochloric acid and the enzyme called pepsin so food can be broken down and its nutrients absorbed. These gastric juices are kept from attacking the smooth, muscular walls of your stomach and duodenum by a protective mucous membrane. It is when this breaks down that an ulcer forms.

A peptic ulcer can cause severe, burning abdominal pain that may be temporarily relieved by eating. It is often worse at night. Other symptoms include nausea, vomiting, belching, bloating and weight loss. In severe cases the ulcer may cause bleeding, triggering anaemia. Severe ulcers may, in rare cases, perforate the stomach lining, leading to peritonitis–inflammation of the abdominal lining.

If there is any doubt about where the ulcer is, diagnosis will be by endoscopic examination (gastroscopy) under short-term general anaesthetic. A flexible fibre-optic tube is passed from the oesophagus to the stomach and duodenum while the doctor views the area on a screen. A piece of tissue will be taken (biopsy) to check for bacteria or cancer.

Who's at risk?

Peptic ulcers affect 1 in 15 women, and are more common in those over the age of 50. Ulcers tend to occur in families, possibly passed through close contact. The primary culprit is a bacterium called *Helicobacter pylori* (*see* box right). Ulcers are also common in heavy drinkers, smokers and people who regularly take nonsteroidal anti-inflammatory drugs (NSAIDs), which are used in the treatment of arthritis. Stress can't cause an ulcer but can make it worse.

The symptoms can often be relieved by avoiding any aggravating foods–milk and hot spices, for instance–by eating regular meals, giving up smoking and drinking less alcohol. The doctor may in addition prescribe drugs to prevent acid secretion, and antacids to neutralize the acid and protect the stomach lining. Surgery is a last resort.

TAKE ACTION NOW!

Here's how to reduce your risk of developing peptic ulcers:
- Limit alcohol consumption
- Avoid tobacco smoke
- Keep intake of nonsteroidal anti-inflammatory drugs such as ibuprofen to a minimum
- Reduce stress as much as possible

Pay attention

Ulcers that are left untreated may bleed, and cause anaemia. A symptom of this is tiredness, as well as dark red, bloody or black stools, which indicate internal bleeding. See your doctor immediately.

THE ENEMY WITHIN

For many years it was thought that stress and diet caused stomach ulcers. However, since the mid-1980s, it has been known that bacteria called *Helicobacter pylori* (*H. pylori*) are involved in the formation of 95 per cent of duodenal ulcers and 70 per cent of gastric ulcers. The bacteria live in the stomach lining, making it more sensitive to acid and causing inflammation. Most people are infected in childhood, although not everyone will have symptoms. Once symptoms appear—the most usual being indigestion, reflux (backflow) and stomach pain—your doctor can arrange a blood or breath test for *H. pylori*. If the bacteria are found, a multi-layer regime will be prescribed, consisting of powerful antibiotics and histamine-blocker drugs to reduce acid production. These drugs will be taken over one to three weeks. It is essential to complete the course of therapy for the length of time advised.

TAKE CARE

Over-the-counter pain relievers (such as aspirin) and NSAIDs (such as ibuprofen) can make an ulcer worse. While paracetamol does not affect the stomach lining, it can relieve pain. If you have an ulcer and develop anaemia, be sure you do not take too much iron in the form of a supplement, since this can irritate the stomach lining. Discuss with your doctor the amount you need to counteract one problem without exacerbating the other.

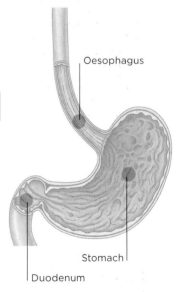

Oesophagus

Stomach

Duodenum

COMMON SITES
Peptic ulcers usually form in the oesophagus, stomach or duodenum, when the protective lining develops raw patches. The ulcers are sensitive and interrupt the digestive process.

CONSTIPATION

Normal bowel habits vary from person to person, ranging from three times a day to four times a week. Medically speaking, however, you are usually considered constipated if three or more days go by without a bowel movement and if your stools are hard, dry and difficult to pass. Chronic constipation occurs most often in women, children and in people over the age of 65.

Constipation usually occurs when the bowel lacks water and works too slowly, causing stools to harden. As food and waste pass through the intestines, the body absorbs water in order to maintain blood pressure at the right level. Other reasons for constipation include eating foods that contain too little fibre or fibrous material, bowel diseases and chronic medical conditions such as multiple sclerosis. It can also be a side effect of some drugs and may occur just before menstruation, with pregnancy or as a result of pelvic floor dysfunction.

TAKE ACTION NOW!

Follow these 3 preventive strategies every day:
- Eat beans and whole grains
- Drink 8 glasses of water
- Exercise for roughly 20 to 30 minutes

Constantly straining to empty your bowels can lead to haemorrhoids (piles), which are swollen veins in the rectal area. The skin in the area is thin and veins may rupture, causing bleeding.

Chronic constipation in people who are elderly or immobile can lead to impacted faeces, when the hard stools are so tightly wedged that they cannot be removed with normal pushing. A doctor may consider it necessary to soften these with oil or enemas. In particularly difficult cases the doctor may remove part of the hardened stool by inserting one or two (gloved and lubricated) fingers into the anus.

Avoiding the problem

You can prevent constipation by eating at least 30 g (1 oz) of fibre a day (beans, wholegrain bread, bran cereals, fresh or dried fruit such as prunes, and fresh vegetables). The fibre adds water-retaining bulk to stools so they don't become hard.

You can make bowel movements easier by drinking at least eight glasses of water a day. Avoid alcohol and caffeine, and limit how much chocolate you eat.

Muscles play an important part in the peristaltic action of your bowels, which propels the waste along. Regular daily exercise will tone your muscles and improve digestion.

Laxatives: only if fibre fails

Laxatives help stimulate the large intestine to contract.

There are different types of laxative. Stool softeners and some gentle laxatives make the stools bulkier, just as food fibre does, while others make them looser. Pills or liquid are taken by mouth; suppositories are inserted in the rectum.

Laxatives should be taken for only a short period of time and only if a change to a high-fibre diet doesn't work. They should not be taken regularly as the colon begins to rely on them to bring on faecal movements. Over a period of time, this can affect the colon's ability to contract. This may cause diarrhoea and interfere with the body's absorption of nutrients. Laxatives also interact with various medicines. For this reason, high-fibre foods are usually a better option.

Constipation in pregnancy

Constipation is common during pregnancy because hormones relax the bowels and slow the action of the muscles, causing the heavy uterus to press against the intestines. Iron pills, which may be prescribed for anaemia, can make matters worse. The best advice is to drink plenty of water every day, eat lots of fresh fruit and vegetables and walk regularly. Sitting on the toilet with your feet raised on a small platform may make passing stools easier.

Laxatives should be taken during pregnancy only on medical advice because they can cause the uterus to contract. Constipation usually disappears after giving birth.

DIARRHOEA

Diarrhoea occurs when the bowels contract too quickly or too much fluid passes into the gut, causing more frequent or runnier stools than usual. It may be an acute attack or an ongoing problem related to a medical condition.

An attack of acute diarrhoea comes on suddenly and can last for three to four days, but tends to clear after 48 hours. The first sign is an urgent need to empty your bowels frequently. You may feel nauseous. If you are vomiting and have abdominal pain, you should suspect gastroenteritis (*see* box below).

Diarrhoea may be caused by a change in routine, anxiety, rich or spicy foods, a reaction to monosodium glutamate and some antibiotics. Traveller's diarrhoea occurs through exposure to foreign viruses and bacteria in contaminated food and water.

What appears to be diarrhoea may also occur after prolonged constipation or use of laxatives, when the colon loses its ability to function. Any involuntary leakage from the rectum needs medical

help. A drug will be prescribed to encourage the nerves and muscles to return to normal.

Feel better fast

After a bout of diarrhoea you should avoid food for the first 24 hours, but sip plenty of boiled or bottled water. You can try weak black tea with lemon or herbal tea, but avoid milk or dairy products or fruit juices since these make diarrhoea worse. Light, bland food can be gradually introduced into your diet as the bouts of diarrhoea become less frequent.

You can take antidiarrhoeal medicines to slow down bowel activity (although some suggest it is better to let the bug leave the body). Severe dehydration can damage the kidneys, especially in children and the elderly. If you have severe symptoms, you should see your doctor. Oral rehydration solutions to replace fluids and mineral salts will probably be recommended. These can be bought from supermarkets and pharmacies or you can make your own by dissolving a generous pinch of salt and 5 ml (1 teaspoon) of sugar in 275 ml (1/2 pint) of water. Observe strict hygiene, making sure to wash your hands after a visit to the toilet.

Oral contraceptives are less reliable if you have diarrhoea for over 24 hours– continue taking the pill, but use other precautions for the rest of the cycle.

Chronic diarrhoea

Persistent diarrhoea should be reported. It may occur in inflammatory bowel disease, diverticulitis, irritable bowel syndrome and food intolerance–such as gluten (in coeliac disease) and lactose. A reduced ability to absorb foodstuffs in the intestine–the result of hormonal changes–will also cause diarrhoea.

SEE YOUR DOCTOR

Consult your doctor if you have severe abdominal pain, vomiting, fever or blood or mucus in the stools. You should also see your doctor if the diarrhoea wakens you from your sleep, if it continues for more than two days, if you are severely dehydrated or if you have recently travelled abroad. If a bacterial or amoebic infection, such as dysentery, is diagnosed or suspected, a doctor will prescribe antibiotics or an amebicide to kill the parasites.

GASTROENTERITIS

Gastroenteritis is the medical term for inflammation of the digestive system. It is often caused by a virus. It may be caused by bacterial contamination of food—known as food poisoning.

The symptoms of food poisoning are sudden fever, vomiting, abdominal pain and diarrhoea. The most common culprits are *Campylobacter*, *Salmonella* and *E. coli* from poorly cooked meat and poultry, unpasteurized milk or dairy products. You may be asked for a stool sample that will be analysed in the laboratory so the doctor can identify the bacterium. If several people are affected by the illness, public health inspectors try to find the source to limit the spread of the infection.

Most cases resolve without special treatment other than the prevention of dehydration, although antibiotics may sometimes be prescribed. Young children and the aged and frail are most at risk and may require hospitalization. Food poisoning can be prevented by strict hygiene in food preparation.

FOOD INTOLERANCE
Wheat products and dairy foods may trigger an allergic reaction in some people, causing diarrhoea.

APPENDICITIS

The appendix is situated at the beginning of the large intestine and is a narrow, tube-like sac that resembles a tail. It contains lymph nodes and may be part of the immune system, although it is thought the body can survive without it.

In appendicitis, the appendix becomes infected, although the cause cannot always be found. The appendix may become inflamed if its opening is blocked by faecal matter. The blockage may be triggered by a lack of fibre, which causes food to pass through the intestines slowly.

Most cases of appendicitis occur in people who are under the age of 30. It is rare in babies younger than two. The condition can be difficult to diagnose in women because the pain that is characteristic of appendicitis can be mimicked by gynecological discomfort from the ovaries or uterus.

During pregnancy, because of the growing uterus, appendicitis may often be overlooked. The tube-like sac is pushed out of place and moves from near the right groin area in the right lower quadrant of the abdomen to a position just under the liver. If the appendix ruptures, the resultant scarring can cause a blockage of the fallopian tubes as the scar tissue builds up, and this in turn can cause infertility. A high-fibre diet in pregnancy is the best preventive measure.

WARNING

If you have symptoms of appendicitis, it is important not to eat, drink or take painkillers or antacids, because these may cause the appendix to rupture. Seek medical help as soon as possible.

THE APPENDIX IN WOMEN
The appendix lies at the start of the large intestine. Discomfort or pain in women may be mistakenly attributed to the ovaries or uterus, which lie to the front of the pelvic area.

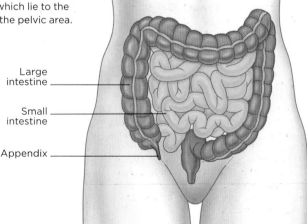

Large intestine

Small intestine

Appendix

A shifting pain

The early symptoms of appendicitis are indistinguishable from many other abdominal disorders. There may be some discomfort in the abdomen, with a dull pain near the navel, loss of appetite, nausea, constipation or diarrhoea and a slight fever. After six to 12 hours, however, the symptoms become more recognizable. Typically, a sharp pain shifts from the lower mid-abdomen to the lower right-hand side and this is aggravated by movement, particularly if the right leg is flexed up.

Pain may also be felt in the back or around the rectum. The pain usually becomes progressively worse, although in some people it may come and go.

A doctor will press the stomach area to establish where the pain hurts the most. If there is tenderness in the right lower abdomen, just under the pelvic bone, the doctor may perform an internal physical examination to establish the cause. The doctor may also examine the rectum with a gloved finger.

Urgent action

Acute appendicitis is a medical emergency. Most doctors operate immediately to remove the appendix, since complications may occur if it is neglected. An appendectomy is a simple, hour-long, laparoscopic operation, usually done under general anaesthetic through a keyhole incision. In women it may be done during a hysterectomy. Antibiotics are given routinely to treat any possible infection.

If appendicitis is not recognized and treated early, the appendix can rupture, releasing its contents into the abdomen. At this point the local pain stops, but urgent help is needed. The escape of the bacteria from the appendix into the abdominal cavity leads to peritonitis–a serious infection and inflammation of the walls of the abdomen. The symptoms of this are pain and tenderness in the abdomen and a fever. Peristalsis (muscular contractions in the gut) ceases and severe dehydration can result.

If the appendix has ruptured, the abdominal cavity will have to be drained of pus and rinsed with a saline solution.

DIVERTICULAR DISEASE

The walls of the lower part of the large intestine (colon) can develop small pouches, known as diverticula, which may be caused by pressure buildup in the bowel as it contracts. The pouches tend to form at weak spots, usually where blood vessels enter the intestinal tract. If hard faecal matter gets caught in them, interfering with their blood supply, inflammation occurs—known as diverticulitis. If it continually recurs it is known as diverticular disease.

Symptoms include pain and severe cramping, nausea, abdominal tenderness, alternating diarrhoea and constipation and, in rare cases, rectal bleeding. If the diverticula become infected, they may bleed profusely or perforate the intestinal wall, leading to peritonitis, which needs emergency medical treatment.

Who's at risk?

It is thought that the tendency to have diverticula can be inherited. However, since diverticular disease mainly occurs in countries in which low-fibre diets are not uncommon it is also linked with lifestyle and eating habits. It mostly affects people over the age of 50. It is most common after the age of 70, particularly in those with chronic constipation, which is both a symptom and cause, since diverticular disease increases the pressure in the colon. Others at risk include those with coronary artery disease, gallbladder disease and obesity.

What can you expect?

As diverticula do not always cause symptoms, they are often found by chance. If there is local tenderness, doctors have three options for diagnosis: ultrasound to look for an abscess; a barium enema to outline the bowel; or a colonoscopy or sigmoidoscopy for an internal examination of the intestines. A CAT scan may also be carried out so that other diseases with similar symptoms, such as irritable bowel syndrome and digestive tract ulcers, can be ruled out.

Diverticula are not generally treated, but the symptoms can be. Constipation

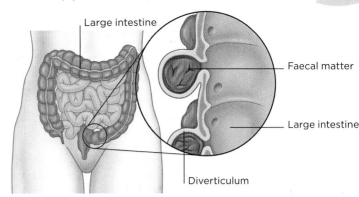

Large intestine

Faecal matter

Large intestine

Diverticulum

may be eased by eating a high-fibre diet or taking bulk laxatives for a short period of time. Some doctors also recommend avoiding foods with small seeds, such as tomatoes, grapes or strawberries, because the seeds can get caught in the pouches. If diverticulitis develops, you will need antibiotics, painkillers, drugs to stop abdominal spasms, and bed rest until the pain and inflammation subside. Severe cases may require a liquid diet or intravenous feeding to give the colon a complete rest. If attacks are frequent or very severe, a doctor may recommend surgery to remove the affected area.

WHY YOUR STOMACH RUMBLES

Stomach rumbling may not be regarded as a medical problem, but it can be a social embarrassment. The noises, which are known medically as borborygmi, are produced when liquid and gas in the stomach are shuffled to and fro by vigorous muscular contractions. This action may be triggered by hunger, anxiety or fright, or it may be the result of eating wind-forming foods such as beans. A noisy stomach can be common in some diseases, such as irritable bowel syndrome, for which antispasmodic drugs may be given. Swallowing air when eating or talking rapidly and drinking too many carbonated drinks are other culprits.

The noises may diminish if you eat regularly and slowly. Having five small meals a day instead of three large ones may help. Loud rumblings with severe abdominal pain should be reported to a doctor. They may be caused by a variety of digestive or other disorders, including gynaecological ones.

TROUBLE SPOTS

In this close-up, diverticula filled with feces can be seen protruding from the wall of the large intestine. They are more likely to occur in the last segment of the large intestine.

CAN LAXATIVES HELP?

Not all laxatives are the same. Bulk-forming laxatives, taken orally, help to retain water and soften faeces, and encourage peristalsis (muscular contractions of the gut, moving food and waste). People who suffer from constipation with diverticular disease, but who find it difficult to increase their intake of high-fibre foods, can benefit from these laxatives. It is important to drink plenty of water when you take them.

IRRITABLE BOWEL SYNDROME

Women are twice as likely as men to report symptoms of irritable bowel syndrome, which is also known as IBS, spastic colon or nervous diarrhoea. Many people never seek medical help, yet it is thought to affect one in five people at some time in their lives, usually at a time of significant change or stress.

There is no established cause of IBS, although nerve changes or genetics may play a role. With IBS, either the bowel is not functioning properly–the muscles work too quickly, too slowly or are out of synchronization–or the bowel is hypersensitive to the normal muscular activity within it. Very often IBS occurs after a bout of food poisoning (also called gastroenteritis) or a stressful life event such as pregnancy or childbirth, marriage or bereavement. For many people, the symptoms may disappear for long periods of time, but the condition usually recurs.

Checking things out

Irritable bowel syndrome is difficult to diagnose because it does not cause any physical changes in the bowel, such as inflammation. No test can give a definitive diagnosis, but a doctor needs to rule out more serious illnesses, such as inflammatory bowel disease, which can have similar symptoms. Women over the age of 50 need to have a thorough investigation, especially if symptoms include weight loss or blood in the stools, which are not typical of IBS.

Your doctor may perform some or all of the following tests: a sigmoidoscopy or colonoscopy to examine the inside of the

WHAT TO LOOK FOR

Symptoms vary from person to person, may be mild or severe and can come and go at different times. They may include:

- Abdominal cramping, especially on the left side of the body or across the lower right abdomen. The pain is often relieved on passing wind or after a bowel movement.
- A feeling of bloating and fullness, which may make clothes feel tight and uncomfortable.
- Excessive flatulence.
- Constipation and/or diarrhoea.
- A sudden urge to rush to the toilet.
- A sensation of incomplete emptying of the bowel.
- Nausea.
- Pellet-like stools, often containing mucus.
- Stomach-rumbling sounds.

Symptoms can be made worse by stress, certain foods and menstruation. Some women may in addition have cystitis-like pain, temporary urinary incontinence, painful periods and pain during intercourse.

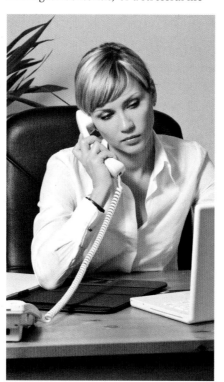

WORKING WOMAN
The constant stress of a busy life can be exciting, but it can also be debilitating. When the "fight or flight" response is a regular event in a day's work, physiological changes occur in the body. These are made worse when personal habits such as eating and going to the toilet are irregular.

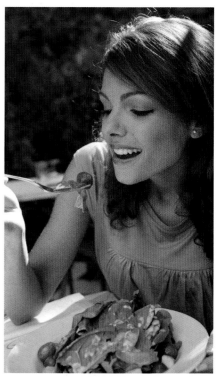

SUPER WOMAN
Trying to do too much—as wife, mother, working woman—can cause the body systems to react. Digestion is particularly susceptible, since little time is available to sit down and relax as you eat. To coax the digestive tract back into working order may require some self-nurturing.

intestine; an ultrasound scan to look at the outer intestine walls; a barium enema (an X-ray procedure that provides a clear picture of the colon and rectum); laboratory testing of a stool culture to check for parasites or rule out other causes; and a full blood count and blood test to reveal whether there is any infection or inflammation.

Healing the gut

IBS does not lead to complications or cancer. However, the symptoms are highly distressing and should be brought to the attention of your doctor. They can normally be kept under control with medication, although there is no single solution and several drugs may be tried. The most commonly used include antispasmodics to reduce intestinal muscle contraction causing diarrhoea and abdominal pain, laxatives to reduce constipation and peppermint oil for bloating and flatulence problems.

When none of these succeeds, a doctor may sometimes prescribe a tricyclic antidepressant to calm the nervous system and so the intestines. If stress is a contributory factor, your doctor may suggest psychotherapy, hypnotherapy or mind/body therapy. Self-nurturing through relaxation techniques and regular exercise can also have beneficial effects.

Changing your diet

People with IBS are advised to eat a well-balanced diet with meals at set times, since this can reduce the symptoms. Knowing what provokes your symptoms is also important, so your doctor may suggest you try an exclusion diet for a few weeks. Common culprits include wheat, dairy products, fatty or spicy foods, beans and pulses, soft drinks, caffeine and some fruits and vegetables such as the brassicas–cabbage, cauliflower and brussels sprouts.

Eating more fibrous foods helps some people, but makes others feel worse because of the wind problem. You can also try a soluble fibre dietary product such as psyllium husks, to encourage bulk forming in your stools.

Tests may be carried out to find out if you are lactose intolerant (meaning you

WHAT DO YOUR BOWEL MOVEMENTS MEAN?

If your stools change colour, odour or consistency for longer than two weeks, you should consult a doctor. Your doctor may ask you to provide a stool sample, which will be sent to a lab for analysis, and may perform a rectal examination (with a gloved and lubricated finger) to discover the source of the problem.

In most cases the changes in stools are harmless, but in some people they may relate to a disorder of the digestive system. Pale, smelly or bulky stools can be a sign of coeliac disease (gluten intolerance), caused by the malabsorption of food. Loose stools with mucus may be associated with constipation or IBS; if blood is also present it may be a sign of inflammatory bowel disease (IBD) or cancer. Dark stools can be caused by eating too much of a food such as beetroot. But if they contain blood, it can be a sign of haemorrhoids, diverticulitis or, rarely, colorectal cancer.

SYMPTOM	WHAT IT MAY INDICATE
Hard, infrequent stools, much straining needed	Constipation
Runny, frequent stools	Diarrhoea
Alternating hard/infrequent and runny/frequent stools	Irritable bowel syndrome, diabetes, misuse of laxatives
Visible blood, blood in stools	Haemorrhoids, irritable bowel syndrome, IBD, colorectal cancer
Thin ribbon-like stools, anal blood	Possible cancer
Pale clay-like stools	Liver disease
Dark metallic-smelling stools	Bleeding in gastrointestinal tract, possibly certain medications
Foul-smelling large stools, abdominal pain	Pancreatic problems, coeliac disease
Light-coloured threads in stools, anal itching	Worm infection
Pale chalky stools, dark urine	Gallbladder-related problems, disorders of the liver

lack the enzyme lactase that metabolizes lactose, a sugar found in milk and other dairy products). Another test that might be suggested can determine if you have an intolerance to gluten, which is a protein found in wheat and some other grains. Both types of intolerance–lactose and gluten–have symptoms that are similar to IBS.

INFLAMMATORY BOWEL DISEASE

Crohn's disease and ulcerative colitis are related diseases that cause inflammation of the intestines. Together they are called inflammatory bowel disease (IBD). Crohn's disease can affect any part of the digestive tract, with parts becoming red and inflamed; in ulcerative colitis there is inflammation and ulceration only of the colon and rectum.

IBD is more common in women than in men. The cause is unknown, although the condition has been linked to a long-term reaction to bacteria or viruses, such as measles. It is not caused by anxiety, stress or psychological disorders. IBD can run in families.

What it looks like

Crohn's disease causes abdominal pain, diarrhoea (with occasional bleeding), vomiting and inflammation around the anus. Children with Crohn's disease may have poor growth. Sometimes leaks, called fistulas, break through the inflamed gut, leading to infections, or scar tissue builds up that narrows and obstructs the bowel. In severe ulcerative colitis, there is frequent diarrhoea with blood and mucus, and abdominal pain. It can also cause skin and mouth ulcers, eye inflammation and joint pain. Both Crohn's disease and ulcerative colitis can lead to fatigue, weight loss and anaemia.

Flare-ups can occur at any time of life. Active disease can reduce fertility in women, who may be advised to try to get pregnant while in remission. Active IBD can also complicate a pregnancy.

People with widespread and severe ulcerative colitis have a high risk of developing bowel cancer and need regular colonoscopies.

A difficult diagnosis

It can take time for a diagnosis to be finally made, as most people feel fine between flare-ups. In addition, the two conditions are alike and they share symptoms with other, more minor, digestive tract problems.

A doctor may choose a range of tests, which can include: a barium enema to show up any intestinal thickening and identify the parts affected; an internal examination by sigmoidoscopy or colonoscopy to assess the disease's severity; biopsies to analyse the intestinal lining; analysis of stool samples; and blood tests to detect anaemia and nutritional deficiencies.

What to expect

Acute mild to moderate IBD affecting the rectum or distal colon (the end section of colon) is treated initially with local application of steroids (liquids or foams) and aminosalicylates, for example mesalazine. More severe conditions or widespread disease that does not respond to local treatment requires oral aminosalicylates (mesalazine or olsalazine) and corticosteroids (prednisolone or budesonide).

Severe disease invariably calls for hospital admission and intravenous corticosteroids and nutrition, because there is a risk of dehydration and the colon bursting. Antidiarrhoeal agents are used in Crohn's disease. Badly diseased sections of the colon can be surgically removed, but the inflammation often returns elsewhere along the digestive tract. Surgery may repair any leaks or widen badly scarred areas. Sometimes surgery can cure the disease by taking away all or part of the colon–a procedure called a colectomy.

QUESTIONS TO ASK YOUR DOCTOR

- What are the side effects of my medicines?
- If I'm on steroids for IBD, am I at risk of osteoporosis?
- Are there any foods that I should avoid?
- Will I need surgery?
- Am I at risk of bowel cancer?

DURING PREGNANCY
Patients with IBD who are pregnant should be monitored carefully for flare-ups.

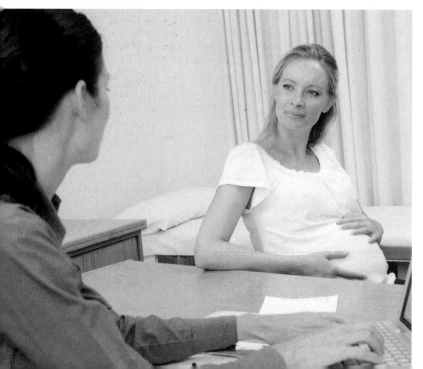

COLORECTAL CANCER

Colorectal (bowel) cancer is the second most common cancer. It often develops when cells in the lining of the colon (the large intestine or bowel) or rectum become abnormal and form small growths called polyps. Although most polyps are harmless, they may sometimes become cancerous.

Who's at risk?

Colorectal cancer is primarily a disease of the Western world, linked to a diet rich in saturated fats and sugar and low in fibre. Excessive alcohol intake, a sedentary lifestyle and obesity also increase the risk. Colorectal cancer can occur at any age but is rare in people under the age of 40 and is common in the elderly. People with IBD (*see* opposite) have a slightly increased risk.

The risk of developing colorectal cancer can be reduced by eating a balanced diet. You should eat at least 30 g (1 oz) of fibre (a minimum of five portions of fruit and vegetables) a day, which aids the passage of food through the body and ensures the elimination of waste. Water also flushes the intestine and helps waste to pass through. Antioxidant vitamins, such as beta carotene and vitamin C, were recently found not to have a protective effect. Avoid high-salt and smoked foods, which are thought to increase the levels of carcinogens in the body.

As many as 10 per cent of those diagnosed have a family history of colorectal cancer. In these families the disease often appears before the age of 45 and may affect two or more close relatives. Hereditary colorectal cancer has been linked to other forms of cancer.

What to watch for

Colorectal cancer often has no symptoms in the early stages. Many of the advanced symptoms are also found in other bowel disorders, such as inflammatory bowel disease. They include a persistent change in bowel habit for three or more weeks (for example, constipation or diarrhoea); rectal bleeding; anaemia with or without tiredness; and sudden unexplained weight loss. The cancer can also block the bowel, with abdominal pain, bloating and vomiting.

Finding out

Colorectal cancer can be difficult to diagnose. Many people are only diagnosed in advanced stages because of a delay in seeking help. If you have symptoms that could indicate colorectal cancer, note down the time and type of your bowel movements or bleeding and consult your doctor, who may refer you to a specialist.

The tests for colorectal cancer include: a rectal examination to check for polyps; a stool analysis to check for blood; a barium enema to check for

TAKE ACTION NOW!

To help prevent colorectal cancer, follow these strategies:
- Avoid salty or smoked foods
- Eat a balanced diet that includes 30 g (1 oz) of fibre a day
- Limit alcohol consumption
- Drink lots of water
- Take exercise daily
- Get a colonoscopy

A study found that a baby aspirin a day reduced the recurrence of colorectal cancer by 17 per cent.

blockages; an internal examination by sigmoidoscopy to look for changes in the bowel lining; a biopsy (cell sample); an ultrasound scan; and a colonoscopy (examination of the inside of the colon).

What to expect

If the cancer is caught in its early stages, the chance of surviving five years after diagnosis is high. When polyps are found, they are removed and examined to see whether they are cancerous. If the cancer has spread, a second operation may be performed to cut out part of the bowel. In advanced cases, the whole bowel may be removed and replaced with an external pouch.

Some people may benefit from chemotherapy or radiotherapy to shrink the tumour before surgery, kill cancer cells at other sites or reduce the risk of recurrence.

In advanced colorectal cancer, cells travel to form a secondary tumour (metastasis), usually in the liver. Treatments may include chemotherapy or surgery to remove further tumours.

GET SCREENED

Doctors recommend that you start screening at age 50. Those with an increased risk, such as a family history will need to start screening at a younger age. Discuss with your doctor your risk and which test is best for you.

Immune System Problems

Your body's ability to protect itself against infections and diseases relies on the healthy and efficient operation of the immune system, which is an integrated system of organs, tissues and their products. In some instances the various white cells that tackle infection are affected by an allergic reaction that makes them unable to cope. The most common reactions are caused by substances and organisms in the world around us.

ALLERGIC ASTHMA

People with allergic asthma become wheezy and breathless when an allergen such as pollen or animal skin scales enters the tiny airways in their lungs, causing the bronchioles (airways) to narrow and fill up with mucus. The bronchioles are hyper-responsive to irritants that would not affect other people. Because the flow of oxygen through the lungs is also restricted, an asthma attack can be life-threatening. People with allergic asthma should always carry an adrenaline injection kit.

YOUR BODY'S DEFENCE AGAINST THE WORLD

Your body has a complex–and usually extremely effective–system of defending itself against attack from organisms such as bacteria, viruses and parasites. However, the system can malfunction in a number of ways.

It may mistakenly attack certain of its own cells or tissues, as in so-called autoimmune disease. The system can also fail partially or completely, for example in AIDS, or in response to drugs that are designed to prevent the destruction of transplanted tissue, such as a new kidney.

But your immune system can also respond to substances that are in fact harmless to most people–such as dust or pollen–causing an allergic reaction. This kind of response, known as atopy, often runs in families.

Allergies come in many forms and most appear before the age of 40. One sensitivity may make you susceptible to others, for example people with asthma often have eczema too. In rare instances, people develop "total allergy syndrome", in which they react adversely to almost everything in their surroundings.

ARE YOU ALLERGIC?

From a medical viewpoint, sensitivity and intolerance are controversial areas. Even if you do not suffer a full immune system response, as with allergies, you may become physically ill from contact with certain foods or ingredients.

Headaches, flushing and numbness occur, for example, in response to monosodium glutamate (MSG), a flavour enhancer. Certain preservatives such as sugar, and additives such as sulphites (found in a range of dried fruit and vegetables, wine, beer, dehydrated soups and baking mixes) may cause reactions in susceptible individuals.

Your doctor may advise you to undergo sensitivity tests in which a tiny amount of one allergen at a time is placed under the skin and your reaction is noted. One recommended treatment may be immunotherapy—also called "desensitization"—which gradually introduces by injection small but increasing amounts of an offending allergen to try to encourage your immune system to learn tolerance.

You can help yourself as well by keeping your environment as free as possible of known allergens. Also avoid cigarette smoke, fuel fumes and other environmental pollutants.

TOP FOUR ALLERGIES

ALLERGY	WHAT YOU CAN DO
HAY FEVER	
Inhaling pollens from a vast assortment of trees, grasses and other plants can set off the misery of hay fever symptoms for millions of people every spring and summer. Watery, sore eyes, a running nose and itchy throat are the result of the immune system reacting to the pollen and triggering an immune response. Nasal steroid sprays can help to suppress the immune response, supplemented with over-the-counter antihistamines (although these may cause drowsiness), eyedrops and nasal decongestants as required.	Wear sunglasses, keep car and bedroom windows closed and stay inside as much as possible when pollen counts peak in the early morning and evening. Take early evening showers to remove pollen.
ECZEMA	
An immune response to allergens in the environment can cause this skin condition in susceptible people. The droppings of dust mites, animal skin scales and pollens are common triggers, causing the skin to erupt in scaly patches and watery blisters that become crusty and may ooze.	Keep the skin cool and wear natural fibres such as cotton, rather than synthetics, next to the skin. Emollients moisturize the skin and help soothe itching, and steroid creams help to get rid of inflammation and encourage the healing process.
STINGS	
Some people develop an allergic response to insect stings, especially those from bees. This response may range from highly unpleasant, with severe itching, dizziness, faintness or vomiting, to potentially fatal if the person goes into anaphylactic shock. This can happen within minutes, and is caused by a massive release of histamine that restricts breathing and causes blood pressure to drop disastrously if urgent action is not taken.	Prompt treatment with an injection of adrenaline is essential. Carry a kit (an Epipen) with you at all times.
FOOD	
A genuine food allergy, rather than a food sensitivity, causes a release of histamine that produces serious symptoms such as hives on the skin, nausea and vomiting, and sometimes asthma. In severe cases it can shut down your airway and cause anaphylactic shock. Common triggers are peanuts, peanut oil and other protein foods.	If the trigger is known, always read labels on prepared foods and ask in restaurants if the ingredient is included. Carry an adrenaline injection kit (an Epipen) with you at all times.

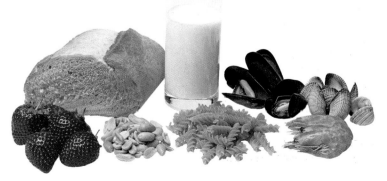

TRIGGER FOOD
The most common foods known to provoke an allergic response are cow's milk, wheat, soya beans, egg white, citrus fruits, strawberries, peanuts and shellfish such as shrimp, mussels and clams.

CHRONIC FATIGUE SYNDROME

No one knows exactly what chronic fatigue syndrome (CFS) is or what causes the condition. Some doctors dispute that it exists at all, believing that it is simply a form of depression or some other psychological disorder.

The confusion is reflected in the variety of different names by which it is known: post-viral syndrome or myalgic encephalomyelitis (ME), chronic Epstein-Barr virus (CEBV) and immune dysfunction syndrome. Although it was once thought to be a type of influenza, it is now considered to be a disorder that is characterized by unexplained persistent fatigue not relieved by rest along with other symptoms including impairment in short-term memory and concentration; sore throat; tender lymph nodes; muscle pain; multi-joint pain, headaches, unrefreshing sleep; and post-exertional malaise. Women are much more likely to contract CFS than men; 80 per cent of those with CFS are women under the age of 45.

Symptoms may come and go and vary both in severity and from one person to another, but some are common to all. The symptoms could be long-lasting (up to two years or more) and may significantly impact quality of life.

How it affects your body

The predominant symptom is fatigue, often to the point of exhaustion, and an overall lack of energy. You may have pain

The ongoing problem of lupus

Systemic lupus erythematosus (SLE) or lupus is a condition affecting the joints, connective tissues and small blood vessels caused by an immune system malfunction. As with other autoimmune diseases, it is not clear why the body's defence system turns against itself, but external factors that may trigger it in a person who has inherited a genetic susceptibility include childbirth, exposure to sunlight, arrival of the menopause and viral infections.

Women between the ages of 15 and 40 make up 90 per cent of cases of lupus. Some women are more severely affected than others and many only have relatively mild symptoms. The disease tends to flare up then subside periodically, with the symptoms often rising and subsiding with the menstrual cycle.

In an active phase, you may feel as though you have flu, with a raised temperature, aching and weakness. Inflammation makes joints in the hands, elbows, knees and ankles swollen and painful, and some people get a red rash—butterfly shaped—across their nose and face.

A common and serious consequence of lupus is a form of kidney disorder. More than half of all lupus sufferers will develop renal failure to a greater or lesser degree.

Steroids keep the condition under control in many people, although they may need increased doses during a flare-up. Drugs used more familiarly as malaria preventives, for example hydroxychloroquine, can also be an effective treatment, while NSAIDs (nonsteroidal anti-inflammatory drugs) can reduce pain and inflammation. Immuno-suppressive drugs and high dose steroids are used in aggressive cases. Mild steroid creams can help with rashes, and sun protection should be used in all seasons. Physiotherapy can help prevent loss of mobility.

Women with lupus would in the past have been advised not to have children. Now, with close monitoring by their doctors, many have healthy, normal pregnancies. There is an increased risk of miscarriage and preeclampsia, and babies are often born small and may be premature.

Areas affected

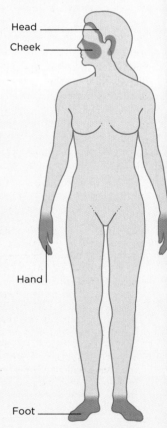

Head

Cheek

Hand

Foot

or aches in joints and muscles, usually in your arms, but without any swelling or tenderness. The lymph glands that are under your jaw and ears may be swollen. Your throat may be constantly sore, and headaches will be frequent. You may be aware that you always seem to have a slight temperature and you find yourself responding to a new allergy, or an old one flares up. You may have difficulty with short-term memory, and you may have problems concentrating for any length of time.

In addition, your sleep pattern can go awry. First there may be insomnia, then waking in the early hours of the morning filled with anxiety. After this, there may be a period of oversleeping–being so tired that you can't wake up at the normal time. You may have dramatic mood swings and generally not feel well.

Can your doctor help?

Your doctor will want to rule out other causes for your symptoms, such as depression, thyroid malfunction, glandular fever, arthritis and cancer, and will arrange tests. If these are negative, your doctor may conclude from your medical history and your symptoms that you are suffering from CFS. Although researchers are developing possible diagnostic tests, there are no reliable ones in use as yet.

Your doctor can prescribe treatment to alleviate some of the symptoms. Since people with CFS can be ultra-sensitive to drugs, any medication will be prescribed in minimum doses at first and can be increased later if it is thought necessary. Acupuncture, exercise and a number of mind-body modalities can also help with symptom management.

A CYCLE OF STRESS?

One theory about CFS is that it may be associated with chronic stress that builds up slowly from pressures at work, problems in relationships, early childhood trauma or dealing with an illness. Stress takes a gradual toll, straining the nervous system so the body is in a constant state of mental and physical readiness for whatever might happen next. The ever-present low-level anxiety that accompanies this adds to the stress, which may then affect the immune system and upset its normal protective role.

TAKING A NAP
Listen to your body and if you need to have a short sleep, then do so. Talk to your boss if you're at work.

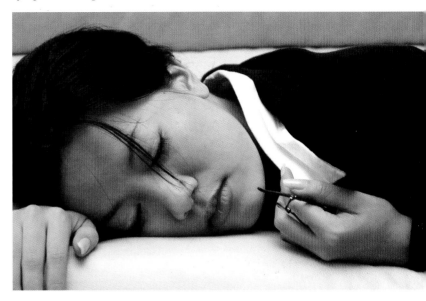

FIVE WAYS TO HELP YOURSELF

You may be told to rest, and when symptoms are severe you will have no alternative. When you have the time and energy available, however, consider some of these other suggestions.

Move An individually tailored programme of gentle, slow-building aerobic exercise may improve low energy levels. Find a gym or personal trainer who understands your needs.

Use your mind Meditation, cognitive–behavioural therapy, breathing techniques, guided imagery, qigong and yoga all reduce stress and may boost your energy levels. Investigate the various Chinese exercise systems that involve little physical movement but stimulate the flow of chi (energy) in the body.

Visualize Join a visualization class. There are six main exercises using the power of visualization to switch off stresses that can exacerbate CFS. You learn in a class until you are self-reliant, but it does require you to practise for 15 minutes, once or twice a day.

Get a massage Therapeutic body massage and reflexology both focus on achieving a state of relaxation. Acumassage is more rigorous: it combines lymphatic drainage massage with acupressure to remove toxins and pep up the immune system.

Nibble well Pay attention to the foods you eat. Include whole grains, good sources of protein and abundant fruits and vegetables. Fresh fruit, vegetables and green tea are good daily sources of antioxidants. Check with your doctor before taking supplements in case they clash with whatever conventional medication has been prescribed.

Nervous System Problems

An extensive nerve network reaches every part of your body, operating by a system of signals and impulses that process information at high speed and initiate action. The nerves are composed of a chain of cells that rely on chemical messengers. Problems arise if nerves lose the ability to carry messages from the brain. Multiple sclerosis (MS) and amyotrophic lateral sclerosis (ALS) are two examples of the result.

MULTIPLE SCLEROSIS

Twice as many women as men get multiple sclerosis (MS), a disease of the central nervous system. Some symptoms are more likely to appear between the ages of 20 and 40, although the disease can strike earlier or later in life, and is more common in people who live in temperate climates. Probably an autoimmune disorder, the cause of MS remains unsolved. Evidence suggests multiple risk factors. In addition to age and sex, there may be an environmental factor, such as a viral agent that operates in a genetically susceptible individual. Epstein-Barr virus, the virus that causes infectious mononucleosis (glandular fever) is a possible trigger.

The symptoms of MS are the result of damage to the myelin sheath–the fatty insulating layer that surrounds the nerves controlling movement and sensation throughout the body. The form that symptoms take and their severity depends on which part of the central nervous system is affected and how badly. This, together with the fact that there is no definitive test for MS, can make the condition difficult to diagnose and it may only be confirmed once a person has had several attacks.

How it works

The course that MS takes varies, ranging from mild, occasional symptoms to a more progressive deterioration. Many people have periods of active disease interspersed with periods of remission when symptoms disappear partially or even completely.

Doctors tend to distinguish between relapsing-remitting and progressive MS, but the difference is not always clear. Some people whose MS starts off as relapsing-remitting eventually develop the progressive form, while roughly 15 per cent do not experience remissions at all. At the other extreme, some people have relatively mild symptoms with long periods of remission.

What to expect

Your medical history and the results of a neurological examination, plus other tests including, ideally, an MRI scan can usually confirm a diagnosis of MS. The doctor cannot tell you, however, what course the illness may take in the future and there is as yet no treatment that can cure it. However, this does not mean that nothing can be done.

The past few years have seen the launch of a new treatment with antiviral drugs known as interferons, which inhibit the multiplication of viruses and may slow the progress of MS in some people. Although the drugs cannot stop MS altogether, they are effective for relapsing-remitting MS. Glatiramer acetate may be prescribed. This mixture of polypeptides may act by blocking immune responses to one of the myelin proteins. It can reduce relapse rate and so significantly affect disability.

Other drug treatments can help ease some of the specific symptoms, such as muscle spasm, and courses of steroids can be effective in relieving or shortening an attack, especially when the eyes are affected. Nonmedical approaches, including physiotherapy, nutritional and occupational therapy and counselling from specialist neurorehabilitation professionals, may also be beneficial.

Find an expert

The amount of support offered by doctors to MS sufferers varies and may depend on where you live. You may need to find out for yourself what is available. Specialized MS nurses are particularly helpful. National organizations and charitable societies dealing with MS specifically can provide information and advice on treatment and suggest other types of help and support available to people with the condition and their families.

Many people who have MS say that one of the worst things about it is its unpredictability and the feeling that they have no control over how it will affect them. This can lead to stress in personal relationships and at work as well as anxiety about the future. It can be almost impossible for other people to understand how you feel, but meeting those who are going through similar experiences can be therapeutic. A number of organizations run local support groups.

Because of the lack of any effective medical treatment for MS, many people look instead to alternative medicine and complementary therapies. While none has been shown to have any long-term effect on slowing the progress of the disease, many people nevertheless feel that they have benefited both physically

and psychologically. Therapies that may help include aromatherapy, massage, acupuncture, reflexology, homeopathy, osteopathy and chiropractic.

It is difficult to assess whether any type of treatment–conventional or complementary–is working because of the way symptoms tend to come and go on their own. Claims for a range of treatments, from pressurized oxygen to gluten-free diets and many others, have been made, but none has so far been substantiated.

AMYOTROPHIC LATERAL SCLEROSIS

ALS–or amyotrophic lateral sclerosis–is a degenerative disorder of the nervous system with no known cure. It is not known what causes the motor neuron cells of the brain and spinal cord (which control voluntary movement of muscle) to die gradually, nor why they should be the only nerve cells affected. During the deterioration, which usually takes between two and five years, the muscles waste away, causing paralysis of the head, lungs and limbs. The mind works as normal and no pain is felt.

ALS is a rare and distressing disease. It affects more men than women. It is believed that between 5 and 10 per cent of cases are an inherited form of ALS, which is the result of a defective gene that normally prevents oxygen molecules called free radicals from damaging body tissue. In non-inherited ALS (the more common form) environmental toxins as well as defects in protective enzymes are thought to play an important role. The inherited form normally appears at the age of 50, whereas 60 is the average age for the onset of non-inherited ALS.

When symptoms appear, a neurologist will carry out various tests to rule out MS and spinal cord diseases, then perform an electromyogram (EMG) to test electrical activity in the muscles and assess nerve damage.

Electronic and other equipment is available to enable people with ALS to eat, talk, breathe and move, but physical assistance from a caregiver may become necessary as the disease progresses.

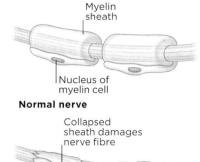

Normal nerve

Myelin sheath

Nucleus of myelin cell

Collapsed sheath damages nerve fibre

Nerve with MS

HOW NERVES ARE AFFECTED

Nerves consist of a chain of neurons along which messages from the brain to all parts of the body travel. Nerves are covered in a myelin sheath that acts as an insulator. When this protective covering is damaged in some way, the messages can no longer travel along the nerve. In multiple sclerosis, this can mean a loss of response in sensitive areas.

DID YOU KNOW?

- There is no established link between high blood pressure and a decline in cognitive or mental function.
- Memory can be impaired at any age—it is not always the first sign of dementia. Other causes include fatigue, stress, grief, vision or hearing loss, excessive alcohol consumption and working too hard.

BRAIN DISORDERS

Some disorders of the brain are more often found in older people and are in some cases linked to ageing, although of course not everyone who lives longer will necessarily be affected.

Dementia

There are various specific disorders collectively called dementia, which display symptoms showing a decline in a person's mental ability severe enough to interfere with everyday life.

Although once known as senility or senile dementia, dementia need not inevitably be a part of ageing. Some illnesses, such as thyroid disease, vitamin B deficiency and depression, cause dementia-like symptoms that can be reversed when the underlying disease is treated. Other causes of dementia, including vascular disease, multiple strokes and Alzheimer's disease, are not curable. But intervention and new drug treatment may help to slow the progress of the disease.

Advanced symptoms may include short-term loss of memory, confusion and non-recognition of people. There may be emotional outbursts, such as anger and irritability, or embarrassing behaviour. Eventually this subsides into a state of non-emotion; personal habits deteriorate and 24-hour care is needed.

Alzheimer's disease

Alzheimer's is the most common form of dementia. Scientists do not yet know the cause of the disease, which affects about 10 per cent of elderly people and causes brain cells to die.

Symptoms characteristic of the disease include problems with reasoning and judgement, changes in mood and behaviour patterns and an inability to manage work and social life. Medications may be given for depression, insomnia and behaviour problems.

One of the hallmarks of Alzheimer's disease is the deterioration of nerve cells releasing acetylcholine, which is the neurotransmitter that carries messages between brain cells. At the same time, the enzyme acetylcholinesterase (AChE) breaks down acetylcholine in the body at an accelerated rate. Several drugs (donepezil, huperzine A and tacrine) are used to try to restore acetylcholine levels by inhibiting AChE activity.

Brain "plaques" are another hallmark of the disease. Protein, called amyloid-beta (A-beta), is naturally made in the brain, but when it clumps and forms plaques it causes inflammation and other changes in brain tissue that eventually rob sufferers of the ability to think and function. Researchers aim to develop a drug that lowers A-beta levels. Research is also being carried out on genetic disposition, and on calcium usage, which is essential for neurotransmission but is affected by Alzheimer's.

People with Down's syndrome (caused by an extra copy of chromosome 21) are at high risk of developing Alzheimer's.

Parkinson's disease

The characteristic symptoms that occur in Parkinson's disease are muscle tremor or stiffness, slow movements, shuffling walk, stooped posture, loss of balance and a fixed expression. It is a progressive degenerative disease of the nerves that generally appears in people aged between 50 and 65. If it is treated, it may not be directly life threatening and its course may vary from mild to severely debilitating. Dementia also occurs in about a third of cases.

There is no cure for Parkinson's disease, but several drugs are available that improve quality of life. Treatment aims to improve morale and mobility. Links with a support group are essential for the caregiver as well as the patient.

BRAIN DEGENERATION
Coloured scans show a normal brain (left) and a brain of someone with Alzheimer's disease (right). Yellow and red areas indicate high brain activity and the normal brain has many of these areas. The blue and black areas show low activity and these predominate in the dementia patient's brain.

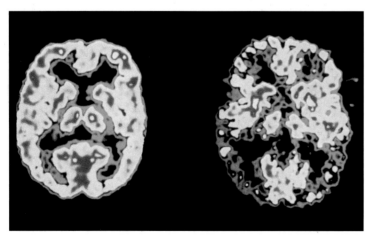

Respiratory Problems

A wide range of diseases affects the nasal passage, airways and lungs. Problems range from contagious illnesses that are spread by viruses and bacteria to occupational hazards that may have long-lasting effects on the airway.

PNEUMONIA

The medical term for inflammation of the tissues and airways of the lungs is pneumonia. Depending on its cause and the vulnerability of the sufferer, pneumonia can range from mild to life threatening. Those particularly at risk include the elderly, the very young, smokers and those who suffer from immune-related disorders, heart or lung disorders, diabetes or alcoholism. To prevent infection these people should be vaccinated against pneumococcal pneumonia. Pneumonia can be a potentially life-threatening complication during the post-operative stage of surgery and can be prevented with early emphasis on deep-breathing exercises.

Bacterial pneumonia

This type can arise spontaneously, but usually results from an infection after another disorder, such as influenza or chronic bronchitis. Generally, the bacterium responsible is *Streptococcus pneumoniae* (which is also known as pneumococcus) though *Staphylococcus aureus* is often implicated in cases when pneumonia follows influenza. Symptoms commonly associated with this pneumonia include a high fever with chills, coloured sputum–possibly blood flecked–and, especially in the elderly, confusion. Pleurisy (inflammation of the lining of the lungs) is a common complication. The usual treatment is antibiotics.

Viral pneumonia

Many viruses responsible for other lung infections, including the influenza virus, can cause viral pneumonia. Its onset is often slower than that of bacterial pneumonia. Initially there is a dry cough with a headache, aching muscles, fever and lethargy. Symptoms progress to a productive cough, often with blood-flecked sputum and breathlessness. An attack may be followed by bacterial pneumonia.

Mycoplasma pneumonia

This type of pneumonia is common among young adults. It is caused by a microorganism called *Mycoplasma pneumoniae*. The symptoms of the condition include a harsh, non-productive constant cough and rapid onset of headache. The high fever and chills seen with bacterial and viral pneumonia are not usually present. The condition tends to progress slowly. The most common treatment is antibiotics.

Lung diseases

Different parts of the lungs are affected by different diseases. Bronchitis affects the main respiratory tubes and pneumonia the smaller tubes and alveoli. In emphysema, the alveoli break down, reducing the area available for oxygen exchange.

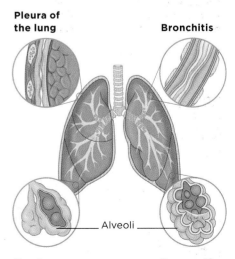

Pleura of the lung

Bronchitis

Alveoli

Emphysema

Pneumonia

PLEURISY

The pleura is a double membrane that lines the cavity of the chest and surrounds the lungs. The space in between the two skins is filled with fluid, which provides lubrication as the lungs expand and contract. In pleurisy, the pleural membrane becomes inflamed, usually following another infection such as pneumonia. The main symptom is a sharp pain felt in the chest when breathing in. Treatment is with antibiotics for the underlying infection and painkillers for the pain.

INFLUENZA

An acute respiratory illness, influenza–flu, as it is popularly known–involves both the upper and lower respiratory tract. It also causes fever, aching limbs, headache, sore throat, weakness and lethargy. These symptoms may be less apparent in milder forms of influenza, but coughs and and nasal congestion are common. The cause is a virus: most commonly influenza A followed by influenza B and C. In type C, symptoms are almost indistinguishable from those of the common cold–no aching muscles or fever and the onset is usually slow.

Influenza outbreaks often begin in late autumn and winter and can last into the new year. However, outbreaks occur any time of year. The severity of symptoms varies according to the precise strain of the virus, which mutates frequently, and the constitution of the sufferer.

The most severe form of influenza is caused by A-type viruses. The virus is spread from person to person through minute droplets exhaled during

Each year there are 3–5 million severe cases of influenza, leading to between 250,000 and 500,000 deaths globally.

coughing, sneezing and talking. In general, symptoms appear suddenly, between one and three days after infection, and last for six to 10 days.

The biggest danger is secondary, opportunistic bacterial infections of the lungs. These range from acute bronchitis to severe bacterial pneumonia, and the young, the elderly and those suffering from diabetes, immune system disorders and heart and lung diseases are particularly at risk.

An ounce of prevention

Vaccination offers good protection against influenza and is recommended for those at risk of developing complications. The vaccine is designed to combat only the specific strain of virus that researchers believe will be prevalent in the coming months. It does not give protection against all strains.

Nevertheless, influenza vaccination is advisable for high-risk groups, which include all persons age 50 years or older, residents of nursing homes and other long-term care facilities, adults and children of 6 months and over who have chronic heart or lung conditions, such as asthma, and women who are more than 3 months pregnant during the flu season.

Other people who need vaccinating include doctors, nurses and other employees in hospitals or medical offices or facilities where there is contact with high-risk individuals. Anyone who wants to reduce their risk of getting the flu should be able to get the vaccination.

Influenza vaccination should not be given to individuals with an allergy to eggs, and those who have had prior severe reaction to the vaccine. During severe outbreaks these people should reduce contact with possible carriers.

Fighting back

The major antiviral treatments, which attack only influenza A strains, are the drugs amantadine and rimantidine. Side effects associated with these medications include nervousness, lightheadedness, difficulty concentrating and nausea. When given early just after the onset of symptoms, they can reduce the severity and duration of symptoms. Antibiotics have no effect against the influenza virus, but may be given to combat any subsequent infection.

Another drug available for treatment of uncomplicated acute illness due to influenza A and B virus in adults and children greater than 7 years of age is zanamivir. It is a neuraminidase inhibitor that attacks the influenza virus directly. It is taken via a nasal spray, and if given within two days of the start of an attack it can reduce the severity and duration of symptoms by 24 hours. The drug is not recommended for people with asthma and chronic lung disease. Side effects include diarrhoea, nausea and dizziness.

Oseltamivir is available as a capsule and recommended for adults and children 13 years and older. It can cause nausea and vomiting.

BRONCHITIS

Bronchitis may be acute or chronic. Repeated attacks of acute bronchitis may develop into the chronic form.

Acute bronchitis usually develops in the winter, coming on suddenly often following a viral infection such as a common cold or influenza. It may also be triggered by air pollution, which causes increased sensitivity of the respiratory tubes. Bacteria invade the bronchi–the tubes that branch off the windpipe (the trachea) in the lungs–and the area becomes inflamed.

Symptoms

Initial symptoms include a mild fever and a dry, hacking cough which, after a few days, starts to produce greenish-yellow sputum, the colour indicating that the mucus is infected. Breathing may be affected by a characteristic wheezing and shortness of breath, and coughing may be painful. There may also be a rise in temperature.

This stage lasts for a few days, then the fever dies down. The coughing may persist for 10 days or so. In chronic bronchitis sputum is coughed up on most days for at least three consecutive months in at least two consecutive years.

Anyone who is at risk from complications of respiratory disease–the young, the elderly and those suffering from diabetes, immune system disorders and heart and lung diseases–should consult their doctor if they develop the symptoms of bronchitis. So, too, should anyone who experiences breathing difficulties, particularly smokers and people living in an area that has a high level of atmospheric pollution.

How to help

Use a humidifier and drink fluids to help relieve the symptoms. Antibiotics may be prescribed to combat bacteria. Call the doctor if you have severe breathlessness after three days, if you cough up blood or have a persistent high temperature.

TAKE ACTION NOW!

To minimize the symptoms of bronchitis:
- Fire up the humidifier
- Rest for as long as possible
- Consider NSAIDs (nonsteroidal anti-inflammatory drugs)
- Ask your doctor about expectorants to ease the cough

ENVIRONMENTAL AND OCCUPATIONAL LUNG DISEASES

The environment and the workplace are responsible for many life-threatening respiratory problems, and more are being recognized each year. Fortunately, preventive measures are also improving. The three main types of problems are: pneumoconiosis, extrinsic allergic alveolitis and occupational asthma.

DISEASE	CAUSES AND SYMPTOMS
Pneumoconiosis	Caused by the inhalation of minute particles of mineral dust, the three main types are: asbestosis (from inhaled asbestos fibres); silicosis (from silicon dioxide, or "quartz", particles); and coalworker's pneumoconiosis ("black lung disease" from coal dust). In silicosis and asbestosis the lung tissue becomes progressively more fibrous with decreased compliance of the lungs over a period of two to 20 years; asbestosis can develop at any time from 10 to 40 years after exposure and commonly people with this develop lung cancer. Breathlessness and oxygen starvation increase until the lungs can no longer operate. The diagnosis and severity of symptoms are evaluated with chest X-ray and pulmonary function tests (PFTs).The conditions are usually fatal and the only treatment is oxygen therapy.
Extrinsic allergic alveolitis	Hypersensitivity to an allergen causes the alveoli at the base of the lungs to become inflamed, with fibrous tissue forming in the area. The allergens are found in inhaled organic dust, and include bacteria, fungal spores and proteins from other organisms. The reaction may be acute, or progress slowly over many years. If acute, there may be fever, tiredness, tightness in the chest, coughing and wheezing; in other cases there may be weight loss, increased coughing and clubbing (rounding) of the tips of the fingers and toes. Treatment involves stabilizing the condition with bronchodilators and anti-inflammatory drugs.

- Breathlessness, especially when walking or lying down, which causes sleeping problems.
- Constant wheezing with production of as much as a cupful of mucus each day.
- Increased weight through lack of exercise.
- A blue colouring of the face and fingers (cyanosis), as a result of the lack of oxygen in the blood.
- Swelling in the ankles, which indicates problems with circulation.

COPD

Cigarette smoking is the main cause of chronic obstructive pulmonary disease (COPD), the most common chronic condition affecting the lungs. COPD (which encompasses previous labels such as chronic bronchitis and emphysema) affects more women than ever before, as a result of the increase in women smoking or living with a smoker. Women who smoke have a significant risk as compared to nonsmokers of dying of COPD. Other less important risk factors include environmental pollution, occupation, diet and genetic inheritance.

COPD is diagnosed from a history of chronic progressive cough–which may occur with or without mucus production– breathlessness and wheezing. In advanced cases when severe obstruction is present in the airways, the blood vessels in the lungs can become constricted. This puts

these tubes. This adds to the permanence and irreversibility of COPD.

Emphysema is the name given to permanent destruction of the alveolar walls and enlargement of the air sacs at the ends of the bronchioles. It can be caused by cigarette smoking. In less than 1 per cent of emphysema cases the condition affects younger people and is caused by the lack of alpha-1-antitrypsin, a protein in the walls of the air sacs that protects the lungs from destructive emphysema. Symptoms of emphysema vary between people but generally include difficulty in breathing with a long expiration phase; severe breathlessness, especially after even light exercise; wheezing; weight loss; a barrel-shaped chest; and tiredness.

Prevention and treatment

Various North American and earlier UK studies confirm that stopping smoking can help lung function. However, the risk of mortality is not back to the same as a non-smoker until 10 years or more after stopping. This emphasizes the need to stop smoking as early as possible.

Inhaled drugs (bronchodilators) can be useful in helping with symptoms of wheezing and reverse the effects of bronchoconstriction. Infections can be treated with antibiotics. Annual influenza and pneumococcal vaccines should be recommended. In severe cases of COPD, oxygen therapy at home is extremely useful. This involves inhaling oxygen from a cylinder by means of a mask, for up to 12 hours a day.

A programme of pulmonary rehabilitation exercises may be suggested by your doctor, in an attempt to maximize lung function and build up exercise tolerance. Some studies have shown that a high intake of antioxidants and eating a lot of fish may reduce the risk in smokers. Corticosteroids are effective in the treatment of acute exacerbations of COPD.

With good management, COPD sufferers can have their condition stabilized. Avoiding cigarettes, having regular exercise and taking the correct medication are essential components of a management plan, as is regular review by a doctor.

10 years or so after tobacco use is stopped, your risk returns to normal.

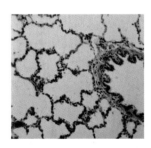
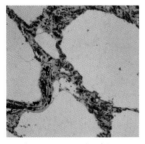

EMPHYSEMA
A section of normal lung (top) shows many alveoli (air sacs). In emphysema (bottom) the walls of the air sacs have broken down.

pressure on the right side of the heart and can lead to heart failure, which can require treatment with diuretics and heart-stabilizing drugs.

Associated conditions

Disorders that are associated with COPD include chronic overproduction of mucus (chronic bronchitis), which in cigarette smokers largely results from mucous gland enlargement in the bronchi (central airways). Progressive obstruction of the airways can also occur, caused by a combination of inflammation and scarring in the smaller airways and loss of elasticity of the lungs because of emphysema. This is measured by tests of airway function known as pulmonary function tests (PFTs) that can specifically assess the forced expiratory volume (FEV). Another condition, bronchiolitis or inflammation of the walls of the bronchioles (terminal smaller airways) can progress to fibrosis–permanent narrowing–of

ASTHMA

Asthma is a respiratory condition in which the small muscles controlling the diameter of the airways have a tendency to go into spasm; this occurs along with inflammation of the lining of the airways. The airways narrow and excessive mucus is produced.

Asthma is particularly common and despite efforts to provide better diagnosis, prevention and treatment, the number of people affected and death from asthma continues to increase. The primary cause of asthma is unknown as yet, though attacks can be precipitated by many environmental and other stimuli such as physical exercise.

Symptoms

Patients with asthma may experience tightness in the chest, coughing, wheezing and shortness of breath which, without treatment, may last for several hours. When asthma is very severe— status asthmaticus, or severe acute

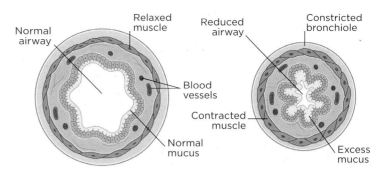

Normal bronchiole

Asthmatic bronchiole

asthma—it is life threatening and hospitalization is usually required.

Because asthma is caused by inflammation of the airways, some sufferers will wheeze most of the time. There is a vicious circle: the lining of the tubes swells and secretes mucus that constricts the airways, reducing the amount of air that can pass through them. At the same time the lining becomes more sensitive to various trigger factors that in turn increases the constriction.

Extrinsic asthma

This type of asthma is triggered by a variety of allergens, most often pollen, dust mite droppings and salivary protein on cat hairs. This type of asthma is also called atopic, meaning that the allergens affect a different part of the body from the point of contact.

Other causes of extrinsic asthma may be irritants such as tobacco smoke, exhaust fumes, household cleaners and burning

WHAT HAPPENS

Breathing difficulties experienced in asthma are a result of a constriction of the respiratory tubes. This constriction is caused by the spasmodic contractions of the muscle in the walls of the bronchioles (airways), or by their inflammation. The tubes may become blocked by the excessive production of mucus.

TAKE ACTION NOW!

If dust triggers your asthma, here's how to minimize the problem:
- Wash your curtains and bed covers frequently in very hot water
- Dust with a damp cloth so that dust is collected rather than spread around.
- Choose wood floors and blinds rather than carpets and curtains.
- Invest in a high-efficiency particulate-arresting (HEPA) or double-filtered vacuum cleaner

USING AN INHALER

It can take practice to use an inhaler correctly and deliver the drug directly to the lungs. A reservoir device, also known as a spacer, can help because you do not have to press and inhale at the same time. The drug is held in the device until you breathe in.

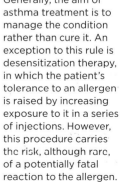

A RISKY FIX

Generally, the aim of asthma treatment is to manage the condition rather than cure it. An exception to this rule is desensitization therapy, in which the patient's tolerance to an allergen is raised by increasing exposure to it in a series of injections. However, this procedure carries the risk, although rare, of a potentially fatal reaction to the allergen.

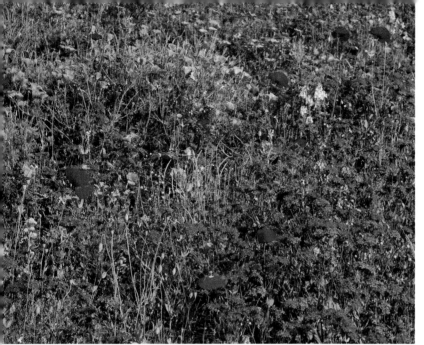

SUMMER ALLERGIES
Many species of plants can trigger asthma attacks, but you can learn to avoid the worst. Wind-pollinated flowers produce more and smaller pollen grains than insect-pollinated flowers. Your reaction to pollen granules will also be worse if they are damp, since the water carries them to the lungs more easily.

fuels; respiratory infections such as acute or chronic bronchitis or a cold; exercise, especially in cold weather; some drugs, typically aspirin and NSAIDs; sulphate preservatives; emotional stress; and chemicals and organic substances found in the workplace (occupational asthma).

Immune cells called eosinophils are activated by the allergen and respond more aggressively the next time it is encountered. They are also more likely to be activated by other allergens as well. This type of asthma usually starts in childhood, and often persists into later life. It is rare for it to develop after the age of 35.

Intrinsic asthma

If no specific allergen is found, the disease is called intrinsic asthma. This type usually develops later in life, possibly after the age of 35, and is more common in women than men. Attacks of intrinsic asthma are triggered by stress, emotional crises or physical exercise. Although the disease is treatable and manageable in most cases, it is still responsible for an alarming number of hospital admissions and around 6,000 deaths each year.

How asthma is diagnosed

The diagnosis of asthma is made based on a typical history of abrupt shortness of breath, with a dry cough and wheezing symptoms. The doctor will arrange pulmonary function tests (PFTs) that measure the amount of air that the lungs can expel. If allergy is suspected to be the cause, allergy tests may also be carried out.

A peak flow meter is an essential tool for home monitoring of asthma and should be used by all patients with asthma. The patient blows into the peak flow meter, which records the maximum rate at which air can be expelled–this is the peak expiratory flow rate (PEFR).

A PFT called spirometry is usually carried out every 1-2 years and measures how much air can be expelled in one second–the forced expiratory volume in one second (FEV1)–and also the time it takes to empty the lungs of air after a breath–this is the forced vital capacity (FVC). These tests are performed before and after a bronchodilator inhalation is given to widen the bronchioles. Asthma is diagnosed if the bronchodilator causes improvement in the results. Skin-patch tests may then be carried out to see if an allergen is responsible.

If skin tests do not reveal any allergies, you will have to identify your trigger factors yourself. The best way to do this is to keep a diary in which you describe asthma symptoms, grading them on a scale of one to ten, and correlate them with outside factors. For example, note if wheezing symptoms increase when walking alongside a busy road, or when using a particular domestic cleaning product. However, bear in mind that individuals often have more than one trigger factor, and that a hypersensitivity to new trigger factors can develop.

What to expect

Once diagnosed, asthma should be monitored by a doctor. One of the most important ways of managing it, however, is to avoid triggers by taking steps to keep yourself away from the substances that trigger an attack. For example, stay indoors on days when the level of a pollen to which you are allergic is high, or wear a mask outside; avoid cats and dogs if you are allergic to proteins on animal hair.

Asthma treatment itself is based on the degree of severity of the symptoms.

Asthma is mild intermittent if the symptoms occur less than two times per week and inhaled low-dose corticosteroids are helpful in decreasing bronchial hyper-responsiveness. Asthma is mild persistent or moderate when symptoms occur more than two times per week along with night-time symptoms. These patients benefit from daily low-dose inhaled corticosteroids. Severe asthma will result in continuous symptoms and requires large doses of inhaled corticosteroids or oral prednisone daily to control symptoms.

Asthma patients will be encouraged to use a peak flow meter at home, as a way of monitoring their health, and should take appropriate action when their condition worsens.

When asthma affects you more frequently, it may be necessary to inhale corticosteroid drugs on a daily basis, to reduce inflammation; oral corticosteroids may be used as well but they tend to produce more side effects than when inhaled.

Metered-dose bronchodilators are also inhaled, either to prevent an attack–before exercise, for example, in exercise-induced asthma–or to provide relief during an attack. A spacer device with the inhaler is useful with metered-dose inhaled corticosteroids.

A new group of drugs known as leukotriene modifiers has proved effective in relieving the symptoms of an attack. In practice, a combination of drugs is likely to be given, tailored to individual needs.

THE TB THREAT

Tuberculosis (TB) is caused by the bacterium *Mycobacterium tuberculosis*, which is spread in the droplets sneezed or coughed out by those in whom the disease is active. More rarely, it can be present in milk (bovine tuberculosis). In most people the bacteria will multiply to form a pocket of infection, but this will be healed by the immune system and surrounded by scar tissue. It is estimated that about 50 per cent of the population in developing countries and around 5 to 10 per cent in the industrialized world harbour the bacteria.

When the immune system starts to falter, as a result of age, infection, immune system disorders such as AIDS, malnutrition, some drug therapies, infections and other disease, the bacteria may begin to spread through the bloodstream, causing fatigue, weight loss, loss of appetite, fever and night sweats. Then tubercles—nodes of affected tissue—form in the lungs and in other organs, and blood-flecked sputum is coughed up. Without treatment, tuberculosis is fatal in about 50 per cent of those affected.

There are several reasons why TB has become a problem once more in the industrialized world:

- International air travel has increased the risk of exposure.

- Both AIDS and the increase in drug use have increased susceptibility to the bacteria (AIDS sufferers, for example, have a 10 per cent chance each year of contracting active TB, while others have only a 10 per cent lifetime risk).

- A new strain of the bacterium has emerged, called multiple drug-resistant TB (MDR-TB) as drugs so far have little effect on it.

The risk of TB is highest among volunteer workers and young travellers in developing countries, who spend long periods in overcrowded, badly ventilated conditions and have not been vaccinated. If you suspect you may have been exposed to TB, you should consult your doctor. Tests include chest X-ray, sputum samples for acid-fast bacillus smear and culture and tissue biopsy if disease is suspected to have spread elsewhere. The PPD (purified protein derivative) skin test is carried out to check for any previous exposure to the tuberculosis bacterium. You may be a candidate for treatment with a drug such as isoniazid to prevent the bacteria from becoming active.

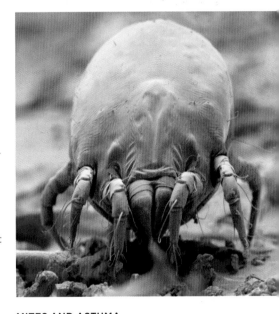

MITES AND ASTHMA
Allergy to faeces of invisible dust mites can trigger asthma attacks.

LUNG CANCER

Approximately 80 per cent of lung cancers in women are the result of cigarette smoking. Lung cancer is the leading cause of cancer-related death in women followed by breast and colorectal cancers–a situation that is regarded as serious by the medical profession. As the number of women who smoke continues to increase so does the number with lung cancer. There has been a noticeable rise, too, in nonsmoker's cancer among women, which may be related to environmental factors.

There is some evidence that women may be more vulnerable to lung cancer: in other words, a woman who smokes could be more likely to do damage to lung cells than a man with the same

As the number of women who smoke continues to increase, so does the number with lung cancer.

smoking habits and history. The length of time and amount a person smokes increases the risk of developing breast cancer. Secondhand smoking (passive smoking) also increases risk.

The symptoms of lung cancer are primarily a cough, especially with the

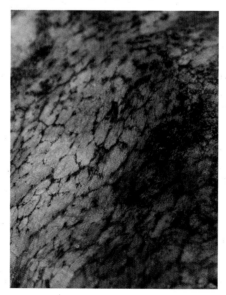

SMOKER'S LUNG
This close-up of a section of a smoker's lung clearly shows the damage that smoking has done. The black deposits between the healthy pink and red tissue is caused by tar deposits from cigarette smoke. Over time the buildup of toxic substances will stimulate the production of cancerous cells in the bronchi or bronchioles leading to lung cancer.

WHAT TO WATCH FOR

You should consult a doctor if you have one or more of the following symptoms:

- A persistent sore in the mouth.
- A constant sore throat.
- A lump, white spot or scaly area on the lip or in the mouth.
- A swollen lymph node in the neck, armpit or groin that remains for longer than three weeks.
- Moles, freckles or warts that change colour or shape, or bleed.
- Unusual bleeding or discharge between periods, especially during or after the menopause.
- Thickening or lumps in the breast.
- Difficulty in swallowing or a lump on or near the thyroid gland.
- Rectal bleeding or changes in bowel habits (which are unconnected to diet or lifestyle changes).
- Urinary difficulties such as pain when passing urine, frequency, weak flow or blood in the urine.
- A change in voice (new hoarseness).

production of sputum, which may be blood-stained. Other symptoms include difficulty in breathing; pain in the chest or centre of the back; difficulty in swallowing; a hoarse voice; and unintentional weight loss.

There is good news for a woman who stops smoking, even if she has been a heavy smoker for years. After 15 years she will reduce her risk of developing lung cancer to nearly the same level as that of a lifelong nonsmoker. However, a nonsmoker who has a partner who smokes runs twice the risk of getting lung cancer.

Living with cancer

Although at present only a minority of people with lung cancer can be completely cured, various research and clinical trials are under way to find different ways of applying the various current treatment methods.

Surgery is usually only possible if an early diagnosis is made and the tumour is fairly small. Some treatments are aimed at easing pain and discomfort rather than curing the disease. For example, laser surgery may be used to shrink a tumour that cannot be removed completely but which is blocking an airway. In some people a small metal tube, called a stent, may be inserted to keep the airway open. There are various ways of minimizing the side effects of radiotherapy and chemotherapy (*see* box below), which may include nausea and vomiting and constipation.

Palliative care for lung cancer, which is designed to improve the quality of life rather than cure the disease, can also be very effective in controlling pain and other symptoms.

Emotional difficulties linked to lung cancer and other types of cancer are not easy to talk about and are often hardest to share with those close to you. You may find the help you need is available from a trained counsellor specializing in cancer. Your doctor should be able to put you in touch with a counsellor or a self-help cancer group, which can also provide support and advice.

Types of lung cancer and treatments

Adenocarcinoma, which affects mucus-producing cells in the airway linings, is the most common type of lung cancer in women. This type of cancer is most frequently found in nonsmokers. Squamous cell carcinoma is the most common in men and accounts for about half of all cases of lung cancer. It develops in the cells that line the bronchi (airways), leading from the trachea (windpipe) to the lungs. Large cell carcinoma is the least common. The three types are often referred to collectively as nonsmall cell cancers, to distinguish them from small cell lung cancer, which accounts for around a quarter of all lung cancer. Small cell lung cancer occurs almost always in smokers and spreads rapidly through the lungs and to other parts of the body. This type of cancer is usually inoperable by the time it has been diagnosed and is therefore treated in a different way.

Steps to diagnosis A chest X-ray will usually show whether cancer is present, but other tests will confirm the diagnosis and give the more detailed information that is required before any decision can be made about treatment. A sample of sputum will be analysed in the cytology lab. A test called a bronchoscopy may be performed under local anaesthetic to allow the doctor to look inside the lung and do a biopsy (take a tissue sample). Alternatively, the doctor may perform a mediastinoscopy, which involves inserting a small telescope via an incision in the neck to look at the chest and lymph nodes and take samples. Lung biopsies may be done with the aid of X-rays or a CT scan.

Surgery The treatment plan will be based on the type of cancer and whether it has spread beyond the lung. An operation to remove the tumour may be the best option for nonsmall cell cancer. This may involve removing all or part of an affected lung. In some treatment trials, radiotherapy and/or chemotherapy may be used together with surgery in various combined treatments. Surgery is rarely the right treatment for small cell cancer, since it is unlikely that the cancer will be confined to the lung and so it would be impossible to remove all the cancer with an operation.

Radiation This can be very useful for relieving pain and in situations where a tumour is causing other problems, such as blocking an important blood vessel or causing a lung to collapse. It is also being used in new ways in clinical trials, such as giving it in several daily doses for people with nonsmall cell cancer or combined with chemotherapy for some people with small cell cancer.

Chemotherapy Anticancer drugs that destroy the tumour cells or inhibit them from multiplying are the best option for treating small cell lung cancer. In many patients combination chemotherapy is recommended over therapy with a single agent.

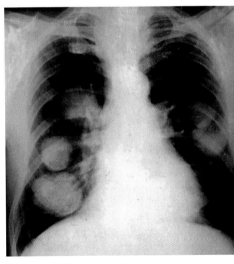

X-ray revealing area of lung cancer (blue) in lungs (black).

Problems of the Senses

The senses are vital to your quality of life. Illnesses or infections that affect the ears, nose, throat and eyes will affect how you perceive and function in the world if they are not treated quickly. Most people will suffer some sensory loss with age, but this can be minimized with care.

EARS

Most people have no problems with their ears until they notice that their hearing becomes less sharp late in life. However, certain illnesses and infections can arise that may affect either your hearing or your balance.

Otosclerosis

A fairly common condition, more often occurring in women than men, otosclerosis affects the three tiny bones in the middle ear, called the auditory ossicles, which connect the ear drum to the hearing part of the inner ear, the cochlea. The innermost of the three bones, the stapes or stirrup, becomes progressively thicker, so that it cannot vibrate as much and therefore transmits less sound. The net result is that you become increasingly deaf.

Other symptoms include tinnitus–ringing in the ears (*see* opposite). The thickening occurs more quickly during pregnancy and may be oestrogen-related. In most people, both ears will eventually be affected. The only available treatment is surgery, in which the stapes bone is replaced by a synthetic graft, but there is a risk of deafness and a hearing aid may still be required. Women who have this condition are usually advised not to use hormone replacement therapy (HRT).

Mastoiditis

The mastoid process is a part of the temporal bone, which is just below and behind the ear. It is honeycombed with air cells that connect with the middle ear. If an infection here spreads inside the bone then it causes the inflammation called mastoiditis. The symptoms are earache, fever, ringing in the ears and hearing difficulties. Antibiotics should clear up pus or bacteria. In some rare cases a mastoidectomy operation will be necessary, which involves draining the pus and removing the infected bone.

Labyrinthitis

The inner ear (labyrinth) includes three fluid-filled, semicircular canals that contain the sensors for balance. Labyrinthitis is an infection of the canals

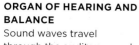

ORGAN OF HEARING AND BALANCE
Sound waves travel through the auditory canal to the ear drum, causing it to vibrate. The vibrations are amplified by the tiny ossicles in the middle ear, causing vibrations in the fluid of the inner ear.

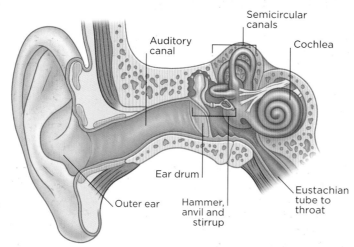

Semicircular canals

Auditory canal

Cochlea

Ear drum

Outer ear

Hammer, anvil and stirrup

Eustachian tube to throat

that may be either viral or bacterial. A virus causing a throat infection may travel up the eustachian tube to the middle and inner ears, causing symptoms such as a loss of balance, vertigo or dizziness, nausea, vomiting and hearing loss. The infection generally clears up by itself in a few weeks. You should have bed rest and take drugs to treat the nausea. Bacterial labyrinthitis is characterized by exactly the same symptoms as the viral type but should be treated with antibiotics immediately as it can lead to deafness and, if it should spread to the brain, to the development of meningitis (p. 258).

Tinnitus

An extremely distressing condition that may be either temporary or permanent, tinnitus occurs when the auditory nerve is subjected to interference so that sounds ranging from a deep roar or buzz to a high-pitched whine are heard intermittently or continuously in one or both ears. The usual cause is damage to the cells in the inner ear, through an infection, a head injury, an underlying health problem such as high blood pressure or even the use of certain drugs (such as aspirin and some antibiotics).

Temporary tinnitus from an infection generally clears up quickly. Tinnitus that will not go away may interfere with all aspects of life, and coping strategies may be learned to "turn off" the unwanted sound, particularly if it affects your sleeping. Yoga and self-hypnosis techniques may ease the irritation of tinnitus, and special masking devices and advice from hearing therapists can be a great help.

Deafness

There are two types of deafness. Conductive deafness is caused by a disruption of the mechanism by which sound waves are transmitted through the outer and middle ear. In sensorineural deafness there is a failure in the transmission of nerve impulses from the inner ear to the brain. This includes hearing loss with age, Ménière's disease (*see* right) and exposure to loud noise (*see* right). A buildup of ear wax in the outer ear is the most common cause of

conductive deafness; the wax should be syringed out at your doctor's surgery.

The other main cause is an infection of the middle ear, called otitis media, which in adult sufferers normally clears up with treatment with antibiotics. Children, however, can develop a chronic buildup of fluid in the middle ear, causing temporary hearing loss. A doctor may decide to drain the ear.

A gradual loss of hearing occurs with age as the inner ear slowly becomes less efficient at translating sound waves into nerve impulses. The rate at which this happens can be increased by circulatory disorders that reduce the blood supply to the ear, such as high blood pressure, heart disease and atherosclerosis. Heredity and exposure to loud noise are other contributory factors. The condition is irreversible, but a hearing aid can be worn to amplify the sound waves entering the ear.

Ménière's disease

Accumulated fluid in the semicircular canals, and sometimes the cochlea, damages the inner ear cells, causing Ménière's disease. It is more apparent in middle age and is slightly less usual in women than men. Symptoms are deafness in one ear, vertigo or dizziness, nausea and high-pitched tinnitus. Drugs may control the symptoms and the condition may be slowed by restricting fluid intake and taking diuretics.

DO YOU GET CAR SICK?

This problem is caused by disorientation of the organ of balance in the inner ear. The following tips can help:

- Drive the car yourself or sit in the front passenger seat. Sit upright with both feet flat on the floor. Make sure the seat belt isn't too tight.
- Don't try to read maps; instead focus on a point on the horizon. A neck cushion will keep your head upright.
- Avoid rich food, alcohol and sweet drinks when travelling.
- Make frequent stops on the journey if possible.
- Keep a window open.
- Breathe in deeply through your nose and out through your mouth.
- Try wearing acupressure wristbands.
- Remember that over-the-counter antinausea pills may make you drowsy.

Blasting your hearing away

Excessive noise permanently damages the nervous tissue and pathways in the inner ear, leading to deafness. The signs of damage are ringing in the ears that fades in a few hours, a reduced ability to hear higher frequencies and ear pain. If you use headphones at high volume, have powerful in-car or home CD systems or spend time in noisy clubs you will be exposed to noise levels well in excess of 85 decibels. You risk injury at a decibel

level over 80. A typical rock concert is about 100, a pneumatic drill at 1 m (3 ft) records 120—which can be felt as actual pain. Operators of all high-noise equipment should be made to wear ear protection.

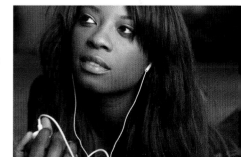

THE NOSE AND THE MOUTH

Although the nose and mouth areas are usually subject only to minor problems, these can make life very uncomfortable and have an effect on your general health and wellbeing.

Crooked noses and perforations

Occasionally, people are born with the nasal septum–the plate of bone and

Women who snore regularly are 33 percent more likely than nonsnorers to develop heart disease.

CLOSE COOPERATION
Lips and cheeks, teeth and gums, the tongue, palate and salivary glands all work together as the first stage of the digestive system. Local infection and structural disorders affect the senses of smell and taste, which in turn may detract from the enjoyment of eating.

cartilage that separates the two nostrils–off centre. This may also arise from damage to the nose later in life. The condition may affect breathing, but it can be corrected surgically.

Long-standing cocaine use or, in rare cases, using steroid nasal sprays over a long period, can cause perforation–a hole in the septum–which can be corrected by surgery.

Stuffy nose

The accumulation of excessive mucus can make breathing difficult and affect your sense of taste and smell. Congestion can occur during pregnancy but for most other people a cold is the usual cause. Persistent congestion, called catarrh, may be allergic rhinitis, triggered by pollen, dust and pollutants. Smokers are more susceptible to nasal congestion, since the smoke destroys the tiny hairs that line and protect the nasal passages. You can ease congestion by inhaling steam over a bowl of hot water with a towel over your head. This loosens the mucus that you can then blow out through the nose. Avoid dairy products, which increase formation of mucus. Decongestant drops or sprays can give relief but should not be used for more than a week, since the mucous lining of the nose may be damaged.

Congestion can spread to your sinuses, causing pain that may be severe. Sinusitis can sometimes be triggered by an abscess in a tooth. It can in turn lead to laryngitis or ear infection and may become a chronic problem. The usual treatment of sinusitis is decongestants and antibiotics but in some cases surgery may be performed in order to improve the drainage of the sinuses.

Nosebleeds

Bleeding from the nose is generally caused by damage to the blood vessels in the delicate lining of the nasal passages. The damage may be caused by trauma–a blow to the nose, for example–or by repeated nose picking, sneezing or excessive nose blowing.

Sometimes a nosebleed can be a sign of hormonal changes in the body–in pregnancy and adolescence–or it may be a reaction to prescribed drugs such as warfarin, which reduces blood clotting to help prevent strokes, allergies and polyps. Atherosclerosis (a disease of the arterial wall) can sometimes cause spontaneous nosebleeds, especially in the elderly. Blood vessels can become enlarged during illnesses that cause a fever, making a nosebleed more likely. Nosebleeds can happen, too, in people with high blood pressure, although this is less common.

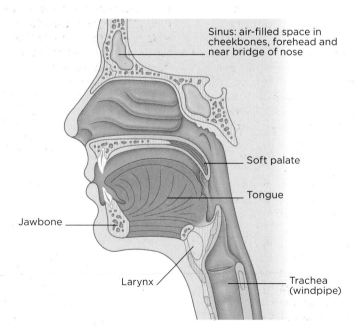

Sinus: air-filled space in cheekbones, forehead and near bridge of nose

Soft palate

Tongue

Jawbone

Larynx

Trachea (windpipe)

To deal with a nosebleed, pinch the nose just beneath the point where the bone turns into pliable cartilage. Hold for at least 10 minutes with your head held tilted forwards and breath through your mouth. Don't rub or blow your nose for several hours or you will dislodge the clot that has formed.

You should consult your doctor if nosebleeds are persistent so that any underlying disorder can be ruled out. The doctor may seal the damaged blood vessel by means of an electrical current (a procedure known as cauterization).

Snoring

Vibration of the soft palate at the back of the mouth is not uncommon but, if someone who doesn't usually snore suddenly starts, it may signify a breathing problem. A congested nose, advancing age, excess weight, smoking, alcohol abuse, use of sleeping pills and general ill health all have a tendency to lead to snoring.

Obstructive sleep apnea (OSA) is an important but under-recognized and under-diagnosed disorder. It increases the risk of neurocognitive problems and other organ dysfunction over years.

The prevalence of OSA increases with age and men have a higher prevalence of this disorder compared to women. Risk factors for OSA include obesity and abnormalites of the soft tissue of the upper airway. OSA itself may cause cardiac arrhythmia and complicate elevated blood pressure, resulting in a feeling of tiredness and reduced attention span during the day. A study of women who snore regularly concluded that they are 33 per cent more likely than nonsnorers to develop heart disease and 46 per cent more likely to develop high blood pressure.

Light snoring can often be prevented by sleeping on the side rather than on the back, or by sleeping without a pillow, which helps to straighten out the airway. Heavy snorers tend to snore in whatever position they sleep.

Nasal polyps

Polyps are soft, jelly-like, benign growths that are attached to a mucous membrane often by a thin, elongated stalk. In the nose, polyps are normally caused by chronic inflammation from an allergy, such as hay fever, although by no means all hay fever sufferers develop polyps. Polyps may be associated with chronic sinusitis and asthma—symptoms include a blocked, full feeling in the nose, a reduced sense of smell, headaches, pain and nasal discharge. Treatment is by steroids, taken by nasal spray.

Dry mouth

Probable causes are thirst, breathing through the mouth and fear or anxiety. Anaesthetics and some prescription drugs–antidepressants for example–may reduce saliva. This in turn can lead to dental problems. Persistent thirst (plus other symptoms) may indicate diabetes.

Mouth ulcers

Small, white, painful lesions with a red margin form in the mouth due to stress, bacteria, infections or occasionally a deficiency of folic acid and vitamin B_{12}. Ulcers can affect women premenstrually and can be treated by a number of over-the-counter preparations.

TEMPOROMANDIBULAR JOINT SYNDROME (TMJ)

The jaw and skull meet at a joint in front of the ear where a disc of cartilage, plus muscles and ligaments, allow the jaw to move. The disc can slip out of place, which produces pain, a clicking sound, headache and earache. TMJ has many causes—whiplash, stress leading to teeth grinding, especially at night, a bad bite (bottom teeth don't meet the top correctly), rheumatoid arthritis—so treatment varies. Relief can be provided with a warm, damp compress to the area. NSAIDS can alleviate pain. For stress, counselling or relaxation may help. Ask your doctor and dentist about preventive appliances.

Caring for your teeth and gums

The aim of tooth care is to remove plaque—the primary cause of tooth decay and gum inflammation. Plaque comes from food. If you have false teeth pay scrupulous attention to cleansing, since plaque buildup can affect your sense of taste and smell.

Brushing your teeth at least twice a day, or after every meal, helps prevent plaque buildup. Use short, up-and-down movements. Don't forget your tongue. Soft-bristled brushes are kind on tooth enamel but need to be changed every three to four months.

A fluoride toothpaste and mouthwash will keep plaque at bay and freshen your breath. Using dental floss will also be beneficial. Floss between your teeth and down to the gum, then form a "C" around the side of the tooth and floss gently up to its top. Repeat on the other side and front and back. Do not over-floss as this can abrade the teeth or cut the gum, allowing bacteria to enter.

You must visit your dentist regularly for checkups.

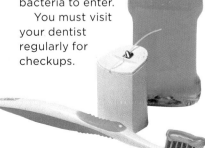

VISION PROBLEMS

Many people are born with eyesight that is less than perfect and most people's eyesight will degenerate with age. Both long- and short-sightedness are errors of refraction–the process by which the surface of the cornea in the eye and the lens bend light rays so that they focus at a point on the retina. If the degree of refraction does not match the length of the eye, the image will not be sharp.

Long- and short-sightedness

In long-sightedness, or hyperopia, the light rays are naturally focused behind the retina because the length of the eye is too short. When you are young, if the hyperopia is not too extreme, the ciliary muscles round the lens can easily change the shape of the lens to adjust this–a process known as accommodation–but as the eye becomes less elastic this ability to accommodate deteriorates. Distance vision may remain good but close vision becomes increasingly difficult. If it is not corrected hyperopia can cause headaches and general blurred vision when the eyes are strained, which is why all those who use computers at work are recommended to have regular eye tests.

In short-sightedness (called myopia) the light rays are focused in front of the retina because the length of the eye is too long. As a result close-up vision is good, but distance vision is deficient. Myopia tends to run in families. It usually becomes evident during adolescence and stabilizes by adulthood.

Both myopia and hyperopia are corrected by glasses or contact lenses that have opposite qualities from those of the lenses in the eyes that are causing the problem: people with myopia have glasses with concave lenses, and those with hyperopia have glasses with convex lenses. Myopia can also be improved with laser treatment, which reshapes the cornea, although it cannot restore elasticity to the eye.

Cataracts

The lens of the eye is made of protein fibres and is normally translucent. With age, or in some other circumstances, the protein fibres undergo changes in structure that make the lens more or less opaque. Around half of people over the age of 60 have some degree of cataract but the effect on their vision may be minor, since the process of opacification may be confined to the edge of the lens. The changes can also be caused by too much ultraviolet radiation, for example from sunlight, cigarette smoking, eye injuries, long-term use of steroids and diabetes. Heredity may also sometimes be a contributory factor. More rarely, children may be born with cataracts.

Cataracts develop very slowly and the effects on the eyesight differ in different people; there may be blurring of the vision, short-sightedness and some distortion in colour perception.

Cataracts are diagnosed by an eye test, in which eyedrops are used to enlarge the pupils and the lenses examined with an ophthalmoscope. They are then treated by surgery. This surgery is very safe; complications, such as infection or retinal damage, occur in only about one in 2,000 cases. A local anaesthetic is given and a small incision is made in the eye. The lens and focal length are measured with ultrasound, then either the whole lens is replaced by

ARE YOU AT RISK?

Check with your doctor if any of these symptoms occur:

- Blurred vision
- Constant headaches
- Haloes of colour around lights at night
- Eyelids that suddenly droop
- Blind spots in your field of vision

SPOTS BEFORE YOUR EYES?

Dark specks, lines or cobwebs sometimes appear to be moving about in the front of the eyes. They are seen more often when you look at a light, plain background, such as the sky.

Floaters are not usually serious and often appear after you have rubbed your eyes. However, the sudden appearance of floaters should always be investigated by an optometrist, especially if you also see flashes of light. This is because the floaters may be a symptom of detachment of the retina—the retina becomes separated from the tissue surrounding it after a tear and vitreous fluid leaks out. The floaters are specks of blood that have escaped into the vitreous fluid.

The problem is not uncommon in the elderly, since the vitreous fluid tends to degenerate with age. It is also a risk for people who are very short-sighted or have had an eye injury.

GLAUCOMA

The damage caused by glaucoma is the result of increasing pressure within the eye. This is created by a buildup of aqueous humour, which is unable to flow away as normal because there is a blockage in the drainage channel. The excessive amount of fluid compresses blood vessels that supply the optic nerve, causing the nerve fibres to degenerate. If the use of medicines fails to lower pressure, surgery may be necessary to unblock the drainage channel or to create an artificial channel for the aqueous humour to flow through.

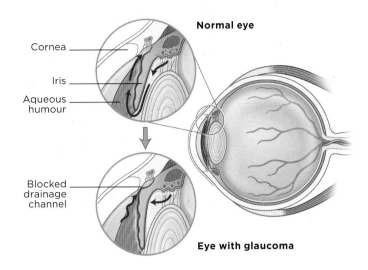

Normal eye

Cornea

Iris

Aqueous humour

Blocked drainage channel

Eye with glaucoma

a plastic one or the implant is fitted inside the lens after the old protein fibres have been removed. Anti-inflammatories and steroids are given as eyedrops, and full recovery is usually within six weeks.

Glaucoma

The main part of the eye behind the lens is filled with a fluid called vitreous humour. The space between the iris and the cornea is filled with aqueous humour. This fluid is constantly renewed and drains away through spongy tissue (the trabecular meshwork) between the iris and the cornea. If this drainage system gets blocked, intraocular pressure builds up and the blood vessels that supply the optic nerve become compressed. The nerve can then degenerate and vision is gradually impaired.

There are various reasons why the drainage system can break down– trauma to the eye, long-term steroid use, diabetes and, rarely, a defect present at birth. However, in most cases the condition falls into one of two main groups: primary open angle glaucoma (POAG) or primary angle closure glaucoma (PACG). POAG is the most common form of glaucoma. It is a slow, progressive condition occurring mainly in the over-50s and rarely seen in the under-40s. It is often not detected until "blind spots" start to appear in vision, usually in peripheral vision.

In PACG, an increase in intraocular pressure slowly closes the angle between the cornea and the iris, forcing the iris against the drainage system. When the system is finally blocked, the intraocular pressure rises suddenly, over a few hours, causing the severe symptoms of an acute attack of glaucoma.

Symptoms may be minor (blurred vision and haloes seen around lights) or severe (intense pain, nausea and vomiting). An acute attack of glaucoma is a medical emergency, since there is a risk of permanent damage to the eyesight. PACG tends to run in families and affects long-sighted people and those of Asian descent more than others; it rarely affects people under the age of 50.

A VISUAL MIGRAINE

A good proportion of migraine sufferers—but not all—experience visual symptoms. Usually these are part of the "aura"—visual and sensory disturbances experienced by about a fifth of migraine sufferers that precede the onset of the characteristic headache. There are flashes of light, bright zig-zag lines in either central or peripheral vision, blind spots and blurred vision. These symptoms normally last for up to an hour until the headache starts.

In some people, however, the symptoms die down and the headache does not follow. This condition is known as ophthalmic migraine, and it is caused by a spasm in the blood vessels supplying the eye. You should consult your doctor if you suffer from visual disturbances—whether or not a migraine headache follows them—to rule out the possibility that another condition may be responsible and to obtain medication to control the problem.

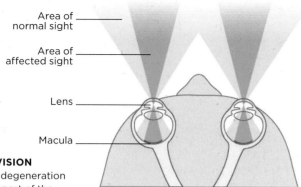

Area of normal sight

Area of affected sight

Lens

Macula

LOSS OF VISION
In macular degeneration the central part of the retina at the back of the eye becomes overlaid with scar tissue. This creates a circular area of blindness in the centre of the visual field. It does not lead to complete blindness since vision is still retained around the edges of the visual field.

COLOUR BLINDNESS

Defects in colour vision are usually inherited. Trauma or conditions such as macular disease may, rarely, be to blame (acquired defective colour vision). Seek medical advice if colour vision deteriorates. Colour blindness affects about 12 per cent of men but only 1 in 200 women. This is because the gene responsible is on the X chromosome. A woman carrying the gene will pass the fault to her offspring. The most common type of colour blindness is an inability to distinguish red and green. The type of colour blindness depends on which colour receptors (cones) in the retina are affected: one group detects red, one green and a third blue. Most sufferers learn to adapt to colour blindness, but driving and navigation can pose problems.

Because glaucoma of both types can progress undetected until a late stage, optometrists routinely check intraocular pressure during eye tests, and it is recommended that all those over age 50 have regular eye tests for this purpose. If glaucoma is suspected, the diagnosis is confirmed by an ophthalmologist.

The treatment of glaucoma depends on the stage that the condition has reached. In its early stages, eyedrops are used to control intraocular pressure: these may be beta-blockers, epinephrine or prostaglandins. Laser surgery is now often used to reduce intraocular pressure by increasing the size of the drainage system, but the effect of this is sometimes only temporary. An artificial drainage duct can be inserted in an operation called a trabeculectomy, but it is usually necessary to continue the use of eyedrops.

Macular degeneration
The macula is the central part of the retina at the back of the eye. Its light receptors distinguish detail at the centre of the visual field–for example, when reading or driving. It is common for the tissues of the macula to degenerate with age and allow fluid leakage–known as age-related macular degeneration (ARMD). However, in some people, ARMD progresses more quickly, leading to a loss of central vision. You will notice a central blind spot, so that reading becomes more difficult and you have difficulty recognizing people's faces.

The risk of ARMD is highest in those over 60, although some younger people who are very short-sighted may be affected. Other risk factors include

gender–women are affected more often than men–a family history of ARMD, smoking and race–white people are affected more often than those of African descent.

ARMD can be detected by an optometrist, so it is important that all those at risk have regular eye tests. The diagnosis will be confirmed by an ophthalmologist. In some cases it may be possible for ARMD to be treated by laser surgery, in which the fluid leakage is sealed off. Other cases may not be treatable but since peripheral vision is unaffected by the condition the eyesight is not lost completely.

Diabetic retinopathy
The high levels of glucose in the blood of people with diabetes can cause a complication called diabetic retinopathy. In the early stages, or background retinopathy, the glucose causes small blood vessels in the retina to become blocked or to leak. The result may be some loss of vision but often there are no symptoms for a long time. However, as the condition worsens, new blood vessels start to grow in the retina–this stage is known as proliferative retinopathy. The new vessels are fragile and tend to leak fluid, and scars may also form on the retina, causing it to detach. Without treatment, these problems can cause blindness. (In people who have type 2 diabetes only the macula may be affected; this causes a loss of central vision that affects reading.)

Once detected, diabetic retinopathy can be controlled by keeping glucose levels under good control. If the condition has progressed to proliferative retinopathy, it may be treated by laser surgery to seal the retinal blood vessels and prevent new ones from growing. However, it is vital that all diabetics monitor glucose levels carefully and have their eyes tested regularly by an ophthalmologist to prevent the condition from developing.

Dry eyes
A condition called dry eye syndrome is now recognized, in which the quantity and quality of the tear fluid that naturally bathes the eye declines.

As a result the eye becomes irritated and feels gritty, it becomes difficult to cry and to wear contact lenses, and over time the sufferer may become very sensitive to light. Eventually the cornea may become scarred, affecting vision. The symptoms are made worse by smoking, dust and exposure to substances to which an individual is allergic.

Dry eye syndrome is extremely common, and it is estimated that about two-thirds of people over the age of 65 are affected to some degree. The condition is most common in women who are either pregnant or who have passed the menopause. In most cases the cause is a reduction in the efficiency of the glands that produce tears—a result of ageing. Other causes include a reaction to drugs, such as antihistamines, that reduce secretions, and also infections of the glands of the eyelids.

However, in a large number of cases—90 per cent of them women—the cause is an autoimmune disorder called Sjögren's syndrome, when the antibodies attack the body's own glands. Some people with the condition only have symptoms of dry eyes and mouth, while others also have symptoms of connective tissue disorders, such as rheumatoid arthritis and lupus (SLE). Although most Sjögren's sufferers are postmenopausal some are younger, and their children have an increased risk of suffering from heart defects. For this reason, symptoms of dry eye syndrome should be reported to a doctor without delay.

The treatment of dry eyes depends on its cause. Antibiotics are given in the case of infection, and artificial tears are used to relieve the irritation. In some cases small plugs can be inserted into the tear ducts in order to retain tears in the eyes to keep them moist. Sjögren's syndrome is treated with a combination of steroids and NSAIDs (nonsteroidal anti-inflammatory drugs) .

Allergic conjunctivitis

The symptoms of conjunctivitis are a reddening and swelling of the membranes of the eyes and eyelids, which often comes on suddenly, together with itching, a burning sensation and a discharge, which may be watery or

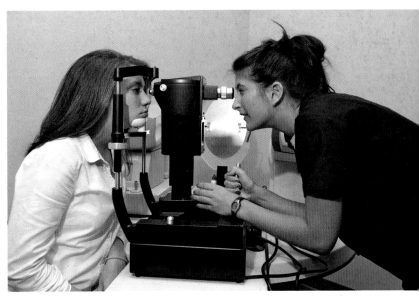

sticky. However, similar symptoms—in particular the itchiness and discharge—can also be caused by bacterial and viral infections (p. 255), so you should consult your doctor to rule these out before starting to use any over-the-counter anti-allergy preparations.

The allergens responsible for causing conjunctivitis are generally the same as those that cause hay fever—pollen, mould spores, and animal or insect proteins, for example from animal hair and the droppings of the dust mite—but may also include certain chemicals found in cosmetics, shampoos, perfumes, contact lenses and contact lens solutions. Eyedrops containing antihistamine will be prescribed or, in severe cases, corticosteroids.

Droopy eyelids

It is not uncommon for the eyelids to start to droop–called ptosis–in old age, as a result of the weakening of the muscles that hold them in place. However, ptosis may also be sign of a number of serious conditions. It may be the result of a muscle weakness caused by a condition affecting the muscles, such as the autoimmune disorder myasthenia gravis, or by a condition that affects the nerves. A brain tumour or cerebral aneurysm (damage to an artery in the brain) may cause drooping eyelids and you should consult your doctor if the condition develops suddenly.

EYE TESTS
You should make sure you have regular eye tests, particularly if there is a history of eye problems in your family. Some conditions, such as glaucoma, may show no symptoms in early stages, and can be detected only by an eye examination.

Skin Problems

Genetics, hormones, drugs, allergies and a wide variety of environmental factors can contribute to the range of afflictions that influence the look, feel and condition of your skin. These can all cause problems for women at any age.

UNCOVER YOUR SKIN

Resist the temptation to try to hide pimples with heavy layers of make-up. This may irritate already sensitive skin. Skin can also become even more sensitive as a result of cover-up medication. It should not be used for more than three months in total, and if there is no improvement in that time, you should discuss the problem with your doctor or dermatologist.

ACNE

The skin condition known medically as acne vulgaris is a very common skin disorder with nearly 85 per cent of all people experiencing acne at some point in their lives. The lesions known as comedomes–blackheads, whiteheads, pimples and deeper lumps (cysts and nodules)–can be very distressing. Acne usually begins in puberty with more boys than girls affected at this age but can persist or develop in the 20s, 30s, 40s and even 50s. For some people, the change in their appearance from the acne lesions can make them self-conscious with psychological consequences. The scarring (skin depressions) that occurs as a result of acne is prominent in those who have a variant of acne called inflammatory acne and can result in permanent skin changes into adulthood.

Acne is most common at times of hormonal upheaval, and the body's sex hormones play a role in triggering the symptoms (except in pregnancy when acne tends to improve). A rise in hormone levels–and in particular the male hormone testosterone–leads to an increase in the production of sebum, an oily substance secreted by the sebaceous glands in the skin, to help keep it moist and supple. Acne results when these glands go into overdrive, producing excessive amounts of sebum that then block a hair follicle. The trapped sebum can form a whitehead under the surface of the skin, or if it reaches the surface, it becomes discoloured on contact with air, causing a blackhead. Infection may set in, making the pimples inflamed with pus and very sore. For some people redness or dark marks may remain even after the acne lesions resolve.

In women who are menstruating the acne skin eruptions can occur for a few days each month just before their menstrual period. Oral contraceptives are helpful in clearing up acne, paricularly if other treatments do not

TAKE ACTION NOW!

To help acne skin:
- Establish a skin-care routine, cleaning and moisturizing twice daily
- Use cover-up cream on red areas
- Use oil-free, nonallergenic products
- Wear a sunscreen every day
- Don't use skin-peeling methods
- Resist the temptation to pick pimples
- Keep a food diary
- Avoid alcohol
- Don't go to sleep without removing make-up

SEBACEOUS GLANDS

The sebaceous glands are found alongside hair follicles in the layer of skin called the dermis, which lies under the epidermis. When they overproduce sebum, they become clogged and a whitehead or a blackhead forms on or under the surface.

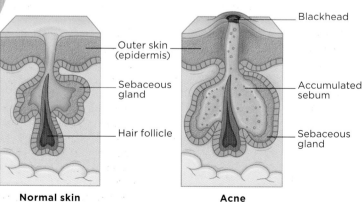

Outer skin (epidermis)
Sebaceous gland
Hair follicle

Blackhead
Accumulated sebum
Sebaceous gland

Normal skin   **Acne**

work and women need to discuss this option with their dermatologist or general practitioner.

Unfortunately, the eruptions tend to be in the most visible areas—on the face and sometimes the neck, the top of the chest, shoulders, upper arms and back. These areas have more sebaceous glands than other parts of the body.

What a dermatologist may do

Your doctor can prescribe different antibiotics (tetracycline, minocycline or erythromycin), which are often prescribed for severe cases of acne. Combination therapies with topical antibiotics (skin creams) may need to be taken for several months for the maximum benefit.

Vitamin A derivatives taken as capsules are one of the most effective treatments for acne, but because they are very powerful and can have serious side effects, they are reserved for severe acne that does not respond to any other treatment. Known as isotretinoin, it is only available by prescription and this treatment should not be used if you are pregnant, since in some cases excess vitamin A can cause birth defects. Usually creams and gels containing vitamin A derivatives will be tried first to reduce the formation of sebum plugs in the follicles and encourage the sebum to drain away.

Because of the hormone content of certain birth control pills, they can improve acne in some women and your dermatologist will help determine if this type of treatment is recommended for you. As a final option, laser resurfacing, dermabrasion and skin fillers may be safe choices to consider

Oral contraceptives can relieve acne.

discussing with your dermatologist for treatment of acne scarring.

Most importantly, do not squeeze, pop or pick at acne spots as this can result in scar formation. Treating acne takes time and patience and it is not going to improve overnight.

Over-the-counter remedies

There are many creams, lotions and gels available to treat acne. They contain substances called keratolytics—usually benzoyl peroxide—that loosen the top layer of skin so that it can be rubbed off and unblock the pores. The remedies are antibacterial and help to suppress the inflammation. Agents should be used once or twice a day after cleaning and drying skin. They may sting and dry out skin, so it is important always to use a moisturizer as well.

Rosacea

Rosacea is a form of acne that mostly affects fair-skinned women and middle-aged people. It is characterized by pustules occurring on a background of redness and telangiectasia (shiny spider veins) of facial skin.

The skin of the nose and cheeks, and sometimes the forehead, eyelids and chin, becomes inflamed. If the inflammation is severe, the swelling on the nose may eventually become permanent. There may also be tiny spider veins on the cheeks or the face may become taut, red and shiny. The cause is unknown, but it is probably genetic. The usual treatment is long-term oral antibiotics, but topical antibiotic creams may be prescribed to keep the condition under control.

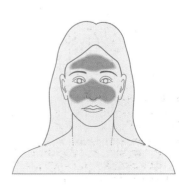

Areas affected

ECZEMA

Atopic dermatitis is the most common form of eczema. The symptoms of atopic dermatitis vary, but generally the skin becomes dry and scaly and unbearably itchy. Blisters may develop and eventually burst, leaving you with red oozing patches that dry into crusts. Scratching the skin tends to make the condition worse and can often lead to infection.

If you have suffered from eczema since you were very young, or if you or anyone else in your immediate family also has asthma, hay fever, perennial rhinitis (year-round hay fever symptoms) or a food allergy, then your skin condition may result from an atopic allergy–an inherited tendency to develop allergies to a wide range of substances in the environment that are normally harmless. Symptoms develop because the immune system reacts to these substances or allergens by triggering a series of defensive actions when the presence of even small amounts of the allergen is detected.

Many people grow out of atopic eczema by the time they reach the age of 30, although it may return. The usual places where it appears are in natural skin creases (such as at the inner elbow or back of the knee, inner ankle), face, neck and on the lips.

There is no cure for atopic dermatitis but the majority of cases can be controlled with appropriate treatment. The treatment includes medication, proper skin care and trigger avoidance and coping mechanisms.

One of the main difficulties with atopic eczema is identifying the allergens to which you are reacting, especially since they may well be substances that do not come into direct contact with your skin. One of the more common allergens are the droppings of dust mites. These mites live in carpets, other soft furnishings and bedding, and feed on your body's dead skin flakes. Other allergens include animal hair and fur; other animal traces such as saliva; feathers or down in pillows; and pollen from grass or trees.

The situation may be made more complicated if you also develop allergies to new substances as a result of long-term exposure to them. Examples of allergic contact dermatitis include nickel, rubber, dyes, preservatives, and fragrances. Contact dermatitis, can occur in people with a prior condition of atopic eczema, but it can also affect people who have not had the condition before.

How do you know what it is?

The fact that most people who have atopic eczema as children eventually grow out of it means that diagnostic tests (including skin and blood tests) are not usually necessary. However, they may be carried out if your doctor suspects your problem is the result of allergic contact dermatitis.

Pompholyx eczema affects the hands and feet, particularly the areas where sweating is prevalent–the palms, sides of the fingers, toes and soles. Small itchy blisters form under the skin. They usually break and ooze, which may lead to a secondary bacterial infection. Outbreaks are common in hot weather and during stress.

Discoid eczema is an adult illness in which round scaly patches form on the skin. It is usually atopic. The patches itch and have the appearance of highly contagious ringworm, a fungal infection that may come from infected animals or people. Discoid eczema is treated with moisturizers and steroid creams.

Varicose eczema may occur if you have severe varicose veins or have had a deep vein thrombosis. The area above the ankles swells, the skin is tense and shiny, then becomes scaly and changes color. It needs medical attention to prevent an ulcer from forming.

Eczema treatment

If you have only a few patches of eczema or they only appear now and again, fairly simple treatment will usually keep them under control.

One of the easiest steps you can take is to avoid cosmetics and keep your skin

TAKE ACTION NOW!

Here's how to ease eczema:
- Apply cold compresses to itchy areas of skin
- Wear natural fibres such as cotton or silk next to your skin
- Pull on lightweight gloves at night to prevent scratching; the liners for ski mittens are perfect

SOOTHING THE SKIN
To ease irritation, use special bath and shower products instead of soap, and apply a cream or gel after washing. Always use products that do not contain perfumes.

Occupational hazards

Dermatitis includes a range of inflammatory skin disorders with symptoms similar to eczema. However, in adults, it is more often the result of a reaction to some substance the skin has come into direct contact with. The skin becomes hot and red, dry, scaly and itchy and may blister then ooze and form crusts. In contact or irritant dermatitis this can be seen on the areas of the skin exposed to the allergen, most often the hands, face, ears, neck and earlobes.

Sometimes you may begin to react to a substance that you have encountered previously without any problems because your skin has become sensitive to it over time. It may happen with cosmetics and skincare products, shampoos, bath and shower additives, perfumes, sunscreens, detergents and fabric conditioners. Other potential allergens include nickel—in jewellery or fastenings in jeans and other clothes—and rubber.

Occupational dermatitis can affect people who work with chemicals over long periods and eventually become sensitive to them. Sometimes these people may develop other allergic conditions such as asthma if they continue to work with the allergen.

If the trigger is not obvious it may be identified through skin-patch testing in a dermatology or allergy clinic. Solutions containing possible allergens are placed on your skin and covered for a few days: itchiness and redness at any site indicates that you are allergic to the substance concerned.

The only real cure is avoidance, but emollients and weak steroid creams can relieve symptoms.

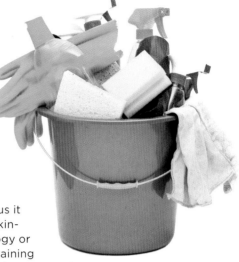

SENSITIVITY
Many household products can cause skin rashes, scaling or blistering. You need to identify which product is causing the problem, and buy an alternative.

well moisturized. There are various products available over the counter as well as by prescription in the form of bath and shower additives, cream and gels, which clean the skin and ease dryness and irritation. You may have to experiment to find the one that works best for you.

To relieve itching symptoms, cold compresses applied directly to the skin can be helpful and effective. You may find it helps to wear natural fibres such as cotton or silk next to your skin (but wool may aggravate the condition). Try to resist scratching the itchy areas. You can scratch yourself unconsciously at night, so it can be helpful to protect yourself by wearing thin cotton gloves when you sleep. Antihistamines to help you sleep may occasionally be prescribed by your doctor.

To reduce inflammation, mild steroid creams, available with or without prescription, can be applied when the skin is irritated. Your doctor may prescribe stronger steroid creams to be used if the eczema flares up badly. Your doctor will stress that they should be used for a limited time only.

Sometimes people with eczema also require antibiotics to treat a bacterial infection that has been acquired. Phototherapy is often a last step in the treatment cycle to relieve moderate to severe cases of eczema.

Tracking down the allergen

Keeping a diary may help you relate your symptoms to specific allergens or stress points. Each day, describe the state of your eczema then note what you ate and drank, the smells you came into contact with, the soap you washed your hands with and other possible triggers. Over time you may see a pattern emerging. If your skin gets suddenly worse or shows no improvement by your late 20s, you may have developed allergic contact dermatitis. You should discuss any such changes with your doctor.

PSORIASIS

Although psoriasis can develop in infancy, it more commonly appears between the ages of 15 and 25, but it can also appear for the first time later in life. For about a third of people there is a hereditary pattern. Although psoriasis cannot be cured, it is a serious medical condition and requires treatment to keep it under control.

When you have psoriasis, you develop patches of raised, reddish skin covered with silvery-white scale. These patches, which may be large or small, are known as plaques and are the result of an abnormality in the way skin cells replace themselves. Although there are other forms, plaque psoriasis is the most common type affecting as many as 80 per cent of people who have this skin condition.

Normally, skin cells are replaced by new ones approximately every 28 days but in people who suffer from psoriasis the turnover happens up to seven times faster than it should, so that the cells reaching the skin surface are improperly formed. The result is itching and flaking, and inflammation of the underlying blood vessels, which causes the skin to look red.

AFFECTED AREAS
The areas of the body most susceptible to plaque psoriasis are the scalp, elbows and knees, but the condition can spread all over the trunk.

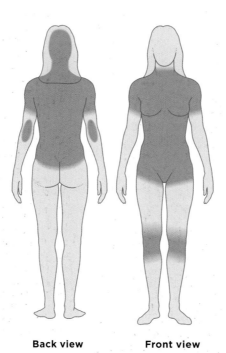

Back view   **Front view**

Types of psoriasis

Plaque psoriasis commonly affects the knees, elbows, trunk, scalp and hairline. About 50 per cent of those affected with psoriasis will experience nail abnormalities. The nails may become pitted and thickened and may separate from the nailbed. Fortunately, psoriasis does not often affect the face. For many people, the most distressing part of the condition is the way the lesions appear on the skin.

Flexural psoriasis appears on the moist areas of the body: under the breasts, in the groin area or on the genitalia. In another type–pustular psoriasis–small pustules develop on the palms or soles of the feet. People with psoriasis usually find that both sides of the body are affected in a symmetrical way. One type of psoriasis starts after a throat infection. This form is called guttate psoriasis and should resolve itself in two or three months.

The causes of psoriasis are not fully understood, although certain triggers have been identified. It may be set off by a streptococcal infection or by hormonal changes brought about by birth-control pills or the menopause. Alcohol and some drugs such as ibuprofen, antimalarials and beta-blockers also seem to act as triggers in some people. Discontinuation of corticosteroids can precipitate or exacerbate psoriasis. Stress may aggravate the condition although it is not thought to cause it directly.

Psoriatic arthritis

This is a complication that affects only a small minority of people who have psoriasis, perhaps 5 per cent. Most of the people with psoriatic arthritis are women between the ages of 40 and 60. Pain and swelling in the hands and feet and other joints, as well as in the spine, are experienced before or after the appearance of the skin plaques.

The activity of the arthritis is usually independent of the skin disease. The inflammation and pain can be treated with NSAIDs (nonsteroidal anti-inflammatory drugs) and in more severe cases with anti-inflammatory agents such as sulfasalazine and methotrexate.

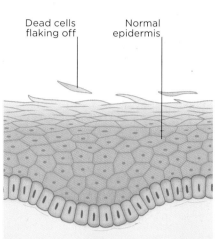

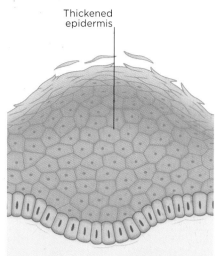

Dead cells flaking off

Normal epidermis

Thickened epidermis

Normal skin

Psoriasis skin

SKIN CHANGES

The epidermis (outer layer of skin) sheds its upper layer of cells continually, but in a psoriasis sufferer new cells reach the surface much more quickly than in normal skin. Dead and living cells begin to accumulate at the surface.

How your doctor can help

There are many treatments available by prescription–including moisturizers, creams, shampoos, scalp lotions and bath lotions containing tar and mild corticosteroid creams, and your doctor will be able to discuss these with you. More intensive treatments, such as skin preparations containing vitamin D analogues or a cream called calcipotriene (not available in Australia) and a topical retinoid, tazarotene, can effectively suppress symptoms. You should weigh the benefits against side effects–skin irritation and more sensitivity–and consider how easy the treatment is to use.

Severe psoriasis that does not respond to medical treatment may improve with a course of ultraviolet (UV) treatment known as phototherapy or a combination treatment involving drugs called psoralens and UV light (known as PUVA). Long-term use of PUVA has, however, been linked with an increased risk of squamous cell carcinoma and melanoma. Methotrexate is used orally to control severe psoriasis, nail psoriasis and psoriatic arthritis. Some of the treatments can be given on an outpatient basis but you may have to stay in hospital for a few days for others.

Drugs that have an effect on the immune system, such as cyclosporin, can help to control the abnormal skin cell turnover, but you will need to be monitored for side effects, which may range from stomach and intestinal problems to skin rashes. Monitoring will involve blood tests and blood pressure checks as the effects of these drugs are not confined to the skin.

New research into the cause of psoriasis has led to the development of target therapies with antitumour necrosis agents (infliximab and etanercept).

Help yourself!

If you only get small patches of psoriasis now and then, you may treat the symptoms yourself with over-the-counter remedies from the pharmacy. If you can, spend time in the sun, which enables the body to manufacture vitamin D. Add oily fish such as mackerel, herrings or sardines to your diet to reduce inflammation, and ask your doctor if rosemary and sage shampoos might help your scalp. Women with psoriasis may also benefit from finding a self-help group where other sufferers meet and share their tips and hints for dealing with the disease.

DOES SUNSHINE HELP?

Very often it does. Many psoriasis sufferers find that exposing their skin to sunshine or to an ultraviolet lamp helps to clear plaques, but for some people it can also make psoriasis worse. Work out a plan for gradual exposure with your doctor. Be cautious. You need to protect yourself against sunburn, especially if you have had any treatment that increases your sensitivity to UV light.

Watch out for photodermatitis (also known as photosensitivity) and urticaria. Photodermatitis is caused by sensitivity to sunlight. Tiny blisters or bumps appear on exposed skin. The skin sensitivity may occur from chemicals in a sunscreen, perfume or an antibiotic, or from exposure to resins from plants such as wild parsley or giant hogweed.

Urticaria, which is also called hives, causes the skin to become acutely sensitive. Cold, heat or sunlight can cause it, or a bite or a sting, or a food allergy. Stress or anxiety or even hormonal changes can make it worse.

SKIN MARKINGS

There are various minor skin disorders that affect the appearance of the skin but that are not serious medical conditions. Some, such as liver spots, are associated with ageing. If they make you feel self-conscious, there are treatments available for those conditions that cannot be disguised with cosmetics.

Spider veins

These tiny, hair-like blood vessels become visible on the upper or lower legs and sometimes on the face. The cause is not known, although they often run in families. Since more women have them than men, the hormones oestrogen and progesterone may play a role in their development. They tend to appear at times of hormonal change such as puberty, the menopause, pregnancy and after childbirth, or when a woman is taking birth-control pills.

The cheeks of fair-skinned people are a common site for spider veins, caused by exposure to weather extremes. Wearing skin protection in the sun or wind can prevent them from appearing. They are harmless and easily covered with cosmetics. If they are unsightly, you may want to talk to your doctor about having them removed by laser therapy or sclerotherapy.

RASHES AND MARKS
Rashes and other skin markings may be a sign of a wide range of disorders. Various infectious diseases, such as German measles, cause a rash. Allergy, as a result of strawberries or shellfish for example, can cause urticaria. The rash may be, for example, mostly on the hands or on moist areas of skin. The appearance and pattern of the blisters or spots may point to a diagnosis as may the degree of itchiness or pain they cause.

WHAT COLOURS SKIN?

Two forms of melanin colour the skin, hair and eyes: eumelanin produces shades of brown or black; pheomelanin is the pigment of red hair. No matter what your skin colour, we all have the same number of melanocytes (cells that absorb ultraviolet rays and convert them to harmless infrared ones). The more melanin you have, the further the melanocytes spread out to protect the skin when it is exposed to sunlight, which is why fair-skinned people (with less melanin) are more susceptible to sunburn than darker-skinned people. The number of melanocytes reduces with age, making the skin more susceptible to ultraviolet rays that damage the genetic make-up of skin cells, and this can cause skin cancer.

Liver spots

Medically called lentigo, liver spots arise where the skin's pigment—called melanin—collects in patches. They look like oversized freckles and develop mostly on the backs of the hands and the face. Since they are most noticeable in middle and later life, they are also known as age spots.

Liver spots are flat, normally light brown in colour and are completely harmless. It is thought that they result

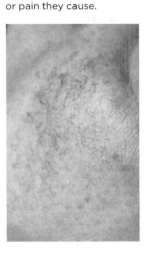

SPIDER VEINS
Spider veins are tiny blemishes that often appear on skin exposed to harsh weather, including cold and wind.

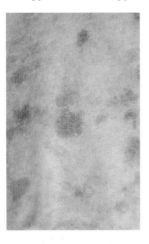

LIVER SPOTS
Liver spots are similar to freckles and develop mostly on the hands, becoming more obvious in middle age.

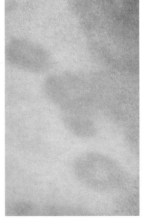

UTICARIA
Commonly known as hives, urticaria leads to itchy, raised red weals on the skin that may last for just a few minutes or several hours.

GERMAN MEASLES
In rubella (or German measles) a rash, which may be faint, develops on the face and then spreads to the trunk and limbs.

from long-term exposure to the sun, and will certainly get darker over time without sunscreen protection. They can usually be covered quite effectively with cosmetics or they can be removed by cryosurgery—a method in which the tissue is frozen with liquid nitrogen.

Vitiligo

Vitiligo is a condition in which some of the melanocytes—the pigment-producing cells in the skin—stop working, and round milky-coloured patches appear. The contrast is particularly noticeable on the face, neck, backs of the hands and arms, although patches can affect the genital area too. It is not known why the melanocytes malfunction in this way, although an autoimmune disorder may be involved.

The pale areas of skin gradually increase making you more vulnerable to sunburn, so you need to use a high protection factor sunscreen and stay out of the sun as much as possible. If you have light skin and can avoid getting a tan, this will make the contrast between the affected and normal skin less obvious. A few people find the condition improves with treatment with UV light, but for some reason this does not work for everyone.

SHINGLES
The rash caused by the herpes virus usually affects one side of the body only, causing painful blisters that are filled with the virus.

FACTS

- Nails can soften if immersed in water for any length of time, so it is best to protect them with rubber gloves when you are washing up dishes or doing similar chores.
- Nails grow faster on fingers than toes and the rate of growth depends on your age, time of year, activity level and even hereditary factors.
- During pregnancy, nails tend to grow more quickly.
- Women's nails grow more slowly than men's.
- Nail disorders seem to increase with age.

SALON SAFETY

Getting a manicure at most nail salons is safe as they are required to follow strict sanitation guidelines. But it is still important to make sure that the salon and manicure stations are clean and that the manicurists wash their hands between clients. Also, do not let the manicurist cut or push back your cuticles as this may allow infection to develop. Consult your dermatologist if you develop itching or burning or an allergic reaction to a nail cosmetic.

What colours nails?

Nails are made of keratin, the same protein that makes up skin and hair. It is normally tough and can resist most things.

There are many possible reasons why nails become misshapen or discoloured. Discoloration or thickening can signal health problems including liver and kidney diseases, and heart and lung conditions. In skin conditions such as eczema or psoriasis nails tend to become loose or pitted. The colour of the flesh beneath the nail, called the nailbed, can be a sign of a circulatory problem. A greenish discoloration of the nail may be a sign of bacterial infection, which is most often due to injury or frequent exposure to water and chemicals.

Melanoma, although uncommon, can grow under the nail and often appears as a dark-coloured streak within the nailplate.

White spots are often a sign of prior injury to the nail. Splinter haemorrhages, which are vertical lines under the nails, can also be caused by nail injury or certain drugs or diseases.

If there is a noticeable change in your nails you should consult your doctor.

HEALTHY NAILS

- Toenails, like feet in general, benefit from wearing shoes that follow the shape of the foot rather than squashing them. This can also help reduce the risk of ingrown toenails.
- To cut thick and hard nails, soak them in warm salt water for 10 minutes and apply an over-the-counter 10 per cent urea cream before trimming them.
- If you are prone to fungal nail infections, use an antifungal foot powder daily.
- Avoid biting your fingernails to avoid the risk of transferring infectious organisms between your fingers and mouth.
- Keeping your nails clean and dry can prevent bacteria from collecting under the nails.

ENJOY THE SUN SAFELY

Although most people enjoy being out in the sunshine, the fact is that ultraviolet radiation from the sun is not good for your skin. According to dermatologists, even a light tan is a sign that skin damage has occurred.

Ultraviolet radiation occurs in various different wavelengths. Virtually none of the shortest wavelength (UVC) reaches the earth's surface and so is no danger to the skin. Although UVA (with the longest wavelength) makes up approximately 95 per cent of the solar radiation that reaches your skin, it is less harmful than UVB radiation, which is what burns the skin. Nevertheless, prolonged exposure to UVA light can cause skin damage such as photoageing and may play a role in triggering some types of skin cancer.

Sun, and how much is good for you, is controversial. The psychological benefits of sunshine and its role in encouraging vitamin D synthesis–essential for strong bones and good health–have to be balanced against the risk of skin cancer.

COVER UP

The message is clear: sun exposure is the most preventable risk factor for skin cancer, and increased awareness about the sun's dangers is helping to reduce the high skin cancer rate. So always remember to slip on a shirt, slap on a hat and slop on the sunscreen. The wearing of sunglasses and skin-protective swimwear has been accepted eagerly by children whose parents grew up in the "tan is beautiful" era and are now suffering the effects. Water, snow and sand can reflect the damaging rays of the sun and increase your chance of sunburn.

TANNING BEDS AGE SKIN

Modern tanning beds deliver only UVA (not UVB) radiation and many people believe that they don't damage the skin. In fact, regular sessions from artificial sources can cause photoageing and may increase the risk of skin cancer in susceptible people. People with fair skin and a lot of moles are at the greatest risk of developing skin cancer and should avoid tanning altogether. Anyone deciding whether to use a tanning bed should be aware that they damage the skin. Safety guidelines should be on display or explained to you by tanning bed operators. Also, be aware that tanning beds and sunlight are not better sources of vitamin D than food or supplements.

Dermatologists generally recommend staying out of the sun. Sunburn can develop within hours of your skin being exposed to the sun. The redness and tenderness are part of the body's attempt to repair damage caused by UVB radiation to the DNA in cells in the epidermis. If the repair is incomplete, it can cause cells to mutate, and if these abnormal cells continue to multiply, the long-term consequence may be the development of melanoma (*see* p. 139).

Check your bottom

Even if you do not sunbathe, skin that is frequently exposed to the sun–on your face and arms, for example–will show signs of photoageing such as thickening, wrinkles and freckles. You can see this for yourself if you compare the way your skin looks on your face with the skin that is normally covered–your bottom, for example. It will have smoother, younger-looking skin (unless, of course, you sunbathe in the nude). Photosensitization is the name given to an allergic reaction that occurs when a cosmetic or perfume you are wearing causes a rash in the sun.

Why a tan is bad news

When your skin is damaged by UV radiation, defensive measures are set in motion by your body to try to prevent further injury. The outer layer of skin becomes thicker and melanocytes

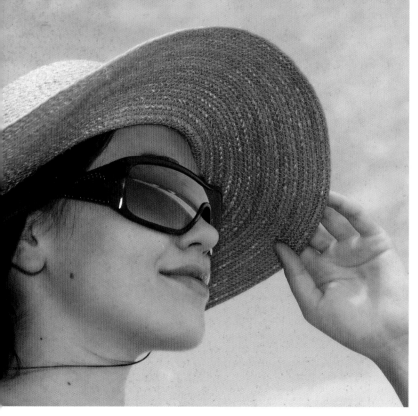

release melanin, which is responsible for your tan. People with dark skin have more of this pigment than pale-skinned people and are therefore better protected against the ill effects of UV light. However, a tan only gives protection roughly equivalent to a low sun protection factor (SPF) sunscreen (about SPF 2 or 3). The tan is not enough to prevent further damage and you can certainly still burn even after you have already developed a tan.

After the age of about 30 you have fewer melanocytes, so you will not tan as easily and you may find you are not able to stay in the sun as long as you once did.

Which SPF is right?

Ideally you should never go out, even on a cloudy day, without wearing a sunscreen that protects against both UVA and UVB, and you should avoid sunbathing altogether. Sunscreens can prevent wrinkles and sun damage. The products are graded by factors, and you will find the higher the SPF, the greater the protection. Daily use of sunscreen on the face and body can help prevent skin cancer and premature ageing. If you can normally stay in the sun for half an hour without burning, a sunscreen of factor 15 could conceivably extend that time to seven and a half hours (15 x 0.5), but always remember that sunscreens are not a substitute for avoiding excessive exposure. The general rule is to use sunscreen if you are going to be in the sun for more than 20 minutes, even on cloudy days, and apply it to dry skin 15 to 30 minutes before going outdoors.

Sunscreens either absorb or reflect UV rays and the chemicals in them differ. Some waterproof types can clog the pores of the skin and can cause adverse reactions, especially for people who have oily skin or acne.

All sunscreens need to be reapplied constantly while you are in the sun, especially after swimming or any exercise that makes you sweat.

You should be aware that SPFs are not standard in all parts of the world. If you are travelling to other countries, take the products that you use at home, and don't rely on being able to buy them on arrival at your destination.

Sun sense

There are many sensible precautions you can take to minimize damage caused by the sun and reduce your risk of developing skin cancer. You should never, for example, sunbathe in the summer months when the sun is at its most intense—between 11.00 a.m. and 3.00 p.m. It is also advisable to put on a sunscreen—at least SPF 15—every day, before applying cosmetics. This will help protect your skin against UVA radiation. Sunscreen should be worn even in the shade, since some UV light will still be reaching your skin. Even on cloudy summer days, UV radiation can penetrate all but the thickest cloud cover and get through the ozone layer. This layer in the stratosphere limits the amount of UVB radiation reaching the earth's surface, but there are areas within it that are being rendered less effective by pollution.

You must be particularly careful at high altitudes where the UV radiation is more intense, and on beaches or by water where the sunlight is reflected on to your skin even when you are in the shade. Wear a long-sleeved T-shirt or shirt and a hat with a wide enough brim to provide shade for your face and the back of your neck. This is particularly important if the hair on the top of your scalp is thinning or if you have had certain types of therapy (see p. 140).

Drink plenty of water to keep your body hydrated in the sun. Don't let sea or pool water dry on your skin after bathing. Dry yourself well and then reapply sunscreen. If you do get burned, apply calamine lotion immediately, to cool and soothe the skin. You may also need painkillers if the burning is very painful.

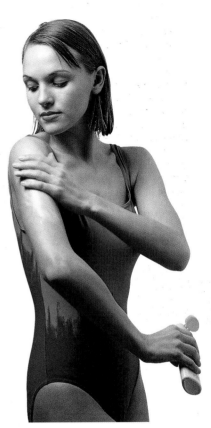

PROTECT YOURSELF
Don't rely on a sunscreen for protection unless you apply it frequently while you are in the sun. Fair-haired, red-haired and fair-skinned people are especially vulnerable to the harmful effects of the sun. Be aware that skin creams and cosmetics for the face may say "protects against UV rays" but if no SPF is given you need a sunscreen as well. Be sure to regularly check your skin for changing moles or bleeding on your skin and bring this to the attention of your doctor promptly. As with other types of cancer, skin cancer is treatable when caught early.

SKIN CANCER

It is estimated that 90 per cent of cancers are caused by ultraviolet light from the sun. Skin cancer is one of the most prevalent cancers in many parts of the world and its incidence is increasing. There are three types–basal cell, squamous cell and melanoma–named according to which cells of the epidermis are affected, and all are related to overexposure to the sun.

Although it is the least common type, melanoma, which is the proliferation of the melanin-producing cells, is the only skin cancer likely to be fatal if not caught and treated in time. Over 75 per cent of skin cancer deaths are from melanoma. The other two types mostly affect older people, especially those who have spent a lot of time out of doors over the years, perhaps because of their jobs or a hobby such as golf or gardening.

All skin changes should be seen by a doctor. Treatment in all cases is likely to involve a skin biopsy of the affected area of skin under local anaesthetic, and sending a sample to the laboratory for analysis to confirm the diagnosis. With basal or squamous cell cancer, this may be all that is done, but additional treatment may be needed for melanoma.

Basal cell cancer

This is the most common skin cancer and you are unlikely to get it before the age of 60. It generally appears on the face, especially in the inner corner of the eye, around the nose and on the neck. The first sign is a slow-growing pearly lump or nodule the colour of normal skin that can persist and even bleed. If it is not treated, over time the affected area grows larger, the tissue breaks down and an ulcer that does not heal forms in the centre. It may eventually reach 6 mm (1/4 in) in diameter. Basal cell cancer is relatively easily to treat, either with surgery or, if it is small, with a skin-freezing technique that uses liquid nitrogen to kill the affected cells. In the rare instances when it spreads, it can also be treated with radiotherapy.

Squamous cell cancer

Squamous cells are flat, scale-like cells and the first sign of this type of cancer is the appearance of scaly patches. Fair-skinned older people are most prone to this skin cancer, which is about four times less common than basal cell cancer and usually occurs in those who have been exposed to the sun over many years. It may also be caused by certain substances used in manufacturing and industry, such as tar, arsenic and petroleum derivatives.

At the start it can look like a scaly, raised, solid nodule that grows quickly–it can double in size in six months–located usually on the face, top of the ears, the scalp (on someone who is bald

TYPES OF SKIN CANCER
The three forms of skin cancer vary both in appearance and severity. They are all caused by exposure to sunlight and can be successfully treated if caught early enough. Basal cell and squamous cell cancers rarely spread, wheras malignant melanoma can rapidly reach other parts of the body if left unchecked. It is important to look out for any skin changes.

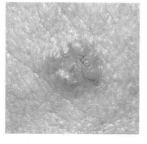

BASAL CELL CANCER
A slow-growing, small, pearly lump or nodule that may be near the top of the nose or between the eyes. Over time, if not treated, this lump will become larger, and an ulcer may form in the centre.

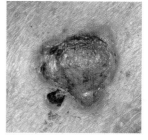

SQUAMOUS CELL CANCER
Although less common, this type of skin cancer appears as a scaly, raised nodule on those parts of the body that have been exposed to the sun. It can double in size in six months.

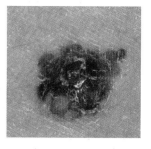

MALIGNANT MELANOMA
An odd-looking mole or freckle is the usual site of a melanoma—in women it may appear on a calf. The edges of the mole are ragged and the colour can be various shades of tan, black or red.

and rarely in women), the back of the hands, the upper chest and the back of the shoulders. The cancer has a high rate of cure when treated at an early stage. Usual treatments are surgical removal, cryotherapy with liquid nitrogen or laser surgery to remove the affected tissue. Radiotherapy may be used if the cancer is in an area difficult to treat surgically.

Solar keratoses

Also known as actinic keratoses, these warty, rough, red scaly patches occur mainly on the face, neck, hands or forearms, and sometimes the scalp, of people who have spent many years working outside. The patches may represent precancerous changes in your skin. Left untreated they may develop into squamous cell cancer, especially if sun exposure continues. They are easily removed with cryotherapy or can be treated with topical medication.

Malignant melanoma

This form of skin cancer differs from others in that it is more serious, and if it is not treated can spread to other organs–notably the liver, lungs, bones and brain–and is then fatal. Malignant melanoma can affect young people, although it is extremely rare before puberty. Melanoma can appear without warning but it can also develop from or near a mole. It is essential that you see a doctor immediately if you notice any changes in appearance in a mole or freckle. The chances of a cure are very much higher if melanoma is treated in the early stages.

Melanoma is found most frequently in men over 50. In women, the most common site of a malignant melanoma is on the calf; in men, it is on the trunk, especially the back. In older people it can also appear on the face. You should be especially careful if you are fair-skinned, have lots of moles or had recurrent blistering sunburns as a child or later. All these factors increase the risk, although melanoma is not always associated with sunburn.

Early signs Skin cancer doctors have devised an alphabetic guideline to help people recognize possible early signs of cancer:

A–Asymmetry or alteration in the appearance of a mole.
B–Border of the mole changes, or there is bleeding from a mole.
C–Colour change, especially if the mole darkens or develops several different pigmentations.
D–Diameter increases to more than that of a pencil end–about 6 mm (¼ in).
E–Enlargement, the mole appears to be getting bigger or seems thicker.

Treating melanoma A doctor may remove a suspicious mole so that it can be examined microscopically in a lab. Treatment will depend on whether the cancer has spread to other tissues. If it is melanoma and it has not spread, it will be surgically removed under a local anaesthetic, although a larger area of skin may have to be removed than with other types of skin cancer. Melanoma that is advanced and has spread may be treated with chemotherapy in addition. This type of tumour does not respond to radiotherapy.

You will be carefully monitored over the following months and years, as about one in three people has a recurrence of melanoma. You will be advised to make sure that you protect your skin very carefully with clothing or sunscreen whenever you are out in the sun.

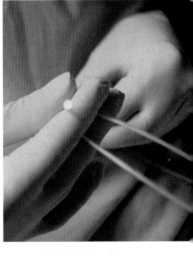

LASER SURGERY
The laser is emitted from a needle-like device controlled by the surgeon. Intense waves of light are aimed precisely onto superficial skin cancers or precancerous growths to cut away or vaporize the tissue.

WHEN CANCER SPREADS

Treatment for many cancers is intended to cure the condition and succeeds in doing so more often than many people realize. Whether it consists of surgery, chemotherapy, hormone therapy, radiotherapy or a combination of these different approaches, the aim of potentially curative (as opposed to symptom-relieving) treatment is to get rid of all the cancerous cells in the body. However, it takes time to tell if this aim has been achieved.

There is as yet no way of identifying and targeting microscopic cancer cells that may have migrated from the original site. This is why anyone who has been treated for cancer must have regular check-ups. If there is any sign of the cancer recurring or the appearance of a secondary cancer in a new place, further treatment will be necessary.

Different cancers tend to spread in different ways. Malignant melanoma can spread everywhere via the bloodstream and lymphatic system. Squamous cell cancer can spread locally to lymph nodes. New tumours that result from an original one somewhere else in the body are known as secondaries or metastases. In those instances when curative treatment is not a realistic prospect, treatment to alleviate symptoms and prolong life is often possible.

HAIR DISORDERS

The importance of hair to a woman may vary but it can play a big part in the way she feels about herself. Every woman has roughly the same number of hairs on her head throughout her life. The look, texture and volume of hair is influenced by a number of factors, including heredity, age, diet and general state of physical and mental health. Studies have shown that women who experience hair loss report loss of self-esteem and feel less attractive. For some women the psychological impact can be severe.

In its natural state, hair is either dry or oily, thick or fine, curly or straight, or any variation of these. It may be affected by how you treat it. Colouring your hair or using a very hot hairdryer may dry and weaken it, for example, and it is likely to split at the ends if you don't have it trimmed regularly.

Each hair, made up of dead keratin-containing cells (the same protein as in nails), grows from a follicle just under the skin and is supplied with oil from nearby sebaceous glands and fed by tiny blood vessels (*see* p. 128). Hair comes and goes constantly–the average growth rate is about 1.25 cm (^{1}/$_2$ in) per month and a hundred or more strands fall out each day. Normally this makes no difference to the 100,000 or so on the average head. As you grow older your hair may become dryer and coarser. After the menopause, you may have less of it.

Pregnancy challenges

In women most hair changes are related to hormones. The dramatic hormonal changes that are a normal part of pregnancy have a noticeable effect on your hair–and not just the hair on your head. As well as becoming drier or oilier, your crowning glory will almost certainly become thicker; this is because pregnancy temporarily interrupts the normal cycle of hair loss and replacement, and you shed much less than you normally would each day.

After childbirth, you compensate by losing hair–sometimes at an alarming rate. This may continue for up to two years. This is normal and does not mean you will end up bald or have thin hair.

When you are pregnant you may notice that your body hair is becoming more profuse or growing where it never did before, and if you are naturally fair it may turn darker. All these changes will reverse themselves.

Are you at risk of hair loss?

A variety of diseases and conditions as well as improper hair care can result in excessive hair loss. If you notice hair shedding in large amounts after combing or brushing or your hair is getting thinner or falling out in clumps you should consult a dermatologist for evaluation and treatment. Abnormal hair loss is associated with a lack of protein or certain vitamins and minerals in the diet, or with a specific health problem such as thyroid disease, anaemia, major surgery, high fever or severe infection. If this is the case, hair loss is unlikely to be your only symptom and you should see your doctor for a proper diagnosis.

Hereditary thinning or baldness is the most common cause of excessive hair loss. Alopecia areata is the medical name for the most common type of patchy baldness and affects all ages. Several patches may occur together. The condition may be precipitated by stress, or by severe shock or trauma. It is generally temporary, although a small number of people lose all the hair from their head and body and it doesn't grow back. Alopecia areata is thought to be an autoimmune disorder. It can be treated by steroids, immune suppressors, minoxidil (*see* box, left) and ultraviolet light therapy. However, these do not all work in every case.

Hair loss or hair thinning can also be caused by illnesses that alter the balance of certain hormones, for example hypothyroidism. The underlying cause will need to be investigated and treated. A mild excess of male hormones can cause hair thinning on the front and top of the scalp, while a severe excess can cause loss of hair from the temples. Either type of hair loss should be evaluated by your doctor. Some drug treatments may cause temporary hair loss, especially chemotherapy for cancer.

A fungal infection such as ringworm can cause hair loss, but it can be treated

TREATMENT OF HAIR LOSS

Treatment of the underlying disease is most important in being able to reverse the symptoms of hair loss. For both men and women, a topical drug, minoxidil, has been used to treat hair loss and has been shown to help in regrowth of hair. Dermatologists are now offering hair transplants for women with thinning hair, for male pattern baldness and for hair loss as a result of burn or scarring injuries to the scalp. This technique utilizes surgery to move existing scalp hair to bald or thinning areas of the scalp.

HEAD CARE
Gentle massage with the fingertips before, during or after hair shampooing, promotes blood circulation to the hair follicles in the scalp. Most people find such head massage very relaxing and soothing.

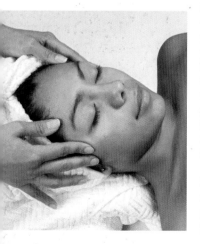

with antifungal medication. Vitamin deficiency and severe undernourishment related to eating disorders, and obsessive hair pulling, most usually from the scalp but also from eyebrows or eyelashes, will need psychological help.

Improper hair care includes excessive use of styling products, such as relaxers, perms, dyes and gels that can cause hair breakage. Brushing too much or too hard can cause some hair loss.

Dandruff

The cause of this irritating condition is thought to be a hypersensitivity to a yeast we all have on our skin. It is not a hygiene or dry skin problem and it can affect anyone. It comes and goes, may be accompanied by itching and may be related to a time of stress or ill health. Antidandruff or dry-scalp shampoos can help but in severe cases your doctor may prescribe anti-yeast shampoos and a topical steroid solution or foam.

An excess of hair

The medical term "hirsutism" means having or developing an excessive amount of body hair and not always on those parts where it is customary. On a woman it can affect the chin, upper lip, chest, stomach, back and thighs. Hirsutism is common and more so among coloured women. This condition will often begin during childbearing years but can develop at any age.

The extra growth may be caused by overproduction of male sex hormones (androgens), which are also present in a woman's body. Just as men have some oestrogen, women have some testosterone. Usually hirsutism is the result not of increased levels of this hormone but an increased sensitivity to even normal levels of it. However, some people naturally have more hair than others–Japanese and Chinese women have very little body hair while Mediterranean women tend to have more. It can also be hereditary– similar excessive body or facial hair may be noticed in mothers and siblings.

If the amount of body hair starts to increase or changes in texture see your doctor, especially if you are also having irregular periods. It could indicate a condition such as polycystic ovary syndrome, needing investigation.

Other rarer conditions might be responsible. Increased body hair and no menstruation are two symptoms of Cushing's syndrome (a disorder of the adrenal gland) or by long-term steroid use (for asthma or rheumatoid arthritis, for example). Women with eating disorders such as anorexia nervosa or bulimia often grow additional hair as they lose weight. This is the body's defensive response to compensate for the absence of an insulating layer of fat.

Sometimes, women may notice a slight increase in the amount or texture of body hair after the menopause due to hormonal changes. In advanced age, hair growth will be noticed around the chin and upper lip. Pulling out individual hairs with tweezers may result in irritation, so you may prefer electrolysis treatment (*see* box, below).

Excess body hair is more obvious in dark-haired women. Cosmetic bleaching or wax removal may help and self-application kits are available to buy.

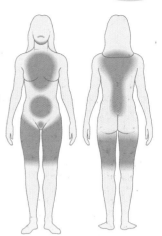

AREAS AFFECTED
The face, chest, stomach, back and thighs may all have excess body hair.

Hair removal treatments

Small amounts of unwanted hair, especially facial, can be removed by electrolysis. This destroys the blood supply to a hair follicle by passing a weak electric current into it. The process is slow and may be uncomfortable. Ask about the likely effectiveness, cost and duration of treatment before committing yourself. Laser hair removal is less painful but very expensive and may result in up to 80 per cent permanent hair loss after multiple treatment sessions. Technology is improving rapidly in this area, but be sure to review the anticipated results, cost and length of treatment. In all cases choose a fully trained specialist experienced in the technique. A new topical cream (Vaniqa), available on prescription, can reduce the rate of excessive facial hair growth. Use of oral contraceptives may alleviate a hormonal problem and help treat excessive hair. Another drug, spirolactone, works by decreasing the production of and blocking male hormone effects in areas of excessive hair growth. It is advisable to see your dermatologist for diagnosis and treatment.

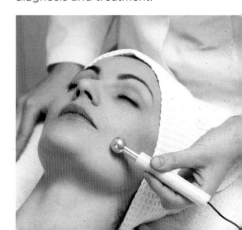

AGEING SKIN

Wrinkles represent skin changes that occur with age. Most women start to notice them in their early 30s. For some women the development of wrinkles occurs slowly as part of the ageing process but for others wrinkles may appear sooner than they would like.

Genetics may also be a factor that determines skin texture and why some women are predisposed to formation of wrinkles, lines and creases.

The key to slowing the process is prevention, which includes avoidance of sun exposure, not smoking, and using moisturizers and sunscreen.

Why skin wrinkles

Wrinkles show up as creases and lines in your skin particularly around the eyes, mouth, nose, forehead and neck.

With age the skin becomes thinner and loses its elasticity. The loss of skin elasticity results in saggy skin and can accentuate wrinkles. Skin also starts to lose its natural oils with age, which contributes to the process. Other factors that help accelerate the formation of wrinkles include:

- Ultraviolet radiation. It causes the collagen and elastin fibres in the skin's connective tissue to break down, which in turn leads to saggy skin and premature wrinkle formation.
- Smoke. Smokers are at most risk of skin damage due to exposure of the skin to heat and alteration in the blood supply to the face. It is one factor that accelerates the normal ageing process.
- Facial expressions. Some people have a tendency to repeat facial expressions, such as squinting, which can result in lines and creases particularly around the eyes and forehead.

New treatments are available to help manage and reduce the appearance of wrinkles but more importantly prevention should be the main focus.

How your doctor can help

A referral to a dermatologist or skin specialist is important if you are looking

---

WHOM DO YOU TRUST?

The best advice for women considering wrinkle treatments is to seek care from a cosmetic surgeon or dermatologist who is specifically trained to provide the treatment you choose and to minimize complications.

THE AGEING PROCESS
Many factors affect how your skin ages, but genetics, hormones and the sun have a major role. Facial expressions, such as frowning, can encourage wrinkles. With age, the skin thins and becomes less elastic. Using a daily moisturizer, applying sunscreens and avoiding smoking can reduce the formation of wrinkles.

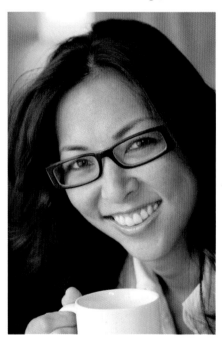

20s
While you are in your 20s your skin is in peak condition and is well hydrated. You are not likely to notice any signs of ageing.

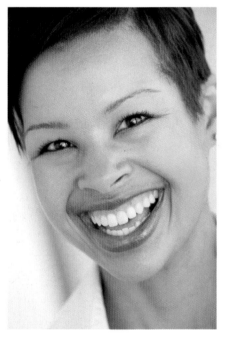

30s
In your 30s you may begin to notice a few fine wrinkles on your face, particularly laughter lines round your mouth and eyes.

for options to eliminate or reduce wrinkle formation.

Your dermatologist will stress the importance of prevention by the use of sunscreens and avoiding smoking.

The specialist may also suggest topical retinoids and nonprescription wrinkle creams. Retinoids are prescription medications and are applied to the skin and help to reduce fine wrinkles. The antiwrinkle creams that contain antioxidants and retinol that are found at your local cosmetic counter have lower concentrations of these agents than those in prescription medications. For this reason, cosmetic counter products are of limited benefit.

The surgical option

A variety of surgical procedures can help with the treatment of wrinkles and some are more effective than others. Your dermatologist will help you determine which is best based on your skin texture and skin condition.

Treatments that involve skin resurfacing include dermabrasion and microdermabrasion, which sand down the surface layer of the skin. These treatments are often repeated and can result in some redness and swelling.

Chemical peels require acid to burn the old layer of skin so new skin can form over time. This technique can also result in redness and swelling.

The most popular and well known treatment is Botox, a botulinum toxin type A that requires an injection into the muscles. There it causes wrinkles to contract and skin appears less wrinkled. The benefits from Botox injections tend to be short lived and need to be repeated at intervals.

Other treatments include laser resurfacing, which burns the outer skin layer to stimulate new skin growth.

The newest treatment includes skin fillers that involve the injection of fat, collagen and hyaluronic acid into wrinkles to smooth them out.

Finally, the most common surgical treatment is a face lift, during which excess skin is removed and muscles and connective tissue are tightened.

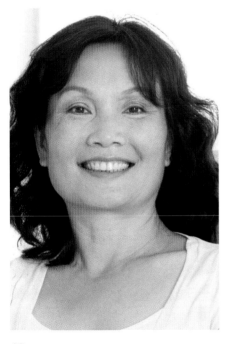

40s
By your 40s skin hydration is reduced and wrinkles and sagging around your mouth and eyes will become apparent.

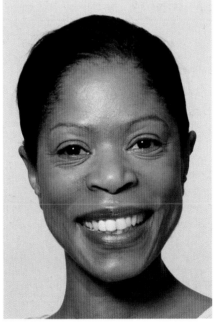

50s
Your metabolism starts to slow down in your 50s, causing weight gain. Skin loses some of its elasticity and is drier.

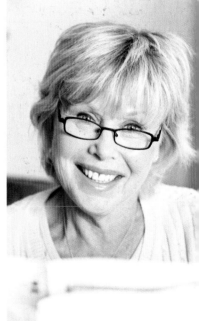

60s
Your skin becomes more transparent and fragile as collagen diminishes.

Urinary System Problems

Disorders of the urinary tract arise from many causes, often linked to a woman's hormonal changes or as a result of the closely related anatomy of the reproductive and urinary systems. Although these problems can cause discomfort and distress, they can often be ameliorated by taking quick action and simple treatments.

INCONTINENCE

Urinary incontinence is a condition that is embarrassing and distressing–and far from uncommon in women of all ages.

It's a condition with many possible causes and not a normal part of ageing or an inevitable consequence of childbirth or changes of the menopause. Some causes are relatively simple and self-limited and others more complex. Too often women do not discuss the problem with their doctor because they feel nothing can be done. For many women, incontinence may be seen as more of an annoyance than a serious problem not realizing that it's possible to restore their ability to control urination. Medications, devices such as a pessary or surgery may help.

Urinary problems can be sorted into types of incontinence. Stress incontinence is the most common type in women (*see* box opposite).

How it is diagnosed

Your doctor will either give you a questionnaire or a voiding diary to complete or ask you a series of questions about your symptoms. These will help determine the bladder-control condition you have. The complete diagnosis will involve a physical examination and a series of simple tests carried out by a specialist–a urologist, urinary surgeon or gynaecologist–to establish the cause of your problem.

Bladder function is tested by asking the patient to drink large quantities of fluid and seeing how much urine is passed in normal circumstances. A second test, called urodynamics, involves several procedures: the pressure in the bladder and the flow of urine are checked, a sample of urine is taken for analysis to detect any infection or bladder stones, the whole urinary system is examined by ultrasound, and a fibre-optic cystoscope may be inserted into the urethra so that the urinary tract can be inspected internally.

The doctor will want to evaluate all the results, since it is not unusual for a woman to suffer both types of incontinence–stress and urge–at the same time. Urinary incontinence may also be a side effect of illnesses such as multiple sclerosis and prolapsed spinal discs in the lower back.

GYNECOLOGICAL PHYSIOTHERAPY

Pelvic floor muscle exercises are aimed at improving the tone and strength of the muscles of the pelvic floor—the muscles that are used to stop urine flowing out. The exercises involve alternate contraction and release of vaginal and anal muscles to restore the neck of the bladder to its correct position. They are taught in antenatal classes and should be used after childbirth or pelvic surgery as a preventive measure. You can do them standing or sitting, when or where you want (no one will be able to tell that you are doing them).

Keep your legs slightly apart and close your anus as if you are trying to avoid passing gas. At the same time, draw the vagina inwards and upwards as if trying to stop passing urine. Count to five, relax for a count of five, then repeat a few times.

Start by contracting the muscles three to five times a day; the goal is to hold the passages closed for 15 seconds. After eight weeks, you should notice an improvement in bladder control.

Range of treatments

Treatment of incontinence depends on its type. Women suffering from stress incontinence may be referred for gynaecological physiotherapy sessions to learn Kegel and other exercises (*see* box opposite). Postmenopausal women may be asked to consider hormone replacement therapy (HRT) (*see* p. 88). If stress incontinence persists, surgery may be done to put the neck of the bladder back in its correct position. The success of this procedure is not guaranteed.

The bladder contractions that cause urge incontinence are treated with anticholinergic and antispasmodic drugs–although these have side effects such as dry mouth and blurred vision–and by treating any underlying condition. With urge incontinence, timed voiding may be suggested. You will be told to go to the toilet at set intervals throughout the day, whether you feel the urge or not. After several days of this, the time between visits is increased. This continues until you can hold urine for three to five hours without leakage. You may be advised to avoid drinking coffee, and to have little to drink in the evening.

If you have urge incontinence, bladder retraining is possible with the use of special devices such as cones, sponges and plugs. The devices have different weights and are held in the vagina to strengthen the muscles.

Which of these apply to you?

A number of symptoms are associated with incontinence. Consult your doctor if you: frequently have a strong, sudden urge to pass urine; go to the toilet eight times or more in 24 hours; get up twice or more in the night to pass urine; are not always able to hold on until you reach the toilet; have a slight loss of urine when you sneeze, cough or laugh; have a loss of urine when exercising or lifting objects; or wear incontinence pads and have to change them two or more times a day.

SEE YOUR DOCTOR

Painful urination is not a symptom of incontinence. Urinating several times at night (nocturia) may be but it is also caused by other conditions. If you suffer from either of these symptoms, go to your doctor for a checkup.

BLADDER-CONTROL PROBLEMS

There are different types of incontinence, which are brought about by different factors and vary in their symptoms and the discomfort or inconvenience they cause. You need to be able to describe to your doctor what happens to you so that he or she can accurately diagnose the cause and try to help.

TYPE	SYMPTOM
Stress Incontinence	Small amounts of urine are discharged involuntarily when pressure is put on the bladder by coughing, laughing or sneezing. It is due to weakness in the muscles of the pelvic floor, perhaps caused by a vaginal delivery, obesity, pelvic surgery, a prolapse or a lack of hormones after the menopause. It is the most common form of incontinence in women.
Urge incontinence	Larger quantities of urine are discharged by involuntary contractions of the bladder muscles. You may need to urinate several times during the night. The causes include bladder infections, alcohol, diabetes and lack of oestrogen after the menopause. Lack of nervous control of the bladder is known as reflex incontinence.
Overflow incontinence	The bladder always feels full, either because of an obstruction caused by a tumour or kidney stones, or some other condition, such as diabetes or a stroke, that affects bladder control. Urine may be forced back up the ureters to the kidneys, carrying serious infection with it.
Functional incontinence	People with this type of incontinence can control urination but are unable, usually because of physical disability, to reach the toilet in time. It is common in older age.
Transient incontinence	Sometimes incontinence is a temporary affliction, the result of an infection of the urinary tract, constipation (faeces press against the urethra, blocking it—which is common in pregnancy) and certain prescription drugs (such as antidepressants and muscle relaxants).

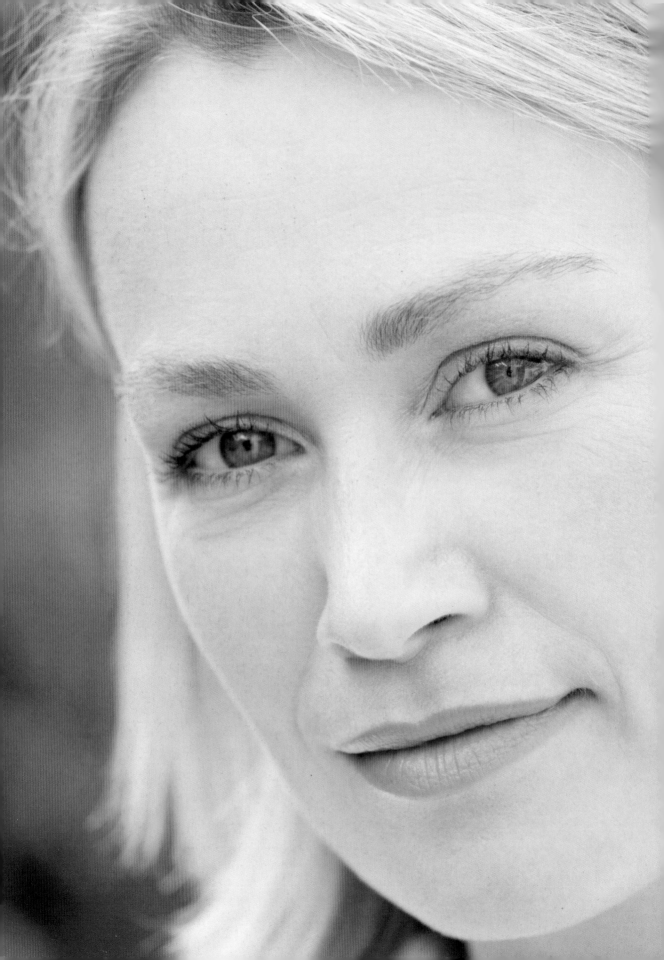

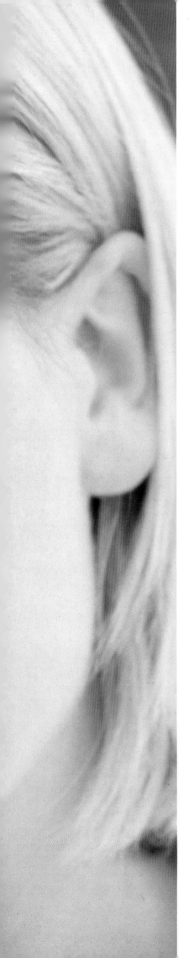

THE HEALTHY MIND

Your mind is beautiful. It holds within so much of what it is that makes you who you are. It gives you power, emotion, thought, compassion, caring, the gift of imagination, and the unique ability to create. This chapter reviews the challenges that can impair those abilities–and offers the strategies that can return the mind to health.

Keeping Your Mind Healthy

Being able to deal with events as they happen without getting stressed, taking things in your stride, and keeping emotions and relationships in perspective are all part of a healthy approach to life. Developing some skills will help you maintain your equanimity. Here's how we suggest you get started.

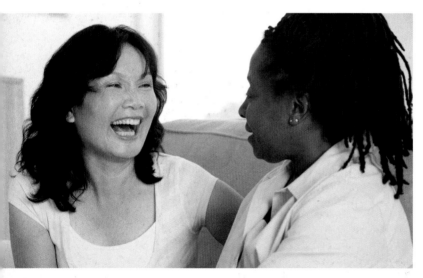

LIGHTEN UP
Laughter is the quickest way to release stress that is building up in your body. Laughter is a simple reflex caused by a chemical reaction that lifts your spirits instantly.

BEAT STRESS

Any life-changing event, even a happy one such as the birth of a baby or a new job, can be the cause of stress. Stress is a normal response and a necessary reaction to many physical and mental challenges. It is only when demands become too much that the stress can be harmful to the body and mind.

Individuals tolerate different levels of stress depending on temperament to a great extent, so there is no indisputable way of measuring when stress reaches the danger zone. What is known for certain is that suffering too much stress over a period of time can be damaging to your health.

There are many symptoms of stress that affect different parts of your body. These include palpitations, digestive disorders, headaches, insomnia, increased urination and irritability. You may experience a reduction in sexual desire or you might notice your periods have become irregular.

There can be even more serious health problems. One of the most common physical symptoms of stress is an increase in blood pressure. When you are challenged or feeling anxious, your blood pressure may rise, and if this occurs on a regular basis the body may adjust the pressure to a higher level. An overstressed person may also smoke, drink too much alcohol or turn to illegal drugs, which cause other problems.

It is important that the symptoms of stress be distinguished from psychiatric disorders such as depression and anxiety. Talk to your doctor about whether professional help is necessary. If this is not the case, you must decide what is making your life so stressful and then what steps you can take to change it.

Pinpoint the problem
Are you trying to fit too much into each day so you never feel on top of things?

You may need to prioritize your workload. This may be easier said than

LEARN TO BREATHE THERAPEUTICALLY

A good way of getting in touch with yourself in stressful situations is by controlling your breathing. When you are anxious, you tend to breathe very shallowly—that is, inhaling and exhaling so fast that very little oxygen-rich air is getting into the lungs and therefore to the rest of the body. This state, called hyperventilation, makes you feel dizzy. Fear and anxiety can also cause you to hold your breath.

To calm yourself you need to slow down your breathing to a rate of six even breaths a minute or less. The best form of relaxed breathing is one that uses the diaphragm, the muscular sheet sited below the lungs.

Lie flat on your bed or floor and put your hands on your abdomen. Breathe in deeply through your nose, counting mentally to four, and feel your abdomen rise. Breathe out slowly through your mouth counting from six to one as your abdomen lowers. Repeat 10 times.

done for many women who are juggling the needs of children or elderly parents, or both, and other domestic issues along with the demands of a full-time job outside the home.

If aiming for perfection is the problem, it is worth trying to strike a balance. You may take pride in having a spotless house, for example, but would it not give you more pleasure to spend time with someone you love rather than concentrating on the household chores?

Perhaps you need to enlist some help. People may not realize how desperate you are feeling unless you tell them that you are finding it difficult to cope. Ensuring that every member of the family shares the chores is a good first step. Even young children can make their own beds, put clothes or toys away or feed the cat.

If the care of elderly parents is making too many demands on you, discuss it with your family. Often this type of responsibility falls on the shoulders of only one sibling, and brothers and sisters need to know you are having difficulties. Also explore the possibility of getting help from volunteer groups. If this isn't available you may have to consider finding paid help—perhaps a cleaner or a nurse for a parent. You must decide whether the extra expense is better than putting your health in jeopardy.

Having too little to do, as in the case of the unemployed or the elderly, can be stressful as well.

If it is your job that is causing you the most concern, don't brood on what you see as your failings, but ask for help. Sometimes even a job you have been doing for years can suddenly become stressful, because there has been a change of personnel or there is a threat of reorganization or redundancy.

Approach your immediate superior or the human resources manager and tell him or her about your concerns. You may be surprised to hear that the company views you as a valued member of the workforce and that your fears have no foundation. It can be difficult to judge your own performance. If there seems to be a gap in your knowledge, perhaps with regard to new technology, request some training.

Too much stress does not always relate to excessive commitments. Having too little to do, as in the case of the unemployed or the elderly, can be stressful as well. Boredom and isolation both play a part. If you find yourself in this situation it is better to accept that paid work may not be an option, and to find out which organization would welcome your help as a volunteer and appreciate your contribution.

TAKE ACTION NOW!

Here are three proven ways to reduce stress:
- Talk: learn to tell other people when you're worried and upset.
- Walk: a brisk walk every day resets your neurotransmitters and alleviates stress.
- Be kind to yourself: a massage here, a flower show there and stress will float away.

CREATE A PEACEFUL SPIRIT
Meditation, yoga and prayer have all been shown to increase the feelings of calm and wellbeing that are an antidote to stress. Take time for yourself and practise one or more of these techniques at home.

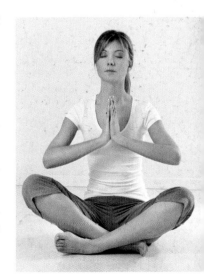

DEVELOPING A POSITIVE ATTITUDE

Women throughout their lives may be vulnerable to the attitudes and the needs of others. The influences come from their earliest years, the culture in which they grew up, the relationships they have throughout their lives and how society puts a perceived value on them and their role.

The reactions you have to irritations and problems in your everyday life can be indicative of whether those early influences were positive or not. If you take difficult situations in your stride and don't let them get out of proportion, you can feel assured that from childhood you were given the tools to deal with

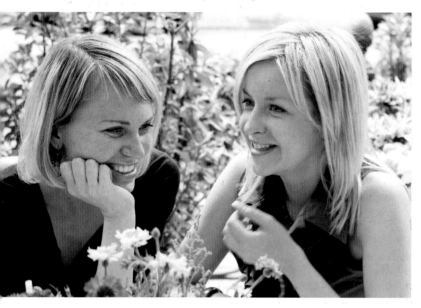

TALK WITH FRIENDS
Being able to express yourself and explain your feelings and fears is a healthy trait. You can talk to a close friend or write your thoughts down to help you gain insight into your emotions.

problems without letting them affect you adversely.

Thoughts determine your emotional state, which in turn can influence your physical health in many different ways. Holding back your emotions time after time increases your heart rate, blood pressure and muscle tension–all of which are signs of stress.

Retrain your brain

To help you uncover negative thought patterns that you may not even know about, you can apply the principles of cognitive therapy.

These principles enable you to reveal automatic thoughts that colour your life without you being aware of them. It's a method of discovery that is especially applicable to women, since they tend to be prone to socially conditioned negative thoughts–about their body or self-worth, for example. The first step is to analyse these thoughts, to recognize where the downturn in your mood springs from and how you may possibly be creating your own lack of self-esteem.

If, for example, you go for a job and don't get it, and say: "I'll never amount to anything", you are in the process of creating an ongoing problem. If you discover your lover is cheating on you and instead of getting angry with him you say: "I don't deserve to be loved", you are putting the blame on yourself.

Identify negative thoughts

The aim of cognitive restructuring is to find out what lies behind these negative thoughts, to get rid of them and to replace them with ones that are truthful and empowering. If your problem stems from your early life–from the attitude of a parent, sibling or teacher–or from your own worst fears at the present time, you can set about trying to change it.

First, identify the negative thought, then ask yourself four questions:
- Does this thought contribute to my stress?
- Where did I learn this thought?
- Is this thought logical?
- Is this thought true?

Take time with your answers. You may want to try and help yourself by writing down your thoughts or ask the help of a close friend or therapist. You may prefer to join a small group where you can talk it through.

Prepare a balance sheet

A lifelong habit of seeing everything negatively is unlikely to disappear immediately, but if you take steps to alter your attitude, you will soon appreciate the results.

Start by making an honest balance sheet of the positive and negative things in your life. You may be surprised to find that there are many more things that you like or enjoy than you had anticipated.

The negative side is that you may not have given them enough time to bring you pleasure. You can now put that right.

Identify all the negative things that you can do something about–getting into shape physically, finding new friends or interests, perhaps getting a new job. If none of these seems to offer solutions, you may be depressed and should see your doctor. Depression can be treated.

Write it down

Writing down your deepest thoughts and feelings can help you gain new insight into yourself. This process, called journalling, may help you release deep emotions, such as anger or fear, that lie frozen in your mind and body. It is a way of finding out whether something hidden is plaguing you and preventing you from being positive about your life.

If you are physically healthy, write about the most stressful event or ongoing problem you face in your daily life. If you believe your current problems are the result of past events, write about the traumatic times in your past. Take 20 minutes to do it. Write about what happened and how you felt then or feel about it now. The facts and the emotions are equally important to help you understand the experience.

Repeat this process for at least three or four days, even a week, if you feel that you are gaining from the exercise. You can use it for decision making, too. If you have come to a crossroads in your life and need to deal with a relationship or a physical problem, writing down how you feel may help you make sense of it. You may find your way through loneliness or unhappiness and gain the strength to make the decision that is right for you.

Assert yourself

Learning to assert yourself, to use anger as an agent for change, especially in your relationships, is a positive process. It is the opposite of passivity but it is not unbridled fury or aggression. It can be applied to co-workers, husbands and partners, children and parents, siblings and friends and people in medical and healthcare situations.

Speak in the "I" language. Learn to say, "I think", "I feel", "I want" instead of

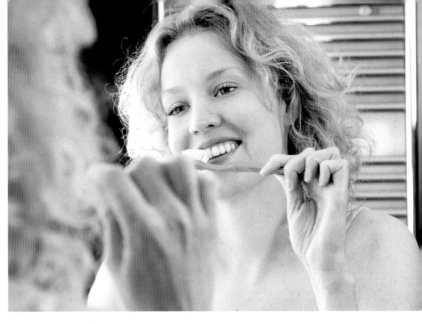

"You are", "You don't". A true "I" statement says something about you without criticizing the other person and without holding the other person responsible for your feelings or reactions. Beware of falling into the trap of telling him or her, "I think you are controlling or self-centred".

Recognize that each person is responsible for his or her own behaviour. Don't blame your mother-in-law because she seems to have a hold over your husband. If you are angry with him about his closeness to her, find another way to make him aware of it. Your husband's behaviour is his responsibility, not his mother's.

Resist telling another person what she or he thinks or feels or should think or feel. If someone gets angry in reaction to a change you make, it is not time to criticize feelings or deny him or her the right to be angry. It is much more helpful to say, "I understand that you are angry and if I were in your shoes I would be angry, too. But I have thought it over and this is my decision".

Remember that there are three ways in which to say no: (1) a simple "no"; (2) "no, because..."; and (3) "no, but how about...".

These offer alternative ways to protect yourself from requests that impinge upon your needs, boundaries or energy reserves. Sometimes it may be difficult, but knowing the ways to say "no" won't inflict hurt or be devastating to relationships that you value and don't want to harm.

TAKE A POSITIVE VIEW OF YOURSELF
Start in a small way and treat yourself well. Before you go to work or to meet friends, breathe deeply, look in the mirror and smile. The act of smiling has a physical effect on your feelings.

COPING SKILLS

Life cannot be lived free of emotional events that may threaten to overwhelm you. Knowing how to cope mentally when you experience personal upheaval can help prevent physical and other repercussions later.

Balancing work and family

Most women spend the greater part of their life in paid work, and an increasing number of young mothers continue to work during pregnancy and their child's infancy. Working full time while raising a family can be demanding on both mind and body.

Survival tactics include learning to compartmentalize your life and being clear about your priorities. It would

If you find you are increasingly angry about almost everything, it may indicate stress levels that are too high.

be rare if you were the only one at your workplace who didn't have similar domestic problems, and discussing them with colleagues may reveal ways to help you deal with conflicts of interest. Having to take work home, for example, can be tricky if it eats into the time you spend with your children. Talk to your employer about the pressure this puts you under and seek another method of dealing with the work. Make sure you have established a good back-up system of friends, relatives or neighbours who can step in if there is a crisis with your children while you are at work.

If you work from home, it is important to prioritize your energies. Isolation can be a problem when you are housebound with young children. It helps to make sure you get to know other mothers in your neighbourhood, who you can spend time with when you are not working.

Deal with anger

Anger is an emotion that can be both positive and negative. If it encourages you to try to improve things in the face of an injustice, anger can be positive. Negative anger, however, can be a destructive force, especially when it tips over into rage and even turns into physical violence. This type of rage is unacceptable. Venting feelings in this way indicates a complete loss of control. If it occurs in a personal relationship irreparable harm may be done.

Parents who feel exasperated by their children should relieve anger by punching a few cushions rather than risk lashing out. If you fear your aggression could harm your child, or you are in a relationship that is violent, you should seek professional help. If you find that you are increasingly angry about almost everything, it may indicate stress levels that are too high.

Some people may not know what the real cause of their anger is. Simmering resentment or hostility may have built up for various reasons and the anger is transferred to something else, often another person. The most serious form of anger is the type that is turned in on the self. This can lead to self-inflicted harm and always needs immediate professional attention.

Facing disease

Most people suffer ill health at some time in their lives, but usually they know that they will get better. Learning that you or a loved one has a serious illness that is life-threatening or will permanently impair physical or mental faculties can be devastating. You may become so preoccupied with the situation that you exclude other aspects of your life.

There is no easy way to cope with a serious illness of your own, but it does help if you have a good relationship with your doctor and other caregivers and are fully involved in your own care. You should keep yourself informed about the nature and implications of the condition so that you can participate in decisions about treatment and remain in control of your life as much as possible. Sometimes knowing what you are up against can remove some of the fear.

Contact with other people suffering similar illness or disability can be helpful and encouraging. Confronting the grief or anger you feel and finding ways to express it may be an important step in the healing process. Mental health backup may be essential for the person suffering the disease but it can be just as important for the caregiver.

Confront death

It is inevitable that at some point in your life you will have to confront the death of someone very close. The most common first experience of such loss is when a grandparent or parent dies, but for some it may be the death of a friend of your own age, a young child, a partner or a sibling. It can leave you feeling stunned by the sense of finality and may cause you to face your own mortality, something you may never have considered before. Whether you have a strong religious belief in an afterlife or see death as the end of any existence, the death of a loved one is always going to be painful.

Under whatever circumstances the death has occurred–shocking and sudden, or the result of a drawn-out terminal illness–the bereaved person must be allowed to go through the grieving process. Grief is a natural and healthy response to a death and helps you to come to terms with your loss, even though you may continue to miss the person all your life.

In some circumstances, a person who does not allow herself to grieve should be cause for concern. A woman who has had an abortion or miscarriage may want to put the experience behind her, but if she hasn't expressed her emotions, it could be detrimental to her mental or physical health. The grieving process has merely been postponed and may surface, possibly years later, in a potentially more harmful way.

Sometimes a bereaved person may refuse to show her feelings for fear of upsetting others. This may be true of a mother who has lost her partner at an early stage but wishes to protect her young children from her distress.

But children need to be allowed to grieve, too, to express their sadness. Crying together can be the beginning of the healing process. Take your own time. Don't allow yourself to be rushed into putting away photographs or disposing

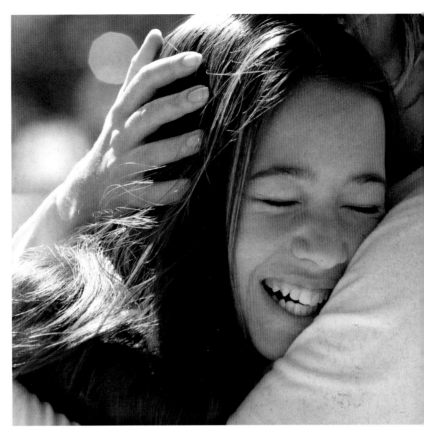

of your loved one's belongings. You can do this when you are ready. Having familiar reminders around you for a while can be comforting and strengthen your memories.

Working for a cause or campaign in the name of the person who has died may help you regain equilibrium. This can be true of parents who have lost a child through an accident or disease and find new resolution in trying to help prevent other parents suffering in the same way.

You may always have a sense of sadness at the loss of people you loved, but you will find yourself able to return to activities you once enjoyed after the hurt you feel lessens. If you find that your unhappiness or depression isn't lifting, or you start getting physical symptoms such as migraine, seek the help of a mental health professional or a bereavement counsellor who will understand your feelings. In some cases, medication may be the best way in the short term of dealing with grief that weighs you down.

CLOSE COMFORT
Sharing feelings at an emotional time can draw mother and daughter or friends closer together. You may not always understand why someone is so deeply affected, but you can sympathize and literally provide a shoulder to cry on.

Challenges to the Mind

Habits may not be recognized as destructive for a long time. They begin in your mind and, once they have taken over your body, they are hard to stop. Addictions to alcohol, smoking and drugs or a lack of control over eating habits have a direct impact on a woman's life, including her relationships, and increase her risk of developing physical illnesses.

ADDICTION

An addiction is an unnatural craving for a particular feeling or sensation and for the food, drink, drugs or behaviour pattern that satisfies it and results in temporary euphoria, excitement, wellbeing or relief from pain.

Causes of addiction

Almost all addictions have harmful, sometimes fatal, physical consequences and can profoundly disrupt the lives of the addict and the people around him or her. Early recognition of growing dependency is the best way to avoid addiction. Once a person is addicted, cures are difficult, painful and expensive.

Why is it that one person who experiments with, or indulges in, occasional substance abuse will become addicted, while another person, from an apparently similar background, doesn't? Four major factors of addiction have been studied. It is unlikely that only one of them is responsible for the tendency to addiction. The more likely situation is that all four factors are involved, with the relative importance of each one varying from one person to another.

Physiology Some experts believe that something akin to an allergic reaction takes place in those people who are predisposed to addiction. This in turn creates the craving for more of the addictive substance.

Genetics There is evidence that addiction–particularly alcoholism–runs in families. However, no specific genetic markers have yet been identified. The role of gender is uncertain. Women seem to be more likely to abuse prescription drugs such as pain medication and tranquillizers, whereas men are more likely to abuse hard drugs and alcohol.

Environment Socioeconomic status, lifestyle, peer pressure and family background have been shown to have an important influence on the development of addiction. Women who have alcohol problems or dependence on other substances may have been physically or sexually abused as children, have a partner who drinks heavily or may be socially isolated. Some professions and ethnic groups are more prone to heavy drinking than others.

Psychological disturbance Addiction may be a response to inability to cope with elements of the outside world, including relationships and employment, or with some aspect of the addict's life history. Low self-esteem, aggression and a refusal to recognize and confront problems are features of addictive behaviour. Problems such as depression and anxiety are common in addicts and need to be treated.

ALCOHOL

Alcohol abuse is a major problem in most Western countries today. Moderate alcohol consumption may be a pleasant and harmless aspect of social life, but excessive intake of alcohol is a much more dangerous matter.

Alcohol abuse is estimated to affect at least one in 10 people and to be directly responsible for long-term liver damage, heart disease and some cancers. It is implicated in about a third of accidents in the home and nearly the same proportion of murders and drownings. It is a factor in nearly half of all violent crime, including incidents of domestic violence and is a major cause of death and injury on the roads.

Women are more susceptible than men to alcohol because one of the digestive enzymes that metabolizes alcohol doesn't work as efficiently in them. Alcohol enters their bloodstream faster, making the risk of liver damage for them greater. In addition, women on average weigh less than men and have more fatty tissue, which contains a lower proportion of water to dilute alcohol. This susceptibility appears to increase during menstruation.

Young women between the ages of 18 and 29 need to be especially conscious of the effect alcohol can have on their lives.

Women in this age group are prone to abuse or dependence and to bouts of binge or social drinking during which the risk of violence, sexual assault or having unsafe sex increases.

When to avoid alcohol

A woman who is trying to conceive or is pregnant or breastfeeding should stop drinking altogether.

If you have liver disease or damage such as hepatitis or cirrhosis, a digestive disorder such as gastritis, or epilepsy, you should not drink.

Certain drugs, such as metronidazole (used to treat some dental and vaginal infections) and some sleeping pills, pain medications, tranquillizers, blood-thinners, and antihistamines react badly with alcohol–or alcohol may negate the effect of the drug. Seek your doctor's advice about alcohol consumption when you are taking prescribed drugs.

Seeking help

It is difficult for alcoholics to give up drinking without some sort of assistance, but there are various kinds of treatment available, depending on the degree of dependency and the extent of physical and mental damage.

In many cases, medical intervention may be required to counteract a range of unpleasant withdrawal symptoms.

DRINKING PROBLEM

You have a drinking problem if:

- You cannot fulfill obligations at work, school or home.
- You have blackouts after which you can't remember how you got home or what you said or did the night before.
- You continue to use alcohol despite possible legal problems (for example, driving under the influence of alcohol) and the disruptive effects drinking has on your personal relationships.
- You need a drink first thing in the morning to "steady your nerves" or get rid of a hangover.

What is safe drinking?

The recommended limit is 14–21 units for women a week. A standard glass of wine, which measures 125 ml (4¼ fl oz), contains 1½ units. One unit is:

- 300 ml (½ pt) beer or cider
- 50 ml (1½ fl oz) of fortified wine (port, sherry, marsala, Madeira)
- 25 ml (¾ fl oz) of spirits such as gin.

Moderate drinking, within these limits, may help protect against heart disease. However, this only applies to postmenopausal women and to men over the age of 40. For women, even moderate drinking increases the risk of breast cancer.

COMPARE DRINKS
The alcohol content of different drinks varies. A small amount of any spirit is stronger than a glass of wine or beer.

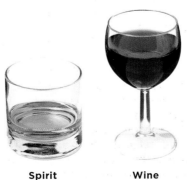
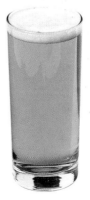

Spirit   **Wine**   **Beer**

BE VIGILANT

Drinking alcohol in social situations is obviously acceptable but, for women, particularly if they are on their own, it is worth being extra vigilant when among strangers. Certain drugs or even a clear spirit can be added to a drink and not be noticed. However, the effect of a spiked drink can be dramatic, causing blackout and memory loss.

Delirium tremens (DTs), hallucinations and seizures require treatment with tranquillizers called benzodiazepines, such as diazepam, possibly administered by intravenous drip.

Vitamin supplements, in particular vitamin B6 and thiamine, may be given to repair liver and nerve damage caused by poor nutrition.

Aversion therapy, in the form of drugs such as disulfiram, which produces a severe and unpleasant physical reaction to alcohol, may be prescribed.

Antidepressants and anti-anxiety medications may be prescribed if there is an underlying psychiatric illness.

Maintaining long-term sobriety can depend on the degree of support available. Alcohol addiction is hard on the drinker's family, and outside support, perhaps psychotherapy or counselling, is vital. Voluntary support groups, notably Alcoholics Anonymous (AA) and its related organizations Al-Anon (for the families of alcoholics) and Alateen (for young drinkers), provide emotional and practical support for recovering alcoholics on a long-term basis.

Heavy drinkers or alcoholics tend to be secretive; they hide alcohol supplies and go to great lengths to disguise their consumption. Being in an environment, such as a support group, where the problem is publicly acknowledged is a big step towards dealing with it.

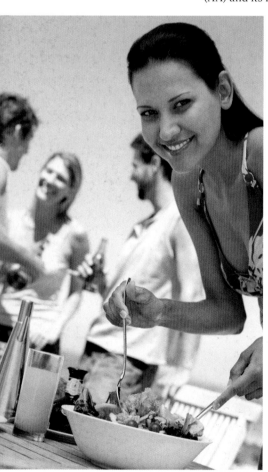

BE ALCOHOL AWARE
Although alcohol can oil the wheels in any social setting, women, in particular, should observe several alcohol-free days each week to rest their livers. For women who find it difficult to resist the temptation of alcohol, it may be best to avoid social occasions on these days.

SHORT-TERM EFFECTS OF ALCOHOL

The first effects are loss of inhibitions—the drinker may become lively, talkative, confident and relaxed. At the same time, however, judgment and coordination are affected. After a period of time, which differs from one person to another, the deleterious effects may dominate. The drinker may become aggressive or full of maudlin self-pity; speech may become slurred and he or she may become clumsy and fall down, bump into things or knock things over.

A bout of heavy drinking may result in a hangover due to a combination of dehydration and toxins building up in the blood. Typical symptoms include acute headache, shakiness, nausea, listlessness and an inability to remember the activities of the night before (known as alcoholic amnesia). In severe cases, there may be nausea, vomiting, mental confusion, visual disturbance, delirium tremens and possibly coma. Death from acute alcohol poisoning, or from the inhalation of vomit while in a coma, could also result.

LONG-TERM EFFECTS OF ALCOHOL

- Cancer of the mouth, throat, stomach, colon, liver and breast.
- Heart and circulatory disorders such as stroke and congestive heart failure.
- Brain and nerve damage, often causing pain in the arms and legs and sometimes leading to permanent intellectual impairment and severe memory loss.
- Organ damage, most notably to the liver (causing cirrhosis and hepatitis), but also to the stomach and pancreas.
- Gastrointestinal disorders such as gastritis, ulcers, pancreatitis, intestinal bleeding, diarrhoea and nausea.
- Malnutrition due to avoidance of food and regular meals in favour of alcohol. This leads to physical weakness and muscle wasting and a variety of disorders related to a deficiency of nutrients.
- Sexual problems, possibly infertility or impotence.
- Fetal alcohol syndrome.

MONITOR YOUR DRINKING

Answer this questionnaire honestly. If you find your ticks fall mainly on the right-hand side of the chart, you have an addictive drinking problem that needs addressing. If you cannot reduce your alcohol consumption, cut it out totally. Talk to your doctor and join a support group.

How often do you drink alcohol?

- ☐ Never
- ☐ Monthly or less
- ☐ 2–4 times a month
- ☐ 1–2 times a week
- ☐ 2–3 times a week
- ☐ 4 or more times a week

How many drinks do you have a day when you do drink?

- ☐ I don't drink
- ☐ 1–2 drinks
- ☐ 3–4 drinks
- ☐ 5–6 drinks
- ☐ 7 or more drinks

How often in the last year have you had four or more drinks on one occasion?

- ☐ Never
- ☐ Less than monthly
- ☐ Monthly
- ☐ Weekly
- ☐ Daily/almost daily

How many drinks does it take before you begin to feel the effects of alcohol?

- ☐ 1 drink or less
- ☐ 2 drinks
- ☐ 3 drinks
- ☐ 4 drinks
- ☐ 5 drinks
- ☐ 6 drinks or more

Have you had any legal difficulties because of alcohol?

- ☐ No
- ☐ Yes

Do you currently use any illicit drugs (marijuana, cocaine, heroin, etc.)?

- ☐ No
- ☐ Yes

Have you used illicit drugs in the past?

- ☐ No
- ☐ Yes

One day at a time

One of the most important things to remember when trying to overcome alcoholism is to take each day at a time and view each alcohol-free day as a triumph. There will be good days and bad days but, if you have a lapse, try to put it behind you immediately and start again. A reward system may work, in which the money you might have spent on drinking can be used more positively and help steer you past temptation.

Most alcoholics find that it is better not to drink at all than to try to limit themselves to one drink, because once alcohol is in the blood it can trigger the craving for more. You have to be honest with other people and yourself and avoid the places, people and occasions that you associate with alcohol.

THE EFFECTS OF SMOKING

Tobacco is the most common of all addictive substances and is one of the most important single causes of premature death. Women who smoke subject themselves to a wide variety of health problems.

As a group, young women represent the biggest increase among users of tobacco. Despite the recognition that nicotine, the active ingredient of tobacco, is physically addictive and carcinogenic (causes cancer), warnings on the packs and elsewhere have not

Women may be more at risk from smoking than men because they have a different chemical response to nicotine.

been successful in deterring tobacco use by this vulnerable group.

Reasons given for this include the stresses of modern living and an increase in the number of women spending evenings in bars, which were previously mainly male environments. Worries about body shape lead young women to smoke as a way of losing weight because it suppresses the appetite.

Women may be more at risk from smoking than men because they have a different chemical response to nicotine. This increases their susceptibility to cervical, lung, bladder and other cancers, and also the risk of starting the menopause up to two years earlier.

Smoking and your body

There are about 3,600 chemicals in cigarette smoke, many of which are carcinogenic. Once inhaled into the lungs, toxic substances cross into the bloodstream and then to the liver. In the liver, enzymes detoxify substances considered dangerous to the body, breaking them down so they leave in the urine or faeces or through the skin in the form of perspiration.

Tobacco smoking can certainly be connected with various types of cancer– most notably lung cancer, pharyngeal cancer and cancer of the tongue, lips and mouth. Evidence connecting smoking with breast cancer remains subject to debate but, for some women at least, a link between smoking and the likelihood of developing breast cancer can be drawn. In women who have a gene called NAT2 the detoxifying enzymes work slowly, giving the carcinogens more time to travel through the body reaching every organ. The same research also suggests that postmenopausal women

Giving it up

The withdrawal symptoms from tobacco are less severe than those from other drugs. But quitting is far from easy since the physical craving for tobacco may persist for months or years. Common complaints include irritability, jitteriness, anxiety and a tendency to gain weight (because eating is used as a replacement for the oral gratification derived from smoking). Techniques that involve mind and body, so that you understand the physical changes and reinforce your strength of purpose, appear to

give the longest lasting results. There are many methods to choose from.

Nicotine skin patches, nasal sprays and gum provide small amounts of nicotine, but take care not to become addicted to these instead. All replacement therapies present this problem.

Hypnosis, acupuncture and similar techniques work on your subconscious desires to encourage your body to reject smoking and to begin the healing process.

Both group therapy and individual counselling are based on behavioural techniques and aim to strengthen your resolve.

The drug called bupropion, available only through a doctor, is useful when part of a smoking cessation programme.

Nicotine inhaler

Skin patches

Nicotine gum

WHERE SMOKING HURTS MOST

Smokers compared with non-smokers are at risk of:

- An increased incidence of cancer, notably of the lungs, but also of the pancreas, bladder, mouth, tongue, larynx and oesophagus.
- Chronic bronchitis, emphysema and susceptibility to lung infections including tuberculosis. The transportation of oxygen by the blood is impaired, resulting in shortness of breath even in the absence of physical activity.
- Heart and circulatory diseases. Smoking leads to an increase in coronary artery disease (angina and coronary thrombosis or heart attack) and to poor peripheral circulation particularly in the legs.
- An increase in dental and gum disorders.
- A perforated ulcer, since the presence of nicotine in smoke prevents ulcers in the stomach and duodenum from healing themselves.

with the slow-acting gene NAT2 who smoke may be more likely to develop breast cancer. Percentages of women who have this gene vary according to ethnic group.

Smoking is also related to increased blood pressure (hypertension), and this in turn increases the risk of stroke, heart failure and coronary artery disease and possibly kidney damage. Cigarettes cause vascular disease (heart disease, stroke and leg gangrene) by increasing the stickiness of platelets in the blood and increasing thrombus formation, leading to narrowing of the arteries.

Smoking and childbearing

There exists a great deal of medical evidence about the dangers of smoking before conception and during pregnancy.

It is known that women who are smokers find it more difficult to conceive naturally. Miscarriages, stillbirths and infant deaths are more common when the mother smokes.

Babies are twice as likely to be born prematurely and the newborn is usually smaller and lighter than average.

WHEN YOU QUIT FOR GOOD

When you give up smoking, the returns in terms of improvements in your health begin almost immediately. If you can focus on these benefits, it will help you stop successfully.

20 MINUTES AFTER

Your blood pressure and pulse rate will fall. The temperature of your hands and feet return to normal.

8 HOURS AFTER

Carbon monoxide in the blood drops to normal. The oxygen level increases to normal.

24–48 HOURS AFTER

Your chance of heart attack decreases. Your ability to taste and smell is enhanced.

2–3 MONTHS AFTER

Your circulation improves. Walking becomes easier. Your lung function increases as much as 30 per cent.

9 MONTHS–1 YEAR AFTER

Coughing, sinus congestion, fatigue and shortness of breath decrease. Lungs are clearer and more resistant to infection. The risk of coronary heart disease is reduced to half that of a person still smoking.

3 YEARS AFTER

Risk of coronary heart disease and stroke decreases to that of people who have never smoked.

5 YEARS AFTER

The lung cancer rate for the average, former 20-per-day smoker decreases by almost half. Risk of cancer of the mouth, throat and oesophagus is half that of a smoker.

10 YEARS AFTER

The lung cancer death rate is similar to that of non-smokers. Precancerous cells are replaced. Risk of cancer of the mouth, throat, oesophagus, bladder, kidney and pancreas decreases.

The risk of congenital abnormalities, including cleft palate and limb deformities, is increased.

The overall physical and mental development of the child of a smoker may be adversely affected. Furthermore, children who become passive smokers because of their parents' smoking habits or because they are taken into smoky environments are more likely to suffer from respiratory problems, such as pneumonia, and ear problems.

DRUG ADDICTION

Substance abuse, in its numerous forms, is a major problem in modern society. Illegal drugs are one of the biggest threats to law and order in all cities, and the cycle of deprivation, addiction, sickness and despair that comes from drug abuse is well documented in the media. It is less well known that abuse of prescription drugs is even more common, especially among women, and harder to detect. Some drugs are physically and psychologically addictive; other drugs are only psychologically addictive or habit-forming.

Women suffer both from being addicted themselves and from concern for their families. Young and vulnerable children have been lured into drug use by dealers or even by their peers. Drugs may provide the adolescent with a means of escape or of rebelling against parental and other authority. Being aware of telltale signs (*see* box left) may help prevent a tragedy.

If drug use is suspected, parents should confront the child and also seek help from the family doctor or a mental health professional who can advise and guide them. The social and personal consequences of drug addiction are as bad as those of alcoholism and the legal implications may be worse.

Age is no barrier

It is not just children or young people who become addicted to drugs. Some adults can also be in danger in certain situations. An adult may begin to take a prescription drug to relieve pain and becomes addicted. Drugs used to treat chronic or long-term illness range from painkillers such as codeine to more addictive narcotics. Pressure of work or stress may lead you to try illegal drugs; adults also can be susceptible to peer pressure if people in their social circle are experimenting with drugs.

What's on the street

So-called recreational drugs usually have less serious long-term physical effects than either alcohol or tobacco. The chief risks for drug users are overdose, which is often fatal, or infection with hepatitis

B or HIV (the AIDS virus) through the sharing of dirty needles.

Narcotics Opium and opiates–including heroin ("smack" and "scag") and morphine ("morph")–are among the most addictive, both physically and psychologically, of all abused drugs. Narcotic drugs act on the body's nerve transmitters and withdrawal symptoms can be severe. Narcotics may be injected (with the attendant risk of HIV infection), taken orally or by smoke inhalation ("chasing the dragon").

Cocaine Cocaine is most familiar as a white powder ("snow", "Peruvian marching powder", "nose candy" and "coke"), which is inhaled ("snorted") through the nose. Cocaine releases a neurotransmitter that distorts the signals in the brain and produces a rush of pleasurable sensations and an increase in alertness. Cocaine is both harmful and highly addictive (particularly in the purified form called "crack"). In the long term, it causes a range of problems, such as irritability, weight loss, depression, personality changes and paranoia.

Hallucinogens Some hallucinogenic drugs (psychedelics) occur naturally, for example in peyote, mescaline and psilocybin ("magic mushrooms"). However, most are synthetic, including LSD ("acid") and PCP (phencyclidine; "angel dust"). Hallucinogens cause sensory, especially visual, distortion, and users experience intense emotions. The pupils dilate and breathing becomes erratic. Hallucinogens may also cause intense feelings of paranoia, confusion and depression, with potential consequences for psychological health. Hallucinogens are habit forming rather than addictive.

Amphetamines In night-time club culture, ecstasy ("E", "adam" and MDMA), ketamine ("K") and other drugs easily made in backstreet laboratories are popular. Some of these drugs can be altered so that they remain outside the category of proscribed substances. Amphetamines are referred to as "uppers" because they stimulate the nervous system, causing alertness, wakefulness and euphoria. They sometimes produce hallucinations. They are psychologically rather than physically addictive. Long-term abuse leads to irritability, personality changes and paranoia.

Cannabis Also known as marijuana, hash or hashish, pot and grass, cannabis is one of the least addictive and most widespread of illegal drugs. It is usually smoked, in herbal form or as a resin, and produces feelings of relaxation, euphoria, disorientation and sometimes causes hallucinations. It can cause sudden food cravings (the "munchies"), sleepiness and, occasionally, paranoia. It is dangerous mainly because it may act as an introduction to drug culture.

Solvent abuse Solvent abuse, or glue sniffing, is most common among young teenagers, particularly boys. The most frequently used solvents are glues containing toluene or acetone, nail polish remover, butane lighter fuels and some aerosols. Fumes are generally inhaled from a plastic bag held over the face. Symptoms are similar to those of alcohol. A visible rash may also develop around the mouth and nose. High doses may cause hallucinations and coma and can, in severe cases, lead to permanent loss of coordination or death. Solvents are not addictive; most abusers grow out of the habit.

Take prescribed pills with care

Drugs that your doctor may prescribe for you can be addictive. These are usually prescribed for acute or chronic pain and for anxiety or depression. You should be aware of this risk when you are prescribed any painkiller or mood-altering medication and ask your doctor about its effects. When you are taking any of these drugs, you should monitor your responses closely to check for signs of dependence.

Narcotic drugs include opium derivatives–morphine, codeine, methadone and other drugs such as oxycodone–and are often prescribed for the relief of severe pain. People with terminal cancer or other illness do not become addicted.

Amphetamines (commonly known as "pep pills") are sometimes prescribed as treatment for depression, chronic fatigue and, because they suppress the appetite, obesity.

Benzodiazepines and barbiturates (otherwise known as sedatives) are used in the treatment of insomnia, anxiety and depression. This group contains some of the most commonly abused drugs including chlordiazepoxide, diazepam, temazepam, secobarbital and phenobarbital. They are known as "downers" from their tranquillizing and sedative effects, producing relaxation, mood-enhancement, occasionally euphoria and, only in rare cases, hallucinations. Large doses can cause confusion, coma and death. PCP (phencyclidine or "angel dust") causes hallucinations and other extreme physical and psychological effects.

Probably the most common mood-altering drugs prescribed for women are antidepressants. Some are selective serotonin reuptake inhibitors (SSRIs) such as fluoxetine. While not addictive in the same way as hard drugs, withdrawal can cause confusion and depression.

Cannabis has been prescribed to control nausea in cancer patients undergoing chemotherapy and in the management of chronic pain, muscle spasm (as in multiple sclerosis) and anxiety (in Parkinson's disease). Many health professionals support its use as a prescription drug and clinical trials are being conducted to assess its effects and safety for medical use.

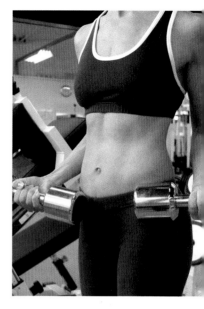

STEROIDS AND HORMONES
The use of drugs in sports has caused controversy worldwide. Anabolic steroids are synthetic hormones taken to increase energy, build muscle bulk and to prolong stamina. Apart from giving the user a physical advantage over the non-user, they may have lasting, adverse effects on the body such as damage to the liver.

WITHDRAWAL AND REHAB

There are two stages in the treatment of a person who is addicted—withdrawal and rehabilitation.

The withdrawal symptoms caused by some types of drugs—notably narcotics and tranquilizers—can be severe. They include sweating, diarrhoea, nausea, vomiting, abdominal cramps, goose pimples, running eyes and nose, yawning, irritability, sleeplessness, confusion, anxiety and depression. Symptoms can last for a week or more, and medical supervision is often necessary. Sometimes a less addictive substitute, such as methadone in the case of withdrawal from narcotics, may be given in decreasing doses to ease the severity of the symptoms.

Rehabilitation and the prevention of relapse require a programme of long-term maintenance. This generally involves counselling or psychotherapy. It is virtually impossible without the active help of family members or a support group and without strong motivation on the part of the former addict. Some form of behaviour therapy, such as aversion therapy, may be effective, so that the addict begins to associate the substance with nausea or disgust. There are many self-help groups, including Narcotics Anonymous, that offer support and therapy often from ex-addicts.

EATING DISORDERS

Overeating and excessive dieting both increase a woman's health risks, but the problem becomes even greater when these preoccupations become obsessive. Women are especially vulnerable to eating disorders involving their weight, self-esteem and self-image.

Anorexia nervosa

Although usually associated with adolescent girls, anorexia nervosa, which means "nervous loss of appetite", can occur at any age and in either sex. However, it is about 10 times more common in women than in men.

There may be a genetic component to the disease, since it tends to run in families. It is associated, too, with a family history of serious depression– nearly half of all anorexics are clinically depressed. Almost as many people show obsessive-compulsive symptoms, which often afflict other members of the family. The condition is particularly common in women whose ideal of female beauty is linked to an image of thinness.

Anorexics often come from families in which the parents are extremely strict or over-protective. They often claim that dieting gives them greater control over their lives, especially during the teen years or young adulthood when it may feel as if other aspects of their lives are uncontrollable. Sufferers may be perfectionists and less sociable than their peers. Dieting to excess may be a form of rebellion, a way to reject their

DID YOU KNOW?

Anorexics do not, in fact, lose their appetite until the late stages of the illness, but their interest in food may be diverted into food-related activities such as cooking for others, hiding food, collecting recipes or obsessive calorie counting.

SIGNS OF ANOREXIA NERVOSA

Anorexics usually deny that there is anything wrong with them. The following are all strong indications that someone is suffering from anorexia nervosa:

- Loss of weight to a level below 85 per cent of normal for the individual's age and height. Most anorexics are usually 25 per cent or more below normal weight.

- Excessive concern over gaining weight or becoming fat. Anorexics have no ability to perceive their own body weight and shape correctly; they see normal weight as fat. Even when they are painfully thin, they insist that they are fat.

- Physical debility due to starvation, including low blood pressure, tiredness, anaemia, constipation, brittle bones (osteoporosis), swollen joints, yellowing of the skin and sensitivity to cold. Anorexics often wear layers of baggy clothes to disguise their thinness and in order to keep warm. Fine body hair called lanugo appears, possibly to retain the body's heat.

- Menstruation may not begin or will cease if body weight is below about 80 per cent of normal. Missing three or more periods in a row is a strong indication of anorexia.

- Anorexics may take laxatives and emetics (which prevent proper absorption of food). They often avoid eating in public and may also exercise obsessively, often at night and in private, where nobody can see them.

WHO'S AT RISK?
Eating disorders are most often encountered in young women who are going through emotional upheavals associated with adolescence or lifestyle pressures in their early 20s. A family history of parental control or emotional starvation can be factors. Often there may be, in fact, a family history of eating problems.

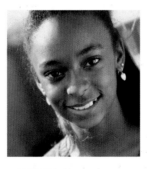

PUBERTY
Anorexia nervosa is very common in teenagers and affects more than 1 in 100 school and university students aged 15 to 25.

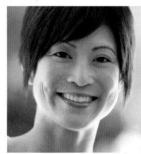

20s
In this age group women may tend to either anorexia or bulimia. Obsession with food can be a substitute for a satisfying emotional life.

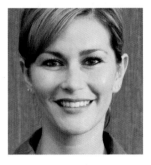

30s–40s
Women in this age group are more rarely affected by anorexia but may be driven by depression to bulimia or compulsive overeating.

parents' care and a means of asserting their own individuality. Since anorexia suppresses menstruation and often begins around the age of puberty, it may also be a way of avoiding the cares and responsibilities of growing up by remaining in childhood. What is clear is that anorexia is a sign of an underlying psychological disorder, often triggered by some stressful life event.

How anorexia is treated

If the condition is life-threatening–if, for example, the anorexic has a pulse rate of less than 40–she may have to be treated in a hospital. Intravenous feeding is often needed, and this requires the cooperation of the patient.

SSRI antidepressants may be prescribed to raise levels of serotonin. Serotonin is a chemical transmitter in the brain that regulates mood). SSRIs can alleviate depression and anxiety.

In addition, long-term counselling or psychotherapy will be necessary, often over many months or years. Therapy may consist of private sessions or include the family, followed by group sessions so that problems can be expressed and shared. The purpose of therapy is to help the anorexic feel deserving of love, enhance her self-esteem and lessen her need to be in control. She can also learn strategies to assist her through difficult times, such as family meals, parties and other social situations.

The outlook for recovery is not good. Only about half of all patients recover completely after four years and about a quarter remain severely underweight. In this group, the risk of suicide, heart attack or starving to death is high.

Binge eating and bulimia

More women than men, particularly young women, suffer from these related disorders. An excess of food is eaten, then it is purged from the body. Binge eaters are seized by an uncontrollable craving for food, which they consume– usually in secret–in vast quantities at a single sitting. As well as inducing vomiting, bingers may use laxatives, enemas, diuretics and excessive physical exercise to control weight. Between binges, most will diet strictly. Unlike anorexics, binge eaters have a realistic perception of their weight and are generally motivated by a desire to lose excess fat. Most binge eaters have a history of dieting. Recurrent episodes of bingeing (two or three a week) over an extended period (three months or more) can be defined as bulimia. The common characteristics of "bulimics" include a stressful event that acts as a trigger, another form of mental problem–such as depression or a personality disorder– or drug or alcohol problems. There may have been sexual abuse in the past.

A family history of depression may be a factor in both anorexia and bulimia. Some physical signs specific to bulimia include grazed knuckles (from sticking the fingers in the throat to induce vomiting), infection of the salivary glands, pitting of the teeth (due to acid in the vomit) and bleeding in the stomach. Mineral imbalances caused by constant vomiting may have serious side effects, such as an irregular heart beat. However, bulimia rarely causes death.

Bulimics are less secretive and less inclined to deny the problem than anorexics and so are more easily treated by long-term counselling or behavioural or cognitive therapy. SSRIs can be useful. Psychoanalysis may be recommended if past sexual abuse is an underlying cause.

Compulsive overeating

Compulsive overeating also involves eating binges, but they are not usually followed by purging. Compulsive overeaters are normally overweight. The condition is associated with guilt, shame, stress, low self-esteem and an obsession with body shape. It may result from fear of having to compete with other women.

When obesity is life-threatening–if blood pressure is seriously high–drastic measures are sought, such as surgically reducing the size of the stomach.

Treatment of compulsive eating generally requires therapy or counselling. Cognitive and behavioural therapies are usually the most successful. Many people also find that self-help groups such as Weight Watchers, where problems are discussed with those who are similarly affected, can help enormously to restore and maintain healthy eating habits.

SIGNS OF COMPULSIVE OVEREATING

- An urge to eat when not hungry—for example, eating to relieve feelings of depression, boredom or unhappiness
- Being constantly preoccupied with food
- An abnormal interest in dietary information in books and magazines
- Alternate episodes of dieting and overeating
- Feelings of guilt at being unable to control the craving for food
- Being ashamed of your weight and body shape

Mind and Mood

Fears, worries, sadness and depression are common and make life difficult. An event that triggers these moods can even be forgotten while the mood itself remains. Fortunately, each of these challenges has a variety of solutions to overcome it.

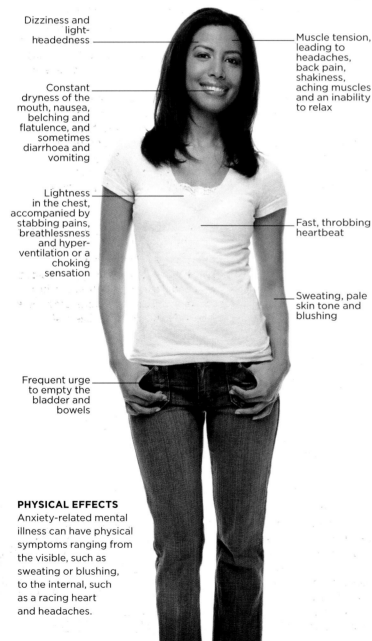

Dizziness and light-headedness

Muscle tension, leading to headaches, back pain, shakiness, aching muscles and an inability to relax

Constant dryness of the mouth, nausea, belching and flatulence, and sometimes diarrhoea and vomiting

Lightness in the chest, accompanied by stabbing pains, breathlessness and hyper-ventilation or a choking sensation

Fast, throbbing heartbeat

Sweating, pale skin tone and blushing

Frequent urge to empty the bladder and bowels

PHYSICAL EFFECTS
Anxiety-related mental illness can have physical symptoms ranging from the visible, such as sweating or blushing, to the internal, such as a racing heart and headaches.

FEARS AND WORRIES

Everyone is familiar with those sensations, such as a dry mouth, pounding heart, rapid breathing and sweating, that occur when you are in a threatening or unpleasant situation. Anxiety is the normal reaction to stress; in fact, its presence is what defines a situation or event as stressful. Anxiety may be harmless or even useful. A reasonable degree of anxiety before an exam or interview is likely to help you perform better. However, if the anxiety becomes so severe that it interferes with everyday life, it becomes an illness that requires treatment.

Who's at risk?

Anxiety appears to affect women more than men and there may be an inherited disposition. It may also stem from early experiences of deprivation—loss of or separation from parents, for example, or a perceived lack of parental attention while growing up. This is particularly the case when current events in an older person's life seem to mirror an earlier traumatic experience.

Personality may be a factor. Some of us are born worriers. Those with rigid and perfectionist personalities or excessively meek and submissive personalities are most vulnerable.

Physiologically, anxiety is thought to be related to an excess of the hormone noradrenaline—a transmitter of nerve impulses—in the brain. There are also some physical conditions, such as disorders of the thyroid gland and oestrogen deficiency during and after the menopause, that can cause or mimic the effects of anxiety.

A feeling of foreboding

Throughout life you have to deal with stressful events that cause some degree of anxiety, for example, if someone you love is ill or a relationship breaks down, if you lose your job or move.

Most people are able to get through the bad time and eventually the anxiety dwindles and ceases. But in susceptible individuals, the symptoms may reach disabling proportions–then known as adjustment disorders–and become persistent. This is genuine mental illness.

There are common symptoms that should be watched for. Prominent is a feeling of foreboding, sometimes amounting to unfounded dread or terror. There may be nervousness, irritability and jumpiness. The person appears to worry constantly, has regular insomnia and subsequent feelings of exhaustion. She shows a fear of physical illness, reinforced by the physical symptoms of anxiety. These may lead to periods of feeling detached from the outside world (depersonalization) or of feeling that the outside world is unreal (derealization).

Obsessions and compulsions

People with obsessions are unable to prevent certain thoughts or ideas from recurring constantly and persistently. Common forms of obsession involve cleanliness, tidiness and doubts about whether particular tasks have been performed. The obsession leads to the performance of ritualized, repetitive actions–compulsions–for example, constant washing of the hands or endlessly checking that all doors and windows are locked, even returning home to do so.

Obsessives are aware that their behaviour is irrational and time-wasting, but are unable to control it. Obsessions are a learned response to anxiety. They also appear to be linked with disorders of brain chemistry, specifically with the serotonin system. Serotonin is implicated in depression and some antidepressant drugs have proven to be useful in the management of inherited obsessive-compulsive disorders.

Coping with a panic attack

One of the most frightening manifestations of anxiety is a panic attack. In this, the anxiety caused by the initial situation is compounded by the fear caused by the symptoms themselves. The increased anxiety further increases the fear, in a vicious circle that rapidly spirals out of control and the person becomes convinced she is having a heart attack or a stroke or that she is going insane.

Panic attacks, however, can be arrested before they reach this stage. Once you recognize the signs, you can take corrective measures.

Mentally, you need to find something to distract your attention from the anxiety you feel. If you're on a street, focus on an advertising board, read every word on it, and think of its meaning. Or concentrate on an activity or conversation going on around you. If you're alone, think of the birthday of every member of your family.

Physically, you need to take action to slow the rate of breathing to combat hyperventilation (overbreathing).

Try deep breathing (see below). Alternatively, breathe in and out of a paper bag held over the mouth and nose for several minutes. This will reduce the intake of oxygen and increase the intake of carbon dioxide. Soon your normal breathing will be restored and your heart will stop racing. Here's how it works:

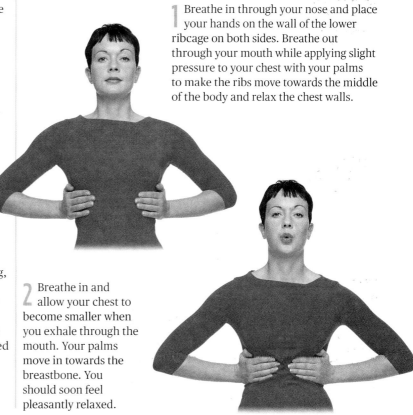

1 Breathe in through your nose and place your hands on the wall of the lower ribcage on both sides. Breathe out through your mouth while applying slight pressure to your chest with your palms to make the ribs move towards the middle of the body and relax the chest walls.

2 Breathe in and allow your chest to become smaller when you exhale through the mouth. Your palms move in towards the breastbone. You should soon feel pleasantly relaxed.

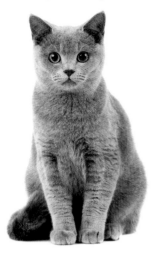

ELIMINATE FEAR TRIGGERS
Anything, even a fluffy affectionate cat, can be the cause of a phobia in susceptible people whose fear may stem from a childhood experience. The best way to learn to cope with such triggers is through desensitization therapy.

Phobias

Irrational fears of objects or situations are phobias. People may be phobic about particular animals, such as cats, spiders or birds, or about specific situations, such as heights, enclosed spaces (for example, lifts) or flying. Most phobias are inconvenient rather than severely disruptive. Some such as agoraphobia (fear of open spaces) and social phobia (dread of being seen by other people), are symptoms of more generalized anxiety and can affect all aspects of life.

Phobias are learned responses to a stimulus. They may result from an unpleasant or traumatizing experience in childhood, being bittten by a dog, for example, or sometimes they may be learnt from parents or other adults.

Mere anticipation of a situation is enough to arouse fear and then failure to confront and deal with it intensifies the anxiety. In the worst cases, the only way the person sees to control the fear is to avoid the situation ever arising. This can give rise to complete withdrawal and can reach the stage of being life-threatening.

Effective stress management can help to reduce anxiety in many situations.

Other disorders

A number of factors can cause anxiety and be a symptom of it. Physical health is one of the most important of these. Some disorders, for example, an overactive thyroid gland, cause anxiety as a direct symptom of the disease. Anxiety is also a fairly common reaction to serious illness.

Difficulties with personal and work relationships and sexual problems are also both a symptom and a cause of anxiety. Conversely, several mental conditions manifest themselves as physical symptoms.

Hypochondria   This is a condition in which people obsessively worry about their health and may display symptoms that appear to have a psychological rather than a physical cause. They interpret minor ailments as symptoms of more serious disease and constantly seek medical advice and help.

Somatization   In some cases, anxiety is experienced and expressed in terms of physical symptoms. These, generally, take the form of vague, unidentifiable illness. Somatization is thought to be the result of an inability to deal mentally with stress and anxiety.

Dissociative disorder   Also called conversion reaction, this used to be known as hysteria. Physical symptoms–often unusual ones, such as temporary blindness or the loss of the use of a limb–have no apparent cause. However, the inability to find a physical cause does not necessarily mean that there isn't one.

Post-traumatic stress

Survivors and witnesses of terrible, violent or shocking events–train or plane crashes, earthquakes, random shootings, battle, terrorism, assault–can often suffer from a form of anxiety known as post-traumatic stress. The condition is characterized by recurrent memories and images of the event, development of phobias about things associated with the event, disturbed sleep and other psychological symptoms of anxiety. There may be feelings of guilt, about having survived when others did not, and depression, which may become severe. The symptoms may develop soon after the event or they may not appear until months or years later.

Treatment may involve various different approaches including psychotherapy, cognitive behavioural techniques, desensitization and psychopharmacological medications. Eventually the person comes to terms with the event and is able to remember it without distressing symptoms.

What can you do?

One cause of anxiety is stress and an important aspect of treatment is learning how to cope with stress. Effective stress management can help to reduce anxiety in many situations, but sometimes professional treatment may be needed. There are two main types of treatment: counselling or psychotherapy, and drugs. The aim of therapy is to unlearn the inappropriate response. Complementary and alternative therapies such as massage and acupuncture may also have a role.

GET IT CHECKED

Sometimes there's a physical cause of some of the symptoms that appear to come from fears and worries. That's why it's always good to discuss any symptoms with your doctor at the earliest opportunity.

Behavioural therapy   Phobias and obsessions may be treated using a specialized form of behaviour therapy that involves gradual desensitization through increasing exposure to the feared object or situation. An alternative technique is flooding: the person is made to confront the situation head-on, with a trained therapist always present to deal with the acute anxiety that may result.

Drug assistance   Behavioural therapy may also be used in conjunction with a course of drugs. Three types of drugs are commonly used. Beta-blockers can help to counteract the physical effects of anxiety. They reduce the activity of the autonomic nervous system, so slowing down breathing and heart rate and reducing tension. Antidepressant and anti-anxiety medications are the mainstays of drug treatment and can be beneficial both for acute situations and chronic cases. A combination of psychotherapy and medication is often the most successful.

Treatment of anxiety disorders has a good success rate. Many cases are completely cured, and most show some degree of improvement.

Harness your mind

Many people find that relaxation training can help with anxiety-related disorders. Trained hypnotherapists induce a state of deep relaxation and then encourage the patient to feel relaxed and stress free. Patients can also be trained in self-hypnosis. In biofeedback, sensors on the body measure various functions such as brain waves, heart rate and muscle tension. The patient can learn to produce changes in these functions first through watching the meters and then gradually without the meters.

BE KIND

It's important to remember that someone whose symptoms are mainly in the mind suffers as much pain and discomfort as she would if there were a genuine physical cause. Both the physical discomfort and the underlying cause need to be treated.

SWITCH OFF STRESS

A form of self-suggestion or self-hypnosis that can be practised at home or at work or whenever you are threatened by stress or anxiety, autogenic training (AT) can help stress-related conditions such as migraine and irritable bowel syndrome. It can also be used to combat addictions such as smoking.

You have to receive training in AT by attending 8 to 10 sessions with a trained practitioner, who teaches you some exercises to switch off stress in the body. In each of these exercises, you suggest to yourself the physical state you want to induce and gradually let it develop.

The exercises are geared to general relaxation as well as your specific needs. So, with phobias, you would concentrate on calming the breathing and heart rate and then suggest to yourself that the object of fear was not too frightening, after all.

Some suggestions of phrases you can repeat to yourself for several minutes to encourage relaxation include:

- My heartbeat is strong and slow.
- My stomach is warm.
- My forehead is cool.
- My breathing is slow and calm.
- My muscles are limp and relaxed.
- My limbs are heavy and warm.
- I'm getting more and more relaxed.

TRY THERAPY

Talking through symptoms, problems and reactions is part of the treatment for anxiety-related disorders. Therapists—particularly those certified in cognitive behavioural therapy or CBT—can provide you with individualized strategies to control fears and worries.

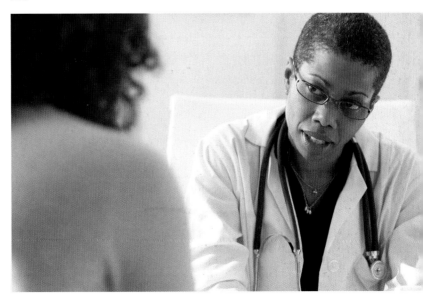

167

WOMEN AND STRESS

Stress acts as a stimulus to performance and makes you more alert and aware. However, there is a point–and that point is different for each person–at which the beneficial effects are outweighed by the anxiety. At this stage the body is stressed by events and, over time, this can lead to serious physical repercussions, one of which is heart disease.

How the body reacts

Within minutes of the immediate release of fight or flight hormones by the adrenal glands other reactions to the situation follow. The hippocampus in the brain activates memory and learning, so that you can remember and deal with the situation if it recurs.

In the immune system, activity shuts down, so that energy can be used for fight or flight. The liver quickly converts stored fat to fuel that can be used by the body and the adrenal glands continue to release hormones.

The problem is that the effects can become chronic and affect health.

STRESS REACTIONS
A stressful situation can trigger the release of adrenaline, which fuels the fight or flight response. However, in modern life we generally do not respond to stressful situations by fighting or running away, but our body may go on reacting, causing chronic effects that can be toxic.

Hair
Follicles react causing hair to stand on end or puff up

Eyes
The pupils dilate to make vision clearer

Lungs
These respond by taking in more oxygen

Liver
Glycogen stored here is converted quickly to glucose (blood sugar) for energy

Brain
To protect the body, the sense of pain is reduced, but thinking and memory improve

Heart
With extra oxygen and glucose to transport around the body, the heart rate increases

Spleen
The spleen releases more blood cells to increase the amount of oxygen the blood can carry

Digestive system
The digestion process stops, so that motor muscles have more available energy to use

Ongoing production of the hormone cortisol by the adrenal glands can be damaging to the brain, the immune system, the intestines and the circulatory system. Infections are not fought, memory and emotions are adversely affected, digestion is upset and blood pressure rises (which can damage the heart and blood vessels).

Measuring stress

Many life happenings can cause stress–and not all of them need be unpleasant. Even propitious events, such as going on holiday or getting married, can cause stress. And stress is cumulative. The stress caused by losing your job is not displaced by the stress of loss of income, it adds to it. Since stress is closely related to anxiety and susceptibility to physical illness, it helps to be aware of situations that contribute to changes in the way your body functions.

In the 1960s, two American researchers Thomas H. Holmes and Richard H. Rahe devised a frequently used scale to measure the impact of stress. They ranked common stress-inducing life events in order of their effects on the body and gave each a score on a scale of 1 to 100–the higher the figure the greater the stress. The theory is that the total score in any one 12-month period accurately predicts the likelihood of future illness.

Apparently straightforward events can turn out to be surprisingly stressful when all factors involved are taken into account. Getting married, for example, may mean moving home, changing financial circumstances, gaining new members of the family which, in combination with other events, result in a high level of cumulative risk.

Women only

Some stressful life events or more long-term problems are specific to women. Infertility or even the lack of children as a result of a conscious decision can cause anxiety and feelings of low self-esteem. Tests have shown that infertility may have as great an effect on a woman's psyche as a life-threatening illness. On the other hand, stress can lead to infertility, probably because the adrenal hormones released by stress affect the reproductive hormones.

Bringing up a family is also a potentially stressful job. This can be worse if trying to work outside of the home as well. When children are very young, if the mother does not have adequate support, she may feel trapped by the situation. She needs to be able to get out of the house, to have childcare taken off her hands every so often and possibly to have the support and company of other mothers. Another time of crisis is when her children are teenagers and she may be worrying about their future or feel that they no longer respond to her care or control.

Girls or women commonly suffer from sexually or physically abusive situations.

This may happen when the child is too young to be able to act for herself and will have repercussions throughout her life. When she is older, a woman may enter an abusive relationship, often

High stress levels carry a 35 to 50 per cent increase to the risk that an illness will develop over the next two years.

because of low self-esteem. Or she may be exposed to sexual harassment in the workplace. These events can cause severe stress or depression which may need long-term therapy to overcome.

HOW STRESSED ARE YOU?

To assess your stress level and the risk of illness developing, check off the events that have happened to you in the previous 12 months, and then add up your total score. Each successive event will add to your stress level. You may have to accept some things, but be able to alter others.

RANK	EVENT	POINTS
1	Death of spouse or partner	100
2	Divorce	73
3	Marital separation	65
4	Prison term	63
5	Death of family member	63
6	Personal injury	53
7	Marriage	50
8	Loss of job	47
9	Marital reconciliation	45
10	Retirement	45
11	Change in health of family member	44
12	Pregnancy	40
13	Sexual problems	39
14	Gain new family member	39
15	Changes at work or in business	39
16	Change in financial circumstances	39
17	Death of close friend	37
18	Change to new line of work	36
19	Change in frequency of arguments with spouse or partner	35
20	Having a large mortgage	33

RANK	EVENT	POINTS
21	Child leaves home	29
22	Trouble with in-laws	29
23	Outstanding personal achievement	28
24	Spouse or partner begins or ends work	26
25	Begin or finish school	26
26	Change in living conditions	25
27	Change in personal habits	24
28	Trouble with employer	23
29	Change in working hours or conditions	20
30	Moving house	20
31	Moving school	20
32	Change in recreation	19
33	Change in religious activity	19
34	Change in social activity	18
35	Having a small mortgage	17
36	Change in sleeping habits	16
37	Change in number of family get-togethers	15
38	Change in eating habits	15
39	Going on holiday	13
40	Christmas	12
41	Minor law violation	11

0 to 100 points
Low stress levels rarely cause problems. At 100 points, there is a small increase to the risk that an illness will develop over the next two years.

100 to 200 points
Moderate levels of stress carry a 10 to 35 per cent increase to the risk of an illness occurring over the next two years.

200 to 300 points
High stress levels carry a 35 to 50 per cent increase to the risk that an illness will develop over the next two years.

300 plus points
With extremely high stress levels, there is a strong probability—80 to 90 per cent—of illness developing over the next two years.

WOMEN AND DEPRESSION

Depression kills. And women are especially vulnerable to it.

For many of us, depression may be transient and mild–a feeling of dissatisfaction, self-doubt, a loss of energy and enthusiasm and a sense that life is pointless.

Many people will suffer deeper symptoms for a while, for example,

Surgery and medication can both have depression as a side effect.

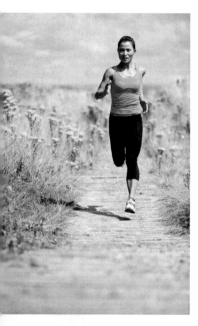

MOVE!
Twenty minutes of daily vigorous physical activity can help beat depression. Outdoor activity is best because sunlight can trigger chemical changes in the brain.

after a bereavement or divorce. However, there are times when these feelings escalate into something more serious–overwhelming feelings of loss, sadness, guilt and despair. There may be physical symptoms, such as loss of weight and appetite, lethargy and fatigue, which become real obstacles to leading a normal life. At this stage, depression becomes a serious brain disorder.

Women and depression

Depression occurs in all age groups, but it is more common from young adulthood up to middle age. In the age group over 65, it begins to diminish. It is twice as common in women as in men and between 10 and 25 per cent of women will at some time in their lives suffer from it. The gender difference is found in severe depression/depressive disorder and in various other types of depression such as dysthymia (mild depression), seasonal affective disorder (SAD) and rapid-cycling bipolar disorder (rapid mood swings).

The difference in incidence of depression between women and men begins after puberty and is probably linked to hormonal changes. Women are also more susceptible to depression at times of hormonal activity such as the premenstrual phase, after giving birth and during perimenopause. Depression at the menopause and later years may be more linked to social factors such as retirement from work or children leaving home, although investigation continues.

The part hormones play in depression is not wholly clear. The hormones oestrogen and progesterone affect the levels of two of the neurotransmitters called serotonin and noradrenaline in the central nervous system. Bouts of depression appear to be associated with low levels of these transmitters. The same hormones regulate the body's cycle of metabolism throughout the day and this may be the reason why some women appear to be much more susceptible than men to SAD–their metabolic rate slows in the hours of darkness.

Women's self-esteem tends to be based on relationships with others rather than having firm foundations in their own personalities. This is also associated with women being less esteemed in society and, especially in more traditional cultures, being given a restricted role to play. Women and men also appear to respond differently to drug treatment with antidepressants, presumably again because of hormonal differences, and women are likely to have recurring depressive episodes.

What causes depression?

Depression can be triggered by various factors separately or a combination of factors. The two main causes of the disorder are traumatic events and inherent predisposition. The genetic linkage to a tendency to depression has been well demonstrated in studies with twins. Traumatic life events may include events in the past, such as loss of a parent in childhood or, even more powerfully, recent events, such as a breakdown of a relationship or the death of a family member. Physical illness can often cause depression, especially if it is long-term or life-threatening, such as multiple sclerosis or cancer. But in addition depression can follow a viral illness, such as flu. It may feature in chronic fatigue syndrome (myalgic encephalomyelitis, also known as ME or post-viral syndrome) and may be linked with another psychological condition such as a panic disorder.

Surgery and medication can both have depression as a side effect. Drugs, including oral contraceptives, some tranquillizers and surgical anaesthetics, can cause depression. Alcohol and drug abuse can be symptoms or causes of depression and, in the extreme, lead to suicide. Anxiety and depression are also common symptoms of withdrawal from drugs or alcohol.

Events in a woman's life can give rise to depressive phases or sometimes a more long-term disorder. Childbirth triggers depression in more than half of all new mothers. Menstruation and the menopause are times when women may feel emotionally low as well as physically uncomfortable. More traumatic events, such as an abortion or a hysterectomy, may be followed by a bout of depression. Infertility, or the inability to have children, can also produce severe depression, which may become chronic.

Generally, older people are less prone to depression, although bereavement or loneliness are common causes of sadness in the elderly.

Lack of daylight can cause SAD ("winter blues"), a form of depression that occurs during prolonged periods of daylight deprivation such as winter. SAD can be treated by antidepressant medication or regular exposure to natural light. There are lights available that simulate natural daylight.

Risk factors

There are several reasons why some people are more likely to develop depression than others.

Genetics Depression appears to have a strong inherited component. With identical twins, if one is depressed there's a 60 per cent chance that their twin will also be. In a family with a history of severe depression, about one in eight of family members are likely to develop the condition. The greater susceptibility of women may be linked to female sex genes.

Abnormal brain chemistry Two substances in particular are known to be involved in depression: the neurotransmitters serotonin and noradrenaline. During intervals of depression, the levels of both chemicals are low and this is thought to lead to the transmission of faulty messages, which is responsible for some of the symptoms of depressive illness. Drugs that increase

ARE YOU DEPRESSED?

See your doctor immediately if you suspect you're depressed. There are a number of observable symptoms that suggest the disorder, which are:

- Lethargy and listlessness—sufferers are sometimes unable to summon the energy to go out or to get out of bed.
- Change in appetite and weight, which demonstrates a lack of interest in food, compounded by constipation, or an increased dependence on "comfort" eating, especially carbohydrates.
- Loss of interest in sex.
- Disturbed sleep and insomnia. Sleep is intermittent and interrupted by constant worrying.
- Depression tends to be worse in the morning (except with sufferers of SAD) with an elevation of mood toward the end of the day.
- Inability to concentrate.
- Anxiety, with possible trembling or panic attacks.
- Low self-esteem, perhaps coupled with irrational guilt.
- Slowing of mental and physical activity. Speech may become soft, halting and monotone, without emphasis or inflection, often tailing off into silence. Movement may be reluctant and requires effort, often with a slow, shuffling gait.
- Mental confusion including forgetfulness, irrational thinking and disorientation occurs particularly in older people. The symptoms may be mistaken for dementia.
- Thoughts of death and suicide.
- Delusions and hallucinations are symptoms of serious psychotic depression.

the brain levels of serotonin and noradrenaline have been used successfully in treating the illness.

Social and environmental factors Social deprivation, poor living conditions and alcohol or drug addiction are all known to contribute to depression. Unemployed single mothers without adequate emotional or physical support from family or friends often become depressed, for example.

Getting out from depression

Anyone who suspects she's depressed should see a doctor.

Many people get through a period of depression simply by talking to friends and relatives, joining a self-help group or reading books and following the advice they offer. People who need more help should make an appointment to see their doctor. Depending on the severity of the symptoms and the type of depression, the doctor is then likely to recommend one or more of three types of treatment.

Drugs   There are various types of antidepressants, including SSRIs (selective serotonin reuptake inhibitors) such as fluoxetine. SSRIs help to maintain the levels of serotonin in the brain and are relatively free of side effects. Drugs are important in relieving mood and physical symptoms, but they do not tackle the underlying emotional or psychological problems.

Therapy or counselling   The long-term treatment of depression normally involves identifying and dealing with the problems that caused it in the first place. The most effective form of therapy is usually cognitive. This is a form of behaviour therapy in which treatment corrects habits of thought rather than patterns of behaviour. Cognitive therapy can replace negative perceptions with more positive accurate ones, so reversing the destructive spiral caused by constant depressive thinking. Psychotherapy or psychoanalysis seek deeper hidden causes of depression, often going back to childhood memories. It is a long process and may not work for everyone.

Electroconvulsive therapy   This involves administering electric currents to the brain through electrodes attached to the head. It is only used in severe depression when other treatments have failed, or when there is an immediate danger to the patient's health, for example from suicide. It is successful in many cases. Treatment is generally only given after full hospital evaluation and there will need to be support facilities available at home or in the community.

Postnatal depression

Mood change after having a baby can be mild and short lived–"the baby blues"–or very severe–puerperal psychosis. Between these extremes lies postnatal depression (PND), which can vary in severity. The risk of postnatal depression is higher in the first few weeks after having a baby. The precise incidence and prevalence of perinatal depression is uncertain. Recent research estimates 13 new mothers in every 100 get postnatal depression. About 1 to 3 in every 1,000 get puerperal psychosis, the symptoms of which are similar to other forms of depression and may include delusional beliefs–that the mother has the wrong baby, for example–and hallucinations. If there is any danger that the mother may hurt her baby or herself, she should seek help immediately. A family member who recognizes the symptoms should not ignore the situation. Tact and sympathy should be used to encourage the mother to see her doctor. At this time, practical and uncritical emotional support from friends and family is essential.

The doctor may prescribe antidepressants or tranquillizers to deal with the more debilitating symptoms. SSRIs may also be prescribed for 6 to 12 months. They have few side effects and can prevent future episodes. Sleep is important and help or medication may both be necessary to ensure the mother gets enough rest. The doctor will also probably recommend counselling to deal with deep-seated or long-lasting effects. In severe cases, in-patient psychiatric treatment may be required, especially where safety issues are involved.

The "baby blues"

Half or more of all mothers experience mild depression, called postnatal depression, after the birth of a baby. They feel generally low, tired and listless. They may cry for no particular reason and they may feel worried and tense. They may also experience unexplained pains and feel generally unwell.

Hormonal changes following childbirth are generally the cause, but other factors may be equally important.

Many mothers are unprepared for the exhaustion that follows childbirth and may not have fully appreciated the impact that a baby, particularly their first, will have on their lives. Any uncertainty about the child's health or problems before or after the birth will be magnified greatly. Psychological and physical support are needed so that the mother gets both help and rest. In most cases the symptoms pass in a few days. However, if they persist or get worse, a doctor should be immediately consulted.

HEADACHES

Many women experience recurrent headaches that may be a response to problems such as tiredness, hunger, dehydration, menstrual problems or a medical condition. Treatment is often more successful than finding the cause.

In medical terms, there are three main types of headache: tension (muscle-contraction), migraine (vascular) and combination (tension and migraine).

In some cases, the symptoms may be due to a disease or disorder, in which case they are known as secondary headaches. Sinusitis, for example, often produces a throbbing headache. It helps to identify which one afflicts you so you can take the appropriate action.

What causes yours?

Tension is one of the main causes of headaches in 90 per cent of people. It affects women three times more often than men. Mental strain produces muscular tension and results in low-level aches, often on both sides of the head, forehead and the back of the neck. They usually last for no more than a few hours, but can continue for as long as a week. Pain is usually moderate.

Hormonal factors may trigger tension headaches from adolescence on. They can appear either before or during menstruation and some women may develop them at and during the menopause. Oestrogen is a known cause for headache sufferers taking the oral contraceptive pill and using some types of hormone replacement therapy (HRT). A gynaecological problem, such as ovarian cysts, may be a cause.

A bacterial or viral infection or parasitic infestation can often have headache as a symptom, particularly where there is fever. Examples include influenza, pyelonephritis and generalized infections, such as measles, ear, nose and throat infections, dental problems and shingles. Headaches may also signal rare but potentially life-threatening conditions.

Infection or inflammation of the lining of the sinuses–the air-filled cavities on either side of the nose–causes a dull pain in the upper cheeks, around the eyes or across the forehead. Sinus headaches may be accompanied by fever and a congested nose. They are made worse by bending over and can intensify when barometric pressure and temperature rise.

Cervical degenerative disease (affecting the upper spine) and neck pain can cause spasm in muscles in the base of the skull and going forwards to the forehead. These muscle spasms can cause headaches.

Temporomandibular joint syndrome (TMJ) is a jaw malfunction that can affect different areas of the head–including the temples, cheeks, ears and the back of the neck. TMJ involves the joint on both sides of the head that connects the jaw bone to the skull. Women aged between 25 and 40 are most prone to TMJ, which usually results from clenching the jaw or grinding the teeth, often while asleep. Malocclusion (when the upper and lower teeth fail to meet properly), other orthodontic problems or dislocation of the jaw are other causes of TMJ.

FEEL THE PAIN

There are many causes of a headache, but when one occurs all you want to do is get rid of it. Pain can be felt in different areas of the head—at the temples, on the forehead, above or below the eyes—and is generally relieved by paracetamol, ibuprofen or other NSAIDS.

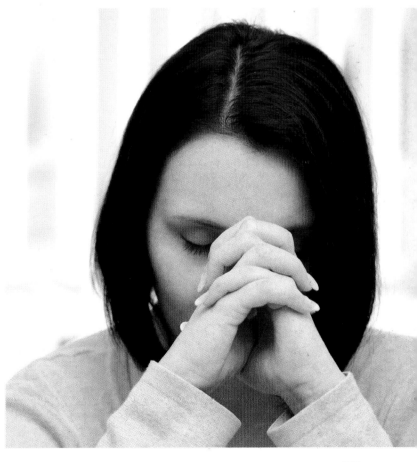

Among the symptoms of TMJ are tinnitus (ringing or other sounds in the head), earache, dizziness, a clicking noise when you chew and pain that gets worse after eating or yawning. People under stress and sufferers of osteoarthritis and rheumatoid arthritis may develop TMJ. It can be treated with muscle relaxants, analgesics or NSAIDs. In addition a mouthpiece can be worn to prevent grinding the teeth during sleep.

Alcohol, drugs and fumes from chemicals can all produce headaches, as can spending too long in a polluted environment, such as lack of ventilation when decorating with paint.

Lifestyle causes of headache

In social terms, headaches can be caused by alcohol (when drunk in sufficient quantities to produce a hangover), tobacco smoke, caffeine (both in excess and when withdrawn) and toxic fumes from industrial chemicals. Lack of food or fluids (especially water), eating ice cream or other cold foods, a sudden change in the weather (impending rain particularly), eyestrain, intense physical exercise, poor air conditioning in the workplace ("sick building syndrome"), fatigue, exposure to intense bright light, continuous loud noise, strong odours and motion sickness can all be triggers of headaches. Stress, anxiety, depression, anger and lack of sleep may also be causes, as can some prescription drugs,

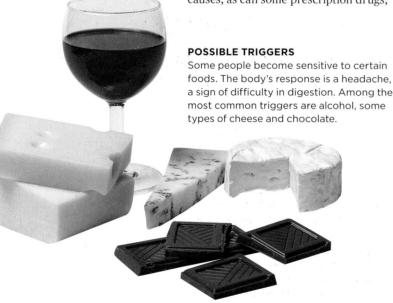

POSSIBLE TRIGGERS
Some people become sensitive to certain foods. The body's response is a headache, a sign of difficulty in digestion. Among the most common triggers are alcohol, some types of cheese and chocolate.

such as nitrates, prescribed for angina, and calcium channel blockers for angina and hypertension.

Simple solutions

The best way to deal with a headache is to prevent it. If the headache is due to posture–for example, working at a desk or computer for long periods of time in such a way that your muscles are tense or strained–change your ways. Alter the way you sit, have frequent breaks and do simple stretching exercises from time to time to release tension.

If a headache does develop, it is best to try to deal with it immediately as the over-the-counter painkillers, such as aspirin, paracetamol or ibuprofen, work best in the early stages. (Note: aspirin should never be given to children under the age of 12 years as it may cause Reye's syndrome.)

Find a quiet, dimly lit corner or darkened room where you can rest for a while with your eyes closed. Cover your eyes with a cold, damp cloth. If you know any relaxation techniques, put them into practice. Otherwise, simply breathe slowly and regularly, close your eyes and think pleasant thoughts. Gently massage your temples and the base of the skull, starting beneath the ears and gradually working round to the back of the neck. Or press your fingers on your forehead above your eyebrows, pressing and moving them gradually up to the hairline (these are acupuncture pressure points). If it is possible, take a warm, relaxing bath.

If a headache responds to over-the-counter remedies and other simple self-help techniques, or if headaches occur only infrequently, there is no need to see a doctor.

Migraine headaches

Many people who suffer from migraines believe that they are merely experiencing severe headaches, but this is not the case. Migraine headaches are a disorder of the nervous system. They affect vision as well as the other senses, and the gastrointestinal system as well. They tend to run in families, although the genetic mechanism involved is not fully understood.

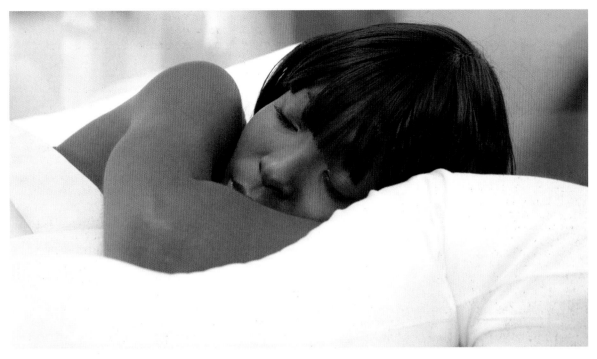

Migraines are three times more common in women than in men. They cause a painful throbbing, usually behind the eye and often on only one side of the head. In severe cases the pain can be intense and completely disabling. Movement of the head tends to make the pain worse as can light, and relief only comes by lying down in the dark until the attack passes–generally after a few hours, but sometimes and in some people an attack can last for two or three days. Migraines may occur as isolated or infrequent attacks, but for some people they strike on a regular basis, as often as once a week.

There are two main types of migraines: common and classical. A third category, menstrual migraine headache, is also identified by some doctors.

With common migraines people have nausea and sometimes vomiting as well as the severe head pain. Some people also experience painful sensitivity to light, noise and/or strong odours. There may be dizziness, confusion, visual and speech disturbance and weakness on the affected side of the body.

Classical migraines are comparatively rare, accounting for as few as 15 per cent of attacks. Sufferers sense an imminent attack through a visual "aura", in which a gradually expanding area of blindness is surrounded by a sparkling halo. It usually disappears after about 20 to 30 minutes. In other respects, the sufferer's symptoms are much the same as in common migraines.

Other migraines are related to hormonal changes. Menstrual migraines occur at the start of menstruation and are thought to affect as many as two out of three women at some stage in their

BED REST
For many people, the best way to deal with a headache is to lie down in a darkened room and rest for as long as possible.

Migraines may occur as isolated or infrequent attacks, but for some people they strike on a regular basis.

lives. Oral contraceptives, pregnancy and HRT may all trigger migraine headaches in some women. Auras are very rare, and symptoms are almost always of the common type. The trigger is likely to be increased production of the female hormone oestrogen, which is thought to be responsible for the greater susceptibility of women to both tension and migraine headaches.

Certain foods are known to have a tendency to cause migraine headaches.

These include: chocolate (although recent research suggests that chocolate may be no more guilty than many other foods); some dairy products, particularly matured cheeses; citrus fruits; cured meats (hot dogs, ham); nuts; onions; pickled foods; the food additive monosodium glutamate; and artificial sweeteners containing aspartame.

It is important for your doctor to distinguish between a migraine and a headache caused by a potentially serious condition. Brain scans (X-rays, CAT or MRI) or blood tests may be required if diagnosis is uncertain.

Inside the skull, your brain cells are fed by a vast number of arteries that are vulnerable to hardening and narrowing (atherosclerosis). Migraine as well as combination headaches are associated with a widening of the blood vessels in the head, and also the tightening of the muscles that surround the head, as can happen during periods of emotional stress or when reading in dim light. Both seem to arise from the brain chemical serotonin that controls the narrowing and widening of blood vessels. It is likely that a wave of electrical activity, stimulated by a trigger factor, crosses the brain and sets off a sequence of events that alters the blood vessels for better blood flow. In the process, the brain is deprived of serotonin, which irritates the nerves and produces the headache.

IS IT SERIOUS?

Headaches may be a symptom of other medical conditions such as meningitis or malaria. You should seek medical advice if your headaches:

- are frequent and very severe.
- become worse over hours or days.
- start suddenly and without warning.
- are present when you wake in the morning.
- came on after a head injury, particularly if there is any degree of mental confusion.
- are accompanied by other distinct symptoms such as high fever, nausea and vomiting, visual disturbance, dislike of bright light, pain and tenderness around one eye, dizziness or signs of mental confusion.
- are characterized by pain in the back of the head, particularly on waking and then lessening during the day. This may indicate hypertension and should be checked by your doctor. High blood pressure that is not treated can lead to heart attacks and strokes.
- do not correspond to the classic pattern. These should be checked by your doctor immediately. This is especially true of a pregnant woman in the last trimester who may have high blood pressure, swelling of the face, hands and feet and rapid weight gain. These are symptoms which may indicate pre-eclampsia and need immediate medical treatment.

Managing migraines

There is no cure but much can be done to alleviate the symptoms of an attack, and to help in long-term management and prevention. Treatment reduces pain, or prevents it from developing after the initial onset. It usually involves one or more of the following:

Over-the-counter (OTC) painkillers Paracetamol, ibuprofen or aspirin may be tried.

Drug treatments If the OTC painkillers are ineffective, more specific drugs that counteract the swelling of the blood vessels in the brain may be prescribed (ergotamine or sumatriptan). An antiemetic, such as metoclopramide, which should be taken before a painkiller, may be recommended for vomiting. Prophylactic drugs such as beta-blockers, tricyclic antidepressants, anticonvulsants, calcium channel blockers and even Botulinum toxin type A injections may be prescribed if you have more than five attacks per month.

Seek out darkness As soon as possible after the onset of symptoms, rest in a quiet, darkened room.

Get in touch Contact a local self-help migraine group, or reach other sufferers online. Find out about exercise routines that generate a relaxation response, relieve stress and depression.

Identify triggers If you can identify what triggers your migraines, you can learn to avoid them. Keeping a migraine diary is an important aspect of this.

What Helps?

There may be times in a woman's life when she needs extensive help and advice, for a long-term problem such as depression or addiction, or a crisis such as having a miscarriage or stillbirth, or being involved in a traumatic incident such as a train crash. The support of friends and family is invaluable in these situations, but sometimes it is important to seek professional help.

There are many reasons why a professional can be the right answer for certain problems. A professional has been trained to listen, to be more objective than family or friends can be, which can give wider scope for discussion. He or she will probably have encountered your type of problem before and be able to use the experience to help you, as well as offering a repertoire of exercises and techniques to support you through difficult times.

How therapy can help

Psychological therapy and similar techniques are not only applicable to overt mental distress. It is now widely recognized that the mind and body interact and that many disorders that manifest through physical symptoms have their primary cause in some psychological problem. This is the case with many stress-related disorders, such

TREATING MENTAL ILLNESS

Psychiatry and clinical psychology are medical treatments for mental illness. Many trained psychoanalysts begin in psychiatry.

Psychology is the scientific study of the mind. Researchers work in a wide variety of fields, including, for example, child development and human behaviour.

Serious mental illness such as schizophrenia, suicidal depression and mania are usually best treated initially with psychiatry. Psychiatrists can prescribe drugs; psychologists can't.

UNWIND YOUR MIND

There are many different ways to help yourself relax. Here are five to try when sitting comfortably in a quiet place where you won't be interrupted. It takes from 15 to 25 minutes to appreciate the benefits.

- As you breathe in, imagine the oxygen-rich air into every nook and cranny within your body. As you breathe out, think of letting go of the old waste-filled air.
- Place your feet flat on the ground. Concentrate on your feet and imagine them growing roots right down into the centre of the earth. As you breathe in, draw up strength from the ground. As you breathe out, send all the unhappiness in your life back down into the earth where it can be transformed into good energy. This takes your focus of attention out of your head so that your mind can rest.
- Think of an inspiring word—like peace, love, trust, joy or pleasure—and repeat the word to yourself as you breathe in and out.
- Imagine yourself in a beautiful place and try to sense everything about it— the sounds, smells, textures and sights.
- Imagine yourself encased from head to toe in a sphere of sparkling white light that protects and heals you.

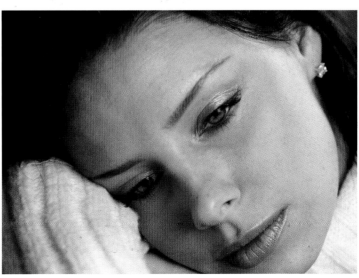

A SUPPORTIVE SPACE
The therapist gives you the time and space in which to explore and express emotions or discuss experiences that are causing anxiety and depression.

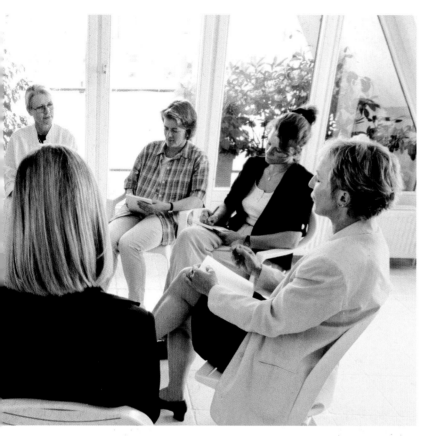

GROUP THERAPY
Group sessions are usually facilitated by a trained counsellor. It can be less stressful to be part of a group of people who have similar problems and can provide an environment of mutual support.

Cognitive therapy This addresses your mental slant–the perceptions of yourself, your life and your beliefs, and helps to restructure your thinking about them.

Behavioural therapy This is based on an analysis of behavioural patterns and on replacing those that are destructive with ones that are positive and purposeful.

Group therapies These include gestalt (focusing on the "here and now"), cognitive, behavioural, psychodrama, transactional analysis and encounter,

as irritable bowel syndrome (IBS) and anorexia. Equally, many physical disorders create mental distress, worry or fear, and the treatment of cancer, heart disease or chronic conditions such as lupus should include counselling from a professional. Finally, counselling should be available for those caring for others, for example coping with a family member with a terminal illness. It is vital that they should be able to talk to someone who is not involved.

Six approaches

Psychological therapy is a blanket term encompassing many approaches. Some of the most common are described below. Your doctor will be able to advise you on what may be the best for you and help you to find a therapist.

Psychoanalysis This technique is based on deep exploration of the unconscious and childhood experiences. It is usually a long-term commitment. It aims to uncover the causes of the person's perceived inability to lead her life successfully.

QUICK TRICK

This is the quickest way to bring about relaxation when you are facing a difficult situation or in an anxious frame of mind. The whole sequence takes about 20 minutes to complete.

- Take a normal breath. Don't change any aspect of how you breathe, but simply take note of your breathing.

- Now take a deep slow breath. Let the air come in through your nose and move deeply into your body. Take note of how the belly expands and don't try to stop it. Using a six second guide can sometimes help. Take six seconds to breathe in and six seconds to breathe out.

- Now breathe out through your mouth. (This is not a rigid rule. Breathe in whichever way is comfortable for you. If you find yourself getting anxious about the air in your lungs, stop the exercise for a minute or two and then try again.)

- Take one normal breath, and follow it with one deep, abdominal breath. Do this several times and note the differences between them, whether one makes you feel more relaxed than the other. Now take time to practise deep breathing, letting your belly expand with each inhalation.

- Then, on a long, slow exhalation, allow yourself to sigh. Repeat for several minutes then begin to imagine that with each out-breath all the tension and anxiety in your body go with it.

- Say to yourself: on inhalation, "I'm breathing in peace and calm"; on exhalation, "I'm breathing out tension and anxiety".

which involves acting out current emotional conflicts and can be confrontational. Creative and movement therapies may be used in conjunction with other therapies. Creative therapies, either as part of a group or individually based, include music, dance, drama and art. Through physical involvement in these pursuits, participants are encouraged to express themselves freely as part of healing.

Counselling Usually aimed at a particular cause of distress, such as losing a loved one or having a sexual problem, this is conducted through sessions of talking and listening. Many organizations such as colleges, hospitals, churches and a range of charities may offer counselling, often without any charge. Counselling qualifications can vary, as can its application.

One-to-one or group?

In addition to the different therapies available, therapists work in different ways–one-to-one, couple counselling, family counselling or in groups. One-to-one is best if you have a specific problem and need close personal attention from an individual session with the therapist. Couples and families often find that talking things through together can resolve difficult situations, although the process can be painful.

Some counsellors have specific training in dealing with particular problems, or special knowledge that can enable you to make difficult decisions. Areas covered include bereavement, rape, finances, dealing with children, physical and mental abuse, assertiveness, drugs and addiction, problems with study or work and medical issues including infertility or cancer.

Counsellors will not tell you what to do or be judgmental. They aim to give you support and to provide pertinent information and helpful techniques that will give you the confidence to deal with your problem yourself. Many people find the presence of others with similar problems in group therapy supportive, especially in treating addictions or, for example, at Alcoholics or Narcotics Anonymous meetings.

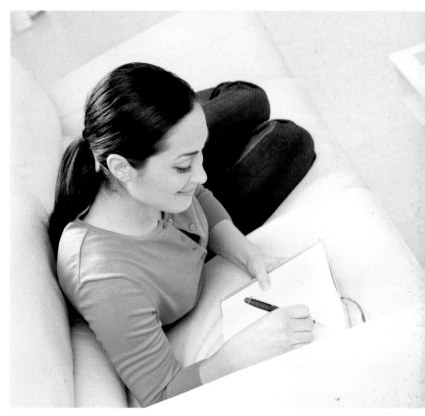

Hypnotherapy

Hypnotherapy (which uses hypnosis to "reprogramme" you through relaxation and concentration) can be useful for pain control (for example, when giving birth), weight control, migraines, blood pressure disorders, depression, skin complaints and addictions. Hypnosis may also be used for nausea control before chemotherapy.

THE WRITE WAY
"Journalling" is one of the most powerful elements of mind and body medicine. Writing down your deepest thoughts and feelings about a traumatic event releases the stress that may otherwise provoke a physical illness.

Soothing body and mind

Aromatic "essential oils", extracted from all the different parts of plants, have been used to soothe the mind in the East for thousands of years.

In the West, they are used to relieve stress-related complaints. Generally, various essential oils —lavender, ylang ylang, basil, rosemary, geranium or sage, for example—are added to an oil base and massaged into your skin. A session takes about an hour.

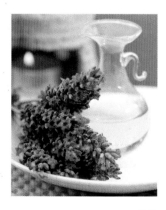

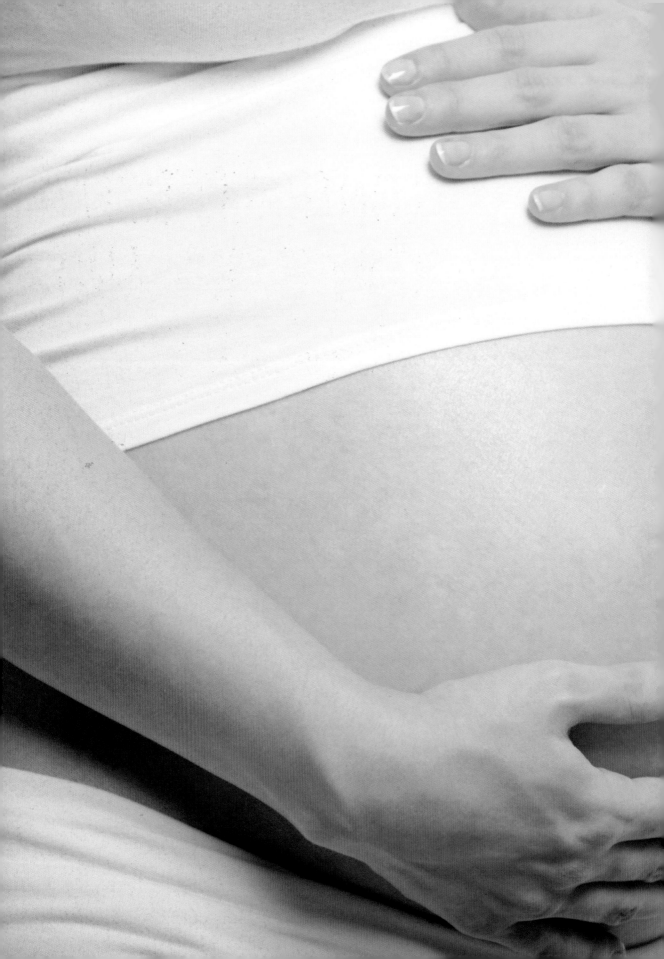

CONTRACEPTION, CONCEPTION AND PREGNANCY

Whether or not to have a child, when, and with whom, are three of the most life-changing decisions a woman will ever make. They will impact both who she is and how she affects the world. The following chapter provides practical information about contraception, conception, pregnancy and motherhood that will help you make those decisions.

Choosing Contraception

The right choice of contraception can be an important part of a happy sexual relationship. Here's what you need to know about the different forms of birth control to help you decide what's best for you and your partner.

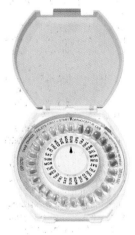

COMBINED PILL
Synthetic female hormones are used in order to prevent pregnancy.

HORMONAL CONTRACEPTION

Your contraceptive needs change during your life; what was suitable for you at the age of 20 may not be right at 40. Your choice may be influenced by whether you have completed your family or hope to have a child in the future. To find the method that's right for you, talk to your partner and doctor about your needs.

The contraceptive pill

Since its invention in the 1960s, the contraceptive pill has been hailed as a revolutionary force for women. It allows effective family planning, spontaneous sex and minimal risk of pregnancy.

Modern forms offer 95-97 per cent protection against pregnancy if taken correctly. The hormone doses have been decreased over the past few years without compromising effectiveness, yet significantly decreasing side effects. A minority of women, for example, may have an increased susceptibility to blood clots. When considering your suitability for the pill, your doctor will assess your risk factors, which you can weigh against the benefits.

The combined pill

What it is The most widely prescribed pill uses synthetic forms of the female hormones oestrogen and progestin. There are different types containing varying levels of hormones. The lowest effective dosage is prescribed.

A "monophasic" pill has 21 identical pills followed by 7 days of placebo pills during which a withdrawal bleeding (similar to a period) occurs. A "triphasic" pill has a constant dose of oestrogen but a stepwise increase in progestin each week for 3 weeks, and then 7 days of placebo.

How it works Oestrogen plus progestin prevents ovulation, so there is no egg for the sperm to fertilize. The progestin changes the uterine lining and thickens the cervical mucus, making it difficult for sperm to travel.

Pros It is convenient, reliable and allows spontaneity; you have lighter, less painful periods and reduced PMS symptoms. It can be taken for years and may protect against pelvic inflammatory disease, benign breast disease, ovarian and uterine cancers and endometriosis.

Cons A few women experience minor cyclic water retention, mood changes, breast swelling, reduced sex drive, migraine headaches, nausea and unexpected vaginal bleeding. You may take some months to reestablish ovulation after stopping it. It may be unsuitable if you're over 35 and smoke, have a history of phlebitis or deep vein clots, have uncontrolled diabetes, high blood pressure or liver diseases such as hepatitis. It may not work if you miss a pill, vomit within three hours of taking a pill or are taking certain antibiotics and drugs such as antiepilepsy medication.

In any of these situations, use other contraception, such as condoms, in addition for the remainder of the pack.

Take note Stop taking the pill if you have migraines for the first time, frequent severe headaches or sudden disturbances of sight or hearing; see your doctor immediately. Talk to your doctor about your options if you are to have major surgery or need long bed rest.

The progestogen-only pill

What it is This pill uses only one hormone–progestogen–a form of progesterone. It is suitable for women who have side effects from oestrogen, are breast-feeding or are unable to take the combined pill for other reasons.

How it works It thickens cervical mucus and changes the uterine lining, preventing sperm reaching the fallopian tubes. It inhibits ovulation in about 50 per cent of women.

Pros As those of the combined pill.

Cons It must be taken at the same time daily (within a 3-hour window), and has a higher failure rate than the combined pill. Irregular vaginal bleeding and breast tenderness may occur. It may be unsuitable if you've had unexplained bleeding or severe depression. It may not work if you have vomiting or diarrhoea. If you miss a dose, take it as soon as possible and continue as usual with the rest of the pack, but use another contraceptive, such as a condom, too.

Contraceptive patch

What it is A small adhesive patch that is applied to the skin weekly for 3 weeks, then is left off for a week to allow a menstrual bleed. It contains oestrogen and progestin that are absorbed into the bloodstream through the skin.

How it works As the pill but you don't have to think about it daily.

Pros You're less likely to forget than a daily method.

Cons Some women experience more breast tenderness than with a pill. There may be an increased risk of blood clots and other cardiovascular problems than with a pill but these are still much lower than those associated with pregnancy. The patch appears to be slightly less effective in women over 98 kg (216 lb).

Contraceptive ring

What it is A small flexible ring that you leave in the vagina for three weeks, then remove to allow a period. It contains low-dose oestrogen and progestin. It may be left in for four weeks and replaced immediately to skip a period.

How it works The same as the pill, but you don't have to think about it daily.

Pros You're less likely to forget than a daily method. It provides a very low level of hormones, minimizing hormonal headaches and breakthrough bleeding.

Cons Some women find it difficult or unacceptable to have a ring in place.

Contraceptive injection

What it is A synthetic progestin, available as an intramuscular or subcutaneous shot given every 12 weeks.

How it works It thins the uterine lining, thickens the cervical mucus and suppresses ovulation.

Pros It lasts for 12 weeks and is about 99 per cent effective. The injection is ideal for women with sickle cell disease or seizures as it decreases the number of sickle cell crises and seizures. Periods are light or absent. It does not interfere with breast milk production.

Cons Fertility may not return for a year after stopping. Weight gain, loss of sex drive, acne or mood changes may occur. It is associated with bone loss (reversible in 2 years of stopping). Consider other methods if you have risk factors for bone loss–smoking, steroid use, eating disorders. It is unsuitable if you want to get pregnant soon.

Contraceptive implant

What it is A toothpick-sized rod placed under the skin of your upper arm. It remains in place and releases progestin into your bloodstream for up to 3 years.

How it works It suppresses ovulation, thins the uterine lining and thickens the cervical mucus.

Pros It is 99.9 per cent effective and you can forget about it for 3 years. It is reversible when removed and side effects are less likely than with the injection since the doses of progestin are lower.

Cons Irregular bleeding may occur. Insertion and removal requires minor surgery under local anaesthetic.

THE NEW PILLS

Would you like fewer and lighter periods each year, as few as only four?

New formulations of the combined pill are available as an extended cycle where 84 active pills are followed by seven placebo pills. You have only four scheduled menstrual intervals per year (instead of the typical 13 intervals). Breakthrough bleeding is expected during the first few months, but this pill is generally tolerated well. Another type offers a small dose of oestrogen only during the placebo interval. This results in lighter periods. It may help with hot flushes and headaches in perimenopausal women.

The combined pill is also available in a continuous form where an active pill is taken 365 days a year, minimizing menstrual bleeding. This pill may help women with menstrual symptoms, such as painful cramping, PMS and endometriosis. It is perfectly healthy not to have a monthly period. The synthetic hormones simulate those created by the body during the intervals of pregnancy and breastfeeding in women not using contraception.

A combined pill that has only four inactive pills in a cycle is the so-called shortened hormone-free interval formulation. It results in a light and short menstrual bleed and suppresses ovulation effectively. It is useful for heavy bleeding and painful ovarian cysts.

BARRIER CONTRACEPTION

Birth control methods that prevent sperm from entering a woman's uterus are known as barrier contraception. The best known types–male and female condoms–are essential for people starting new relationships and when practising safer sex. They help prevent HIV and other sexually transmitted diseases (STDs) from being passed from one person to another. Condoms should be used until you and your partner are familiar with each other's sexual history, are monogamous with each other and have been tested negative for STIs.

Male condom

What it is A thin latex sheath with a nipple-shaped tip, the condom is unrolled on an erect penis. Polyurethane condoms, which are thinner and provide more sensation for the man, can be used with oil-based lubricants.

How it works It covers the penis and collects the semen in the tip, so sperm are prevented from entering the woman's reproductive tract. A new condom has to be used with every act of intercourse. It must be put on right from the start. As soon as the man has ejaculated, the penis must be withdrawn from the

vagina, and care should be taken to hold the base of the condom so no sperm are able to escape.

Pros It is very easy to obtain, protects both partners against STIs and is easily disposed of. Fertility is normal when the condom is not used. There are no side effects unless you are allergic to latex. If used properly, the failure rate can be as low as 10 per cent; when used with a spermicide, a condom is even more reliable. It may be used in addition to other methods of contraception for safer sex.

Cons The condom can come off or break during sexual activity, leaving you at risk of pregnancy and STIs. It should be put on before any penetration occurs (because sperm may leak out before ejaculation) and you have to stop during lovemaking to put it on. There may be reduced or altered sensation for both partners. It is wise to make sure you always have a supply.

Female condom

What it is A polyurethane tube that fits inside the vagina, with a retaining ring on the outside.

How it works Semen is contained inside the condom and doesn't enter the vagina. The failure rate is approximately

LATEX ALERT

Barrier methods of contraception use latex or polyurethane to protect one set of genitals from the other. Those made of latex can be delicate, and you should avoid using oil or petroleum jelly in conjunction with these types. Do not let massage or body oil come into contact with them. You can use a water-based lubricant if you find additional moisture is required.

THE CHOICES
Many factors are involved in choosing contraception, but the advantage of barrier methods is that they are readily available.

Female condom

Male condoms

Spermicide

Applicator

Diaphragm

Spermicide suppositories

10 per cent. A new condom has to be used with every act of intercourse.

Pros It is available from pharmacies and has no side effects. It is under the woman's control and protects against STIs. Unlike the male condom, it can be inserted well before sex. Fertility is normal when the condom is not used.

Cons There is reduced vaginal sensation and the ring protrudes outside the vagina. It may be difficult to insert and must be inserted correctly. It has to be obtained in advance.

It may not be suitable if you find it hard to insert or you or your partner find it physically unsatisfactory.

Diaphragm or cervical cap

What it is A soft latex or plastic dome that fits inside the vagina covering the cervix and is used with a spermicide. There is a range of sizes and types, and it must be fitted to the individual by a trained professional (at your doctor's office or a family planning clinic). You need to be taught the correct way to insert and remove it. After removal, a diaphragm should be washed in warm water, dried and stored in its container. It should be checked regularly for signs of wear and tear; if you have long fingernails, take care not to rip holes in it.

How it works It prevents semen from entering the uterus; any sperm that do bypass the cap are killed or disabled by the spermicide. To make sure that no sperm survive, the diaphragm needs to be kept in place for 6-8 hours after intercourse.

Pros It works well for women who only want contraception when required– that is, infrequently rather than all the time. You have to remember to insert it, but it can be put in up to 2 hours before intercourse. Fertility is normal when it is not used. It offers some protection against STIs and cervical cancer. Side effects are rare.

Cons It is messy. You can't be wholly spontaneous as it needs inserting before sex. You need to put in more spermicide with every act of intercourse. The diaphragm must fit over the cervix, and if you gain or lose more than 8 kg (20 lb) and after pregnancy you should be reassessed by a health care professional

as a new size may be needed. A diaphragm can sometimes become dislodged and some women find it

The "morning after" pill prevents pregnancy. It does not terminate one that already exists.

difficult and messy to insert correctly. It needs to remain in place for 6 hours after sex. It should not be left in place for more than 24 hours because infection may result.

If an unplanned pregnancy would be very difficult to deal with, this method may be unsuitable as the failure rate is about 10-15 per cent if fitted correctly (higher if fitted incorrectly). Also, it is not the best method if you are prone to bladder, vaginal or urinary tract infections (a diaphragm may increase their frequency), if you have poor pelvic muscle tone or vaginal and uterine abnormalities.

Using spermicides

Spermicide are used with barrier contraception to kill any sperm that escape the condom, diaphragm or cap. There are various forms (cream, foam, jelly, suppository) and you may need to experiment with different types until you find the one that suits you. Spermicides may cause an allergic reaction in some women. It is important to remember that used on its own a spermicide is not a reliable contraceptive (even at perimenopause when fertility is low) and a fresh amount must always be used with each act of intercourse.

THE FACTS ABOUT EMERGENCY CONTRACEPTION

What it is Commonly called the morning-after pill, it can decrease the risk of pregnancy for up to 5 days after unprotected sex although it is most effective if taken as soon as possible after contraceptive failure (forgotten pill or diaphragm, condom accident, sex without contraception or sexual assault. This method is now available over the counter from pharmacists if you are over 18 years old. If you are younger, your doctor will need to prescribe it.

How it works One or two higher dose progestin pills are taken as soon as possible after unprotected sex, followed by another one, 12 hours later. Alternatively, both pills may be taken at the same time. They help prevent ovulation so that an egg will not be released. It is not effective post-ovulation and does not affect a pre-existing pregnancy. Use a barrier method of contraception until you have your next period.

Pros Prevents pregnancy in an instance of contraceptive failure or accident. Decreases the pregnancy rate following an episode of midcycle intercourse by about 80 per cent.

Cons Side effects of the morning-after pill can include nausea or vomiting. This method should not be used as a primary contraceptive method.

Alternatively, a copper IUD may be inserted up 5 days after unprotected sex, and left in place for primary contraception. It does not have any hormonal side effects, and the failure rate is very low.

ALTERNATIVE CONTRACEPTION

Other methods of contraception are available if hormonal or barrier methods are unsuitable.

Copper intrauterine device (IUD)

What it is A small T-shaped plastic device coated with copper fitted through the cervix into the uterus (hence its name, intrauterine device). It has a nylon thread attached that hangs down into the vagina so the user can check it is still in place. After discussion with your doctor (and occasionally tests to check that you have no sexually transmitted disease), the IUD will be inserted in the early part of your menstrual cycle. It is effective

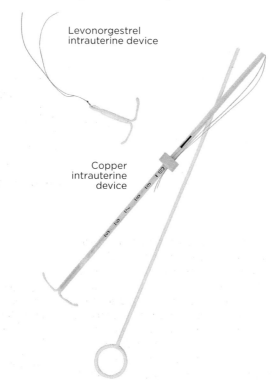

Levonorgestrel intrauterine device

Copper intrauterine device

THE IUD
Intrauterine devices are usually made of plastic wrapped with copper. They are inserted into the woman's uterus by a doctor and provide almost certain contraception. They do not, however, protect against STIs and barrier contraception should be used for safety.

immediately and can be kept in place for 10 years. If it becomes necessary, it can be easily removed.

How it works The IUD acts as a spermicide via its copper coating and also prevents implantation of the fertilized egg by causing a sterile (non-infectious) inflammation in the lining of the uterus.

Pros It has a very low failure rate, less than 1 per cent. After each period you should check for the strings although the expulsion rate is very low. Otherwise you don't have to think about it.

Cons It is not first choice in women who are at risk for STIs. Insertion may be uncomfortable. There is a slight risk of perforation of the uterus during insertion. In rare cases, the IUD may migrate to a different part of the body and surgery may be necessary to remove it. Periods may be heavier and more painful.

This type of IUD should not be used if you have painful or heavy periods, pelvic inflammatory disease, anaemia or Wilson's disease.

Levonorgestrel (hormone-releasing) IUD

What it is An intrauterine system (IUS) that is designed to stay in the body for five years.

How it works As well as acting as an IUD, it releases low doses of the hormone levonorgestrel. It works by thickening cervical mucus to prevent sperm from reaching the uterus and thinning the uterine lining to prevent implantation.

Pros Periods become lighter, and 20 per cent of women don't have periods after 1 year of use, 70 per cent after 2 years of use. Therefore, it is especially useful as a contraceptive for women with heavy periods and severe cramping. Failure rate is less than 1 per cent. A woman can avoid the need for surgery such as endometrial ablation (destruction of the uterine lining) or hysterectomy for heavy bleeding. Since the level of progestin is very low, side effects are much lower than with contraceptive injection or pills.

Cons There is a low risk of ectopic pregnancy. It may be difficult to insert in women who have not had children.

A Permanent Fix

Male and female sterilization are surgical methods of contraception and should be used only by people who have completed their family or who don't want children. Sterilization should be viewed as final—although occasionally, at high cost and with difficulty, it can be reversed. It is the most popular form of family planning for women after the age of 35 years.

Tubal ligation for women
How it works The fallopian tubes are cut or banded via laparoscopic surgery. Eggs from the ovaries cannot reach the uterus.

Pros There is less than 1 per cent chance of pregnancy. Sex can be spontaneous afterwards. Apart from the surgery, there is little risk to health. It is effective immediately.

Cons General anaesthetic is necessary. There is a slight risk of pregnancy. Up to 40 per cent of resulting pregnancies are ectopic. It does not protect against STIs.

It may be an unsuitable option if you're not sure you have completed childbearing. It may be difficult to adjust psychologically.

Vasectomy for men
How it works The two tubes (the vas deferens) that conduct the sperm from the testicles to the penis are cut and then the ends are tied or heat-sealed.

Pros It is 99 per cent effective. It is a short procedure, done under local anaesthetic. It does not affect the ability to have erections and ejaculate (the semen will not contain sperm).

Cons It does not become effective for up to three months after surgery so it is important to use another method until your partner has had two sperm-free semen samples confirmed by his doctor. It does not protect against STIs.

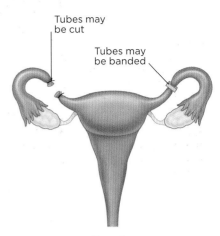

Tubes may be cut
Tubes may be banded

Female sterilization

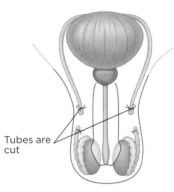

Tubes are cut

Male sterilization

Natural family planning
What it is A woman learns how to use a menstrual calendar. This charts her temperature and changes in vaginal mucus to indicate on which days she is fertile and likely to become pregnant. Most women are fertile a few days before and a day or so after ovulation.

How it works By finding out which days in the month you are fertile, you can avoid getting pregnant by not having intercourse at that time or by using barrier methods.

Pros Your fertility is not affected. Religions that do not approve of artificial birth control accept it. There are no health risks. If strictly adhered to, the failure rate can be as low as 10 per cent (but it is usually higher).

Cons If the method is not followed correctly, failure rates can be high–up to 35 per cent. You need to be extremely motivated to follow this system, as does your partner. It can be complicated to learn and to follow. Each menstrual cycle has to be plotted separately, since the day of ovulation can vary from one month to the next. Illness may affect your temperature, and vaginal infections change vaginal mucus.

It may not be a suitable technique if you are not in a long-term relationship, if you or your partner want to have spontaneous intercourse without having to watch the calendar, if you must not get pregnant for health or other reasons, or if only one of you is committed to the method.

FACT

If you have had tubal ligation and develop pelvic pain and vaginal bleeding, you should do a pregnancy test. If positive, you may have an ectopic pregnancy.

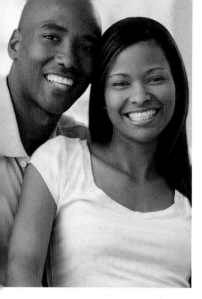

Conception

From the moment you become pregnant, your body, relationships, feelings and life will be forever changed. Learning all you can about pregnancy, childbirth and raising a family will help prepare you for the different aspects of giving birth and being a parent. You will see your doctor during the first trimester of pregnancy. Follow any recommendations specific to your health and work together with your health care team throughout your pregnancy.

TIME OF ADJUSTMENT
Preparing yourself for pregnancy is both physical and emotional. Reducing risk factors and airing any concerns with your partner is essential.

PREGNANCY PLANNING

The ideal situation is to be in the very best of health before attempting to conceive so that you can maximize your chances of a safe and successful delivery of a healthy baby. In essence, this means:

Stop smoking By far the single most important thing you can do to increase your chances of a healthy baby.

Ditch toxins Cutting out alcohol and illegal drugs and limiting caffeinated beverages to one or two a day.

Eat right Plenty of nutrient-rich foods such as fruit and vegetables.

Add folic acid Eating foods rich in folic acid, and taking a dietary supplement, to lessen the risk of bearing a child with a neural tube defect (also called spina bifida or anencephaly) by up to 75 per cent. Taking 800 mcg daily is advised, ideally for 3 months prior to conception.

Watch weight gain Eating to gain weight if you are underweight, and cutting down on high-fat foods as well as improving the overall quality of food that you eat if you are overweight. The old adage of "eating for two" is far from accurate. A woman of normal weight needs only 300 extra calories per day (the equivalent of a small meal or two snacks) in order to maintain healthy fetal growth.

Move Getting plenty of exercise, about 30-45 minutes, at least 3-4 times a week. You should avoid heavy lifting, high impact exercises and activities that put you at risk of falling or of abdominal trauma (for example, horseback riding, volleyball, scuba diving).

Sleep Getting at least 8 hours of sleep per night, and naps as needed.

Stay hydrated Drinking at least 8 glasses of water every day in order to encourage the elimination of toxins from the body and prevent bladder infections.

Check your immunity Checking your immunity for rubella and varicella (chicken pox) by means of a simple blood test is helpful. If you find out you are not immune to these infections, it's best to be immunized prior to pregnancy, as both can cause serious problems in the developing fetus. These vaccines cannot be given during pregnancy.

Check for STIs Getting tested for chlamydia, gonorrhoea, herpes, syphilis, hepatitis B and HIV is reasonable prior to pregnancy. It is generally routinely done during the first prenatal visit. Any treatable STI can be safely treated during pregnancy.

Tend to your teeth Having any necessary dental work done prior to pregnancy is advised, so that you can limit the need for X-rays or anaesthesia while you are pregnant. Good dental hygiene is important as inflammation of gums, called periodontal disease, has been linked to increased risk of preterm delivery. You should continue having your teeth professionally cleaned by your dental hygienist twice a year even during pregnancy.

Check out your past Your personal and family medical history are significant in prepregnancy planning, as is the personal and family medical history of your partner. In your case, menstrual problems, infections, STIs, pre-existing health problems (for example, epilepsy, hypertension, diabetes) will need to be discussed with your doctor, nurse or midwife as part of your care.

If you or any of your family has any inherited condition, for example cystic fibrosis, you may want to see a genetic counsellor recommended by your doctor to discuss and assess the level of risk for you and your baby and the screening options available.

Emotional changes

Having a first baby involves an enormous life change, and in the months before conception you should take the opportunity to talk through possible issues or attitudes with your partner. It is perfectly normal to experience a range of emotions, some of which may be conflicting. Both the mother and the father may need to rework old relationships (with their mothers and fathers, for instance, friends who don't have children, with work colleagues), and their feelings may vacillate from excitement and elation to anxiety. Both of you may enjoy knowing that you are carrying on the family line, but you may also have concerns about finances, job security and personal freedom.

As a couple, over the months that lie ahead, you may make new discoveries about each other. You will be sharing the joys and discoveries of being parents but more negative feelings will also arise, and you should be prepared for them. Not feeling well physically or emotionally during pregnancy may take a toll on your relationship. Worries and hidden anxieties about meeting the demands of parenthood may surface. There may be unhappy memories from the past to deal with. Your feelings for each other may be tested by crises, such as problems with the development of the fetus.

Antenatal groups provide an excellent forum for airing feelings and raising a variety of subjects that concern new parents. The range of information and friendship that is provided by support groups can contribute longstanding help and support to both the new mother and her partner.

WHAT CAN PUT YOUR BABY AT RISK?

The following factors should be discussed with your doctor. Remember that over 97 per cent of pregnancies result in the safe delivery of a healthy baby. If you attend the early antenatal care appointments, your health care team can identify and address any risk factors, such as:

- Age: are you younger than 18 years or over 35 years?
- Have four or more children
- IUD in place
- Vaginal bleeding after last period
- Previous stillbirth or neonatal death
- Previous Caesarean delivery or myomectomy
- Previous small—under 2.25 kg (5 lb) or large—over 3.6 kg (8 lb) baby
- Previous preterm delivery (before 37 weeks)
- Two or more miscarriages before existing pregnancy
- History of premature labour, cervical stitch (called cerclage), late miscarriage or abortion, or two or more abortions
- Congenital abnormality in previous baby
- Antibodies in your blood that could harm the fetus,
- Preeclampsia, hypertension, proteinuria in a previous pregnancy
- Severe bleeding after giving birth or removal of placenta in previous pregnancy
- History of short labour (under 2 hours) or long labour (over 18 hours)
- Postpartum depression after birth of previous baby
- Uterine problem such as fibroids or cysts
- Blood disorder
- Family history of diabetes or congenital fetal abnormality
- Smoking
- Drinking 2 or more units of alcohol a day prior to pregnancy
- Inability to stop drinking while pregnant
- Illegal drug taking by either parent
- Several different sexual partners, anal intercourse, bisexual partner
- Hepatitis B, HIV, AIDS
- High blood pressure (over 140/90 mmHg, after you have been lying down for 5 minutes)
- Over- or under-weight or less than 1.5 m (5 ft) tall
- Protein in urine or other kidney or liver disease
- Heart murmur
- Pelvic or abdominal abnormalities
- Vaginal bleeding late in prior pregnancy

Conception Challenges

The average woman has on average a 15 to 25 per cent chance of conceiving a baby each cycle and about 85 per cent of fertile couples will be successful within 12 months of having regular unprotected sex. For some, getting pregnant, sustaining a pregnancy and achieving a live birth proves to be more difficult.

MAXIMIZING FERTILITY

Taking these steps before trying to conceive will maximize your chances of pregnancy:

- Completely stop all intake of alcohol.
- Stop smoking and avoid smoky rooms.
- Practise good hygiene to avoid infections.
- Maintain a healthy weight for your height.
- Get rid of excess stressors in your life.
- Practice anti-anxiety techniques—deep breathing, prayer, meditation or yoga.
- Give your body a chance to re-establish natural periods before you try to conceive, especially if you have recently taken hormonal contraception..

INFERTILITY

Infertility is the inability to become pregnant after more than one year of regular, unprotected sexual intercourse. It is estimated that just over 10 per cent of women of reproductive age have problems conceiving. In one-third of cases, the problem lies with the woman's reproductive system and in another third the problem lies with the man's reproductive system. In the remaining third the problem is with both partners or is not known. After a specialist's investigation of both partners and treatment, 30–40 per cent of couples achieve a pregnancy within two years.

What triggers infertility?

Why some people are infertile is not yet fully understood, but some causes have been identified. In women, it may be because the ovaries are not producing eggs (anovulation). Endometriosis and pelvic inflammatory disease can damage or block fallopian tubes. In some women, mucus in the cervix may be hostile to the partner's sperm. In men, a common cause is defective sperm (in quantity, motility or function). In couples, the genetic make-up of one partner may prevent the couple from achieving a pregnancy naturally, or in some cases occupational hazards (such as chemicals and working practices) are involved.

What's causing the problem?

To determine the cause of any infertility, your doctor may see you and your partner, both separately and together.

You will have a physical examination and a detailed personal history will be taken. Obesity, acne and menstrual irregularities will be noted, and you may be asked about eating disorders, stress, occupational hazards (working with toxins, for example), exercise methods, sexual pattern, previous contraception and lifestyle habits such as alcohol, smoking and prescribed or illegal drugs. Blood tests may be carried out to seek known reasons for infertility–an excess of prolactin (a hormone regulating menstruation), excess or deficiency of thyroid hormone or an excess of androgens such as testosterone.

If you have endometriosis, uterine fibroids, polyps or ovarian cysts, the doctor may refer you to a gynaecologist or endocrinologist for assessment.

For your partner, the doctor may suggest sperm analysis. Finding out early on that he has too few sperm, no sperm at all or slow-moving or misshapen sperm may lessen the chance of you having to undergo invasive tests (although if you have other physical symptoms, you may still need investigation as well).

If the doctor suspects that sexual problems could be the cause, a sex therapist may be recommended.

Searching for an answer

Various methods may be used to assess the condition of your reproductive system. Laparoscopy is a minor operation involving a small incision in the abdomen through which a special endoscope can be inserted to view the uterus, fallopian tubes and ovaries. Dye is passed through the neck of the uterus (cervix) into the tubes to check for blockage or constriction. Abnormalities may be treated laparoscopically by one of several methods–laser vaporization, electrocautery or excisional biopsy.

Hysteroscopy can be done in the surgery or operating theatre. No incision is required. A tiny tube–a hysteroscope–is passed through the cervix into the uterus to check for adhesions (scar tissue) and other possible problems.

Hysterosalpingography, an X-ray technique, uses a contrast (radio-opaque) medium injected into the uterus to outline the reproductive organs. It may identify abnormalities in the uterine cavity and tubal blockages. It should be done in the first 10 days of your cycle, when you are least likely to be pregnant, because radiation may harm a developing fetus. It may cause abdominal cramps.

The solution

If ovulation is the problem, medication can help induce ovulation. Disorders such as polycystic ovaries, endometriosis and PID can be treated. Damaged fallopian tubes can in some cases be repaired by surgery or in vitro fertilization can be used to bypass them.

Intrauterine insemination with your partner's or donor sperm is a treatment option in cases of infertility where sperm are too few or are insufficiently motile.

Optimize your chances

It is vital to understand your own monthly menstrual cycle so you know when you ovulate and which days are optimal for sexual intercourse. You can identify these by observing changes in vaginal mucus, by making a temperature chart and by calculating over several months the cycle's length.

There are three vital stages. Fertilization occurs within 48 hours of ovulation and implantation occurs some

When do you ovulate?

To find out whether you are ovulating, you may be asked to keep a basal body temperature chart (BBT) on which you record your morning temperature on waking, along with the day of the menstrual cycle. You mark the days when bleeding occurs with a cross, and the days when intercourse occurs with a circle. During the menstrual cycle, the BBT is higher once ovulation occurs—confirmed by a 0.4°C (32°F) rise in temperature for three consecutive days.

Over-the-counter ovulation kits can be used to detect luteinizing hormone, which surges immediately before ovulation occurs.

A blood test to measure progesterone levels can also confirm ovulation—the hormone is secreted around day 22 of a 28-day cycle, about a week after the egg is released, to stimulate the thickening of the uterus lining. The doctor may do an endometrial biopsy towards the end of the menstrual cycle but before bleeding begins, to check that thickening of the uterus lining has occurred. The simple procedure is usually carried out in the doctor's surgery and requires no anaesthetic.

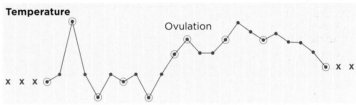

seven days after fertilization. Ovulation takes place 14 days before the expected next period. This is not the same as saying that it takes place 14 days after the last period as menstrual cycles vary in length from 24 to 35 days–hence the need to identify the usual length of your own cycle. In a 28-day cycle, the optimal time for conception is on days 11 to 17 of the cycle, where day 1 is the first day of the menstrual period. Daily intercourse during this time is generally advised.

You should become familiar with the changes in your vaginal mucus. Just before ovulation the mucus increases in quantity and becomes thinner and more elastic, like raw egg white, and transparent–a drop can be stretched into a long strand without breaking. After ovulation, it becomes thicker and whiter.

A BABY IS BORN
Modern advances in reproductive techniques mean that women and men who have difficulty conceiving a baby naturally can be helped to start a family. Ask to see a clinic's successful birth rates before agreeing to treatment there.

ASSISTED REPRODUCTION TECHNOLOGY

Reproduction specialists today have a wide range of options that they can employ to help previously infertile people to have children. Known as assisted reproduction technology (ART), the techniques include using the eggs and sperm of the prospective parents, the mother's egg fertilized by sperm from a donor, or a donor's egg fertilized by the father's sperm.

The procedures are costly and require frequent visits and significant commitment on the part of the couple. Counselling about the procedures is usually made available by an infertility unit. Issues to be discussed should include side effects and risks of treatment, the recommended number of treatment cycles and the legal implications of using donor eggs or sperm. Help may be needed to cope with your feelings should you fail to achieve conception or a live birth.

A range of techniques

AI (artificial insemination) This technique involves a woman using a syringe to place her partner's sperm in her cervix during the time she is ovulating. This method is useful for couples who experience sexual difficulties such as erectile dysfunction and is also used in some cases of unexplained infertility.

DI (donor insemination) This is a similar procedure to AI, but in this case the syringe contains donor sperm. This method is used for erectile dysfunction or defective sperm.

IUI (intrauterine insemination) In this procedure, sperm is introduced directly into the woman's uterus through the vagina and cervix. These measures enhance the chances of conception and are used when the woman's body makes antibodies to her partner's sperm, for erectile dysfunction, male factor infertility, or unexplained infertility. Donor sperm can also be used if the partner's sperm is defective.

IVF (in vitro fertilization) The so-called "test tube baby" procedure that fertilizes the woman's eggs with her partner's sperm outside the body. First the woman's ovaries are stimulated to produce several eggs. These are collected in an operating theatre under light sedation and mixed with sperm.

If fertilization occurs (it takes several days) some of the embryos may be placed in her uterus and the remainder frozen for later use. This technique is

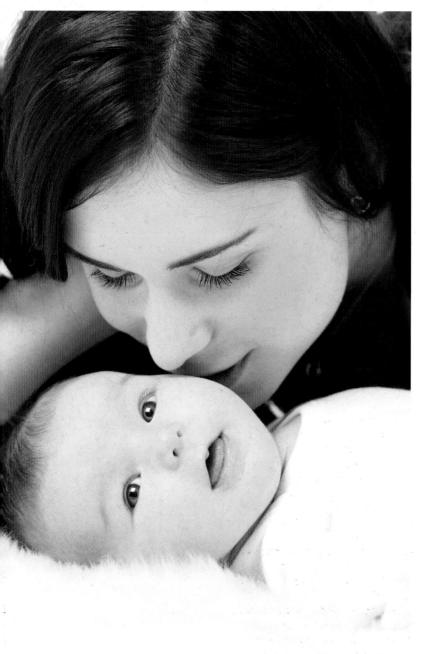

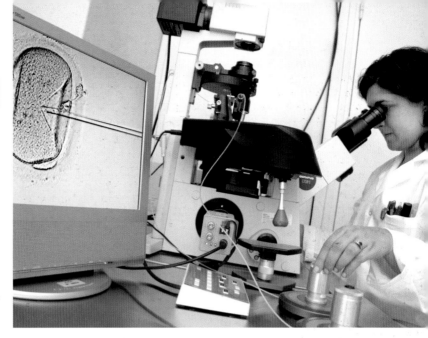

FREEZING EGGS, SPERM AND EMBRYOS

The techniques of ART and the pursuit of a family are made possible by having a supply of eggs and sperm or embryos that can be used at any time. The medium is liquid nitrogen that "freezes" for storage at a fertility unit. Before use their quality is tested and only healthy ones are chosen.

Donor sperm is automatically frozen for six months while it is screened for HIV, the virus that causes AIDS. The freezing method is also important in screening embryos for identifiable inherited diseases such as cystic fibrosis. Genetic testing in this way allows selection of a disease-free embryo.

Freezing sperm or eggs is an option for men and women undergoing treatment such as chemotherapy that may make them infertile.

mostly employed in cases where there is poor quality sperm, when the woman's body makes antibodies to the sperm, unexplained infertility, blocked or scarred fallopian tubes.

ICSI (intracytoplasmic sperm injection) In cases of male factor infertility, a sperm is directly injected into an egg that has been retrieved from the woman in the same way as in IVF and

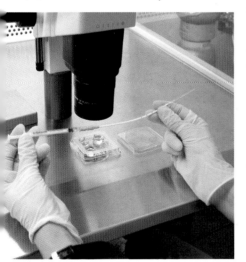

EMBRYO TRANSFER CATHETER

This fine catheter—a flexible tube that is inserted into the body—is used to transfer an embryo that has been fertilized in a laboratory to the uterus, via the cervix.

the resulting embryo is placed in the woman's uterus. This technique may be especially suitable for those couples in whom sperm is of poor quality, has little movement (motility) or is unable to penetrate the egg.

Egg donation This procedure is key to conception when a woman cannot produce her own eggs or her own eggs are not fertilizable. Donor eggs from a woman under age 35 have the highest success rate. This technique is also used to reduce the risk of age-related chromosomal problems such as Down's syndrome in women over 35 years of age. The eggs are fertilized by the male partner's sperm as in IVF and the embryo is placed in the female partner's uterus. She is given hormones to support the pregnancy.

Surrogacy This procedure allows one woman to give birth for another who is unable to carry a baby to term or who cannot conceive. The surrogate carries either the other woman's fertilized egg or her own (after it has been fertilized by the father's sperm) to full term and then hands over the baby at birth. This option involves legal issues–including adoption of the newborn child–and loopholes. It is essential that all parties be fully aware of the implications of this option.

Adoption Welcoming a child who needs parents into your home is a wonderful experience. The legal situation surrounding adoption is much clearer than that of surrogacy.

NEEDLE ACCURACY

Two common causes of infertility concern the inability of eggs and sperm to fuse and create an embryo. With modern help they are brought together to fertilize with ICSI, in which sperm are injected directly into an egg.

Pregnancy and Motherhood

There is no doubt that being pregnant, giving birth and motherhood will change your life in many ways. They are all challenging and enriching experiences—and best approached by knowing what you're getting into.

BABY'S FIRST PICTURE
Ultrasound scanning is a painless procedure and gives you an opportunity to see your child as he or she develops. The scan is done when you have a full bladder which pushes your uterus up so the technician gets a clearer image. You and your partner will be able to see the monitor—and may be given a printout of what you saw.

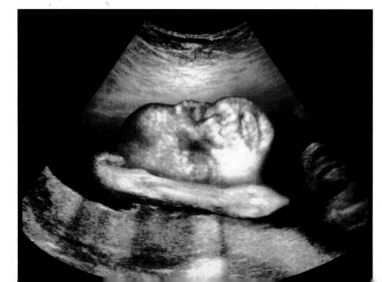

STAGES OF PREGNANCY

Some women know very quickly whether or not they are pregnant, but most may need something more than a missed period to be sure.

You can obtain a pregnancy test at your doctor's surgery, at a family planning clinic or you can buy one over the counter from a pharmacy—although these test kits are not fully reliable as they can provide false-negative results and false-positive results. Pregnancy testing can be carried out six weeks after your last monthly period. Pregnancy can be confirmed by a positive pregnancy test result, a physical examination or an ultrasound scan.

By this stage you may be experiencing common early signs of pregnancy, which include feeling sick, tired, needing to urinate more frequently than usual, swollen and tender breasts, constipation, disliking foods that you normally relish and craving foods that you don't usually much care for, and a significant absence of the irritability associated with PMS.

The first trimester
In the first 13 weeks of pregnancy, the changes occur at an astonishing rate:

Weeks 3-4   The embryo is no more than the size of a grain of rice, as it attaches to the uterus.

Weeks 4-5   The body structures are starting to develop.

Weeks 5-6   The head is beginning to form and the heart is beating. This can be seen on an ultrasound scan.

Weeks 6-8   All internal organs are formed, and the embryo is now about 2.5 cm (1 in) long. The limbs, no more than tiny buds at first, are now visible.

Weeks 10-11   The fetus moves around (although you will not be able to feel it yet); eyes are formed, and fingers and toes are in the process of forming.

Weeks 12-13   External genitals are formed; facial features are distinguishable; muscles increase in strength and movements are becoming more vigorous. Length is 7.5 cm (3 in).

What you can expect
The first antenatal visit is usually scheduled for around 12 weeks. An ultrasound scan may be done to confirm the age of the fetus, check for a heartbeat and for more than one fetus. Antenatal

care in the first three months involves a range of tests (*see* box, left) and is intended to identify any risk factors. Your doctor will discuss the results with you and your partner.

You will experience fatigue and more fatigue. Do everything you can to rest your body and give it the fuel it needs for the developing baby. Eat regularly and well at least three times a day, and avoid junk food and alcohol. If you can, eat five or six smaller meals a day rather than three big ones. Avoid danger foods that may harbour organisms: unpasteurized milk, soft mould-ripened cheese (brie, camembert, blue-streaked), soft ice-cream from machines, fish and meat pastes stored unwrapped at a deli, precooked or preroasted poultry, ready-prepared frozen foods.

ANTENATAL TESTING

Your prenatal care will probably include a variety of tests including:

- Blood tests to see if your baby is at risk of any of a large number of disorders, which include sickle-cell disease, B-thalassaemia, cystic fibrosis, Down's syndrome.
- Blood tests to find out what your blood group is (in case you later need a blood transfusion) and to determine whether you are rhesus positive or rhesus negative).
- Blood tests to see if you are anaemic, have had rubella, are free of hepatitis B, HIV and syphilis.
- Urine tests to check for kidney disease, diabetes and urinary tract disease such as cystitis.
- A cervical smear to check for infections and cancer.

LOOKING FOR TROUBLE

Your doctor may suggest one of the tests below. Before you agree, discuss the risks to your baby of each procedure—and the implications if your baby is found to have a problem.

PROCEDURE	WHEN	TO IDENTIFY
Chorionic villus sampling	Between weeks 10 and 13	Chromosome abnormality
Alphafetoprotein blood test	Between weeks 15 and 22	Fetal abnormality, including spinal cord defects
Amniocentesis	Between weeks 15 and 20	Chromosome abnormality
Ultrasound scan	From 18 weeks	Defects of spinal cord, other fetal abnormalities; check growth and wellbeing
Cordocentesis (fetal blood sampling)	From week 20	Rhesus-negative mother with antibodies that may destroy baby's blood cells

A TIME OF CHANGE
Some days you won't feel or look your best, on others you'll be blooming. Keeping in touch with what's happening to you and your body helps you work in partnership with your doctors.

BE AWARE

No sushi!
No rare meat!
No cat litter!
The organism that causes toxoplasmosis may be present in uncooked or undercooked fish or meat and in cat faeces. You may already have immunity, which will protect your fetus, but if you catch toxoplasmosis while pregnant, the effects on your baby can range from jaundice to blindness and mental disabilities.

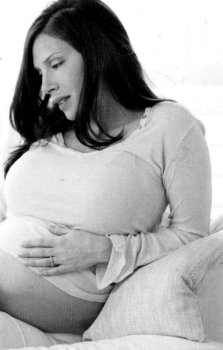

The second trimester

Weeks 14-16 The fetus is fully formed, has all vital organs and is gaining weight fast. It can stretch, turn its head, open its mouth, yawn and frown.

Weeks 16-18 First movements may be felt as the fetus kicks, bumps, twists and turns, and pushes against the springy uterus wall.

Week 20 Teeth are starting to form in the jawbone, and head hair is growing. The fetus is now about 25 cm (10 in) long.

Week 24 Fingernails have formed, thumb-sucking and hiccups begin (to coordinate sucking and swallowing needed for feeding after birth).

Getting ready for birth

When the baby's head moves into the pelvis in preparation for birth, there is less pressure on your ribs and more on the bladder. In some women, the baby's head does not fully engage until labour starts. You may have mild "practice" contractions (Braxton-Hicks)—short, intermittent and relatively painless. Breast lobules enlarge as protein and fat accumulates in the widened milk reservoirs.

Seek medical help immediately if:

- You don't feel movements for more than several hours.
- You lose weight.
- You have vaginal bleeding.
- You have severe abdominal pain.
- You have continuous and severe headache.
- Your temperature is 38.5°C (101°F) or more.
- You have blurred vision.
- Your feet and/or hands swell.
- You are vomiting.
- Your waters break.

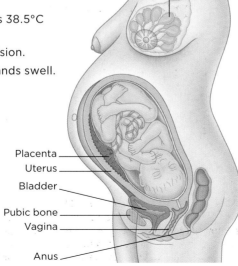

Milk duct

Placenta
Uterus
Bladder
Pubic bone
Vagina
Anus

The eyes open occasionally. Length is now 33 cm (13 in).

Week 27 Body fat is forming, the body is coated with waxy vernix, which protects fetal skin constantly bathed in the amniotic fluid. Length is about 37 cm (14½ in).

What you can expect

Indigestion and constipation may occur as in earlier months, although choosing foods carefully will help, as will allowing plenty of time for meals. Digestion will take longer now. Take some time every day to do something that gives you pleasure, but remember that you will feel very tired very easily, and so should have regular rests. Start pelvic floor exercises and continue to walk and swim. Stretch marks may start to appear at this stage. There is no sure cure for these, but keeping the skin well moisturized and limiting weight gain to recommended amounts may help minimize them.

The last trimester

Week 28 The fetus almost completely fills the uterus and may turn head down. You feel much kicking, and fluttering of feet and hands.

Week 32 All parts are now developed, and the lungs are maturing.

Week 36 The baby's head will probably come down and engage in the pelvis if this is your first baby. You may feel more pressure in the pelvis, but less shortness of breath. Baby gains weight for an efficient heat regulation system after birth. Irises are blue; hair may be as long as 2.5 cm (1 in). The umbilical cord is about 51 cm (20 in) long, resilient and slippery, making it unlikely to knot during fetal movement. Length is about 46 cm (18 in).

Week 40 By this time, there's less space for the baby to move about, but movement does continue. The eyes are sometimes open and the baby is able to discern light through the uterine wall and sense sound vibrations. Its length is now about 51 cm (20 in). Most babies will be pointing head down by this time because the head is the heaviest part of the body. The pressure of the fetal head on the cervix may help you with dilation in early labour.

LABOUR AND BIRTH

The waiting is over. It is time to ease through the contractions and work with the medical team to ensure the health and wellbeing of you and your baby.

How do you know when it's time?

Regular, painful contractions Once labour starts, abdominal cramping and tightening become regular (every 10 minutes or so) and last for 40 seconds or more. During active labour, contractions are frequent, every 2 to 3 minutes, and last up to a minute each. This is not only painful but exhausting, since it may not allow the mother to prepare for the next contraction. Use breathing techniques and pain relief (*see* opposite).

Show A discharge of pinkish blood, indicating the loss of the gelatinous mucus blocking the cervical canal during pregnancy and the stretching of the cervix. The source of blood is maternal, not fetal, and is no cause for alarm.

Breaking of the bag of waters A painless leakage of amniotic fluid, which varies from a slight dribble to a heavy gush. It indicates that the membranes surrounding the baby in the uterus have ruptured. This may precede or follow the onset of contractions.

Vaginal delivery

The birth process consists of three stages:

Stage 1 The uterus contracts at regular intervals until the cervix dilates to about 10 cm (4 in) in diameter. This is the longest stage of labour and may begin weeks before active labour starts.

Stage 2 After the cervix is fully dilated, contractions and the mother's bearing down efforts propel the baby down through the birth canal. This is usually a shorter stage, lasting several hours. It ends with the baby's birth.

Stage 3 After the birth of the baby, the placenta separates from the lining of the uterus and further contractions expel it. This usually takes less than an hour.

Assisted delivery methods

If complications develop and the baby's birth must be hastened, forceps or vacuum are used to assist delivery during the second stage of labour. If the mother does not have adequate anaesthesia, such as an epidural, a local (pudendal) block may be given for comfort. Both forceps and vacuum are safe methods for delivery in experienced hands and often safer and more expeditious than a Caesarean section. Your doctor will discuss specific options and their risks and benefits with you.

A Caesarean birth is chosen if the cervix is not completely dilated, or if forceps or vacuum are not appropriate.

THE BABY'S POSITION
Most babies are lying head down by the time they are about to be born. Some, however, remain head up in what is known as a breech presentation. A baby positioned this way can be delivered vaginally, but your doctor is quite likely to recommend that it be delivered by Caesarean section.

A MULTIPLE BIRTH

If you are carrying two or more babies, you may begin labour earlier and may need to decrease your activity or even be hospitalized to minimize your risk of premature delivery. You may also be at greater risk of high blood pressure and for smaller babies. You will probably see your doctor more often during pregnancy and will have additional testing including ultrsounds, non-stress tests, and/or biophysical profiles to ensure the continued adequate growth and wellbeing of all babies. Twins may be born vaginally if they meet certain criteria. If you have triplets or more babies, Caesarean delivery is safest.

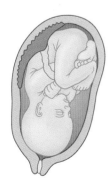

ROP: RIGHT OCCIPUT POSTERIOR
The baby is head down, facing towards the maternal abdomen.

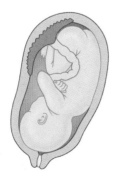

LOA: LEFT OCCIPUT ANTERIOR
The baby is head down, facing towards the maternal spine.

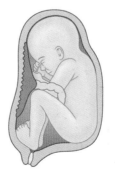

FOOTLING BREECH
The baby is sitting in the pelvic cavity with a foot or both feet extending towards the cervix.

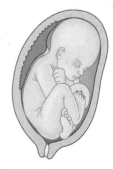

BREECH
The baby is sitting in the pelvic cavity with bottom down towards the cervix and legs crossed.

COPING WITH CONTRACTIONS

Your doctor may suggest one or more of the methods below. Before you agree, discuss the risks to your baby of each procedure—and the implications if your baby is found to have a problem.

Treatment	Action
NATURAL	
Controlled breathing	Between contractions, relax and breathe in. On exhaling make an effort and imagine all the air in your lungs being emptied. As you feel a contraction coming, inhale then exhale while saying "hee hee ha". As the contraction ends, exhale slowly, blowing all your air out.
Relaxation	Close your eyes and imagine yourself in a peaceful place, contract and relax every part of your body, starting from your toes and work up to your head. Focus on something that makes you feel good and brings a sense of achievement. You may choose a favourite photo, object or music. It doesn't matter what it is as long as it holds your concentration and helps you relax.
PHARMACOLOGICAL	
Intravenous analgesia	A variety of pain relievers such as morphine, fentanyl and others can be administered through an intravenous drip to help with labour pain. They are most often used during the first stage of labour and have a short effect. They can also cross the placenta and make the baby sleep when born. They are safe, however, and have no long-lasting effect on the baby.
Local anaesthetic	Lidocaine or its derivatives are used to numb the vaginal opening for an episiotomy, a cut made in the perineum between anus and vagina to widen the exit area for the baby, or for the repair of the episiotomy or any tears to the birth canal. A local anaesthetic can also be injected near nerves inside the vagina to provide adequate relief for assisted vaginal delivery with forceps or vacuum.
Epidural	A tiny catheter is placed in the epidural space outside the membrane surrounding the spinal cord, and a mixture of narcotic and local anaesthetic is infused for as long as is needed. During stage 1 or Caesarean section, an epidural takes away all feeling below the waist. It can be adjusted during the second stage of labour to allow for effective pushing.

The procedure involves making an incision along the bikini line and through the layers of the abdomen and the uterus. The baby is then gently lifted out. The mother's uterus and abdomen are carefully sutured together, layer by layer. A Caesarean is major surgery performed under epidural, spinal or general anaesthesia and lasts about an hour. Your partner may be present if you are awake during the operation.

An elective Caesarean is decided upon and scheduled in advance in certain situations, such as when the baby is breech. An emergency Caesarean is performed when there is an urgent need to deliver the baby quickly. A labour Caesarean is performed while the woman is in labour.

There are many reasons for labour Caesarean, including the baby's intolerance of contractions, failure of labour to progress during the first stage, severe preeclampsia or eclampsia, or when delivery is not brought about using forceps or vacuum.

The great majority of babies are successfully born vaginally. Once the baby is born, the umbilical cord is clamped and cut and the placenta peels off the uterine wall. The placenta is examined by the medical team to ensure that it has been removed in its entirety.

A subsequent vaginal delivery is possible after a woman has had one Caesarean delivery. You should discuss this option with your doctor.

Incision

CAESAREAN SECTION
Some women are not able to give birth vaginally or may need help during delivery. In this safe surgical procedure a lateral incision is made through the abdomen into the uterus. It is possible to deliver another baby vaginally after having had a Caesarean; your doctor will be able to advise you on what is best.

MOTHERHOOD

You are at last handed your newborn baby and the joys and irritations of pregnancy and the pain of labour are behind you. In these first few minutes in the delivery room as you hold the baby close, a new stage of adjustment begins: the start of the bonding process. In the last stage of labour or after delivery, you may be given an injection of oxytocin. This stimulates the uterus to contract strongly to push out the placenta, stop bleeding, and later stimulates milk production.

What's next?

Immediately after birth, an episiotomy or tears will be repaired. The sutures are absorbable and will dissolve over the next few weeks. The baby will be dried, weighed, measured and dressed to keep him/her warm. He/she will receive an antibiotic eye ointment to prevent eye infection, and a vitamin K injection to help with blood clotting. If you plan to breastfeed, this should begin as soon as feasible after birth. A baby's sucking reflexes can be strong in the first hour after birth, and the sucking action stimulates the release of oxytocin from the pituitary gland, which helps your uterus to contract and return to its normal size.

During the first few days after the birth your breasts will produce colostrum, a yellowish watery liquid rich in proteins, sugar and antibodies (lymphocytes and immunoglobulins). It may not seem much in quantity, but it is rich and nourishing and helps to protect the baby from infection.

A mix of emotions

It is quite normal to experience an array of emotions during birth and just after, responses brought about by excitement and hormones, and it may take some time to come down to earth. For the first-time mother especially, there may be a new intensity of feeling, balanced perhaps by the physical effects of childbirth that can leave you tired, sore and overwhelmed. Give yourself time. The adjustment process–of bonding with your baby, and becoming a family–is gradual and evolves as you recover and gain confidence.

Fluctuating hormone levels may cause you to feel dejected between 3 and 7 days after the delivery. This is called the "baby blues" and commonly occurs as your body recovers and you are tired from the unaccustomed routine and demands.

THE APGAR SCORE FOR YOUR BABY'S HEALTH

Your baby is assessed for the five factors shown below and then weighed. A baby scoring 7 or more points is in good general health. A week or so later, a blood sample from the baby will be analysed for vitamin K deficiency—phenylketonuria.

SIGN	0	1	2
Respiratory effort	None	Weak cry, slow breathing	Strong cry
Pulse (heart rate)	None	Slow, under 100 beats per minute	Fast, over 100 beats per minute
Colour (pallor)	Blue-pale	Pink body with blue fingers and toes	All pink
Muscular tone	Limp	Some flexing of fingers and toes	Active, fingers and toes flexing well
Response to stimuli (reflexes)	No response	Grimace	Cry

No one will think less of you for feeling weepy or irritable. Don't hesitate to talk about it. If these feelings persist, see your doctor. You may need some help to get you through this time.

You may start walking or gentle exercise shortly. Do your postpartum exercises, including the pelvic floor exercises for strengthening the pelvic floor. Use pads not tampons. You will have a postpartum check-up at six weeks, but your health visitor or midwife can address any concerns that you may have before this appointment.

Breastfeeding

Putting your baby to the breast as soon as possible after delivery introduces the baby to your nipple and the surrounding dark area (the areola). When the baby takes most of this into the mouth, called "latching on", a vacuum is created with the tongue. In the first few days, colostrum is sufficient, and it soon gives way to mature breast milk–delivered at the right temperature and full of nutrients–stimulated by the baby's suckling. Initially you should place the baby at your breast about every 2 hours and offer both breasts each time.

If you have difficulties positioning the baby, or with latching on, ask your midwife, nurse, or a lactation consultant to help you. While breastfeeding may be natural, it may take a week or two for feeding to get going and perhaps longer

NIPPLE HEALTH

When you are breastfeeding, take good care of your nipples. Express some milk after feeding and allow it to dry; it will act as a natural moisturizer. If you need to wear pads inside your nursing bra to catch leaks, change them as frequently as you change the baby's nappies.

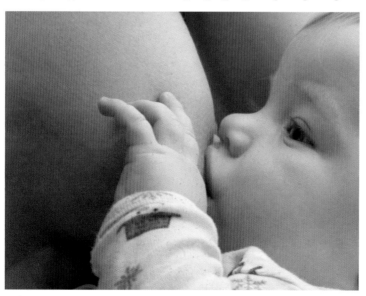

for a pattern to be established. The baby's weight and mood are the best indicators of whether or not he or she is receiving enough food.

If your baby cries a lot and is not producing 6 to 8 wet nappies a day after the first 5 days of life, he/she may not be getting enough milk. Allow about 20 to 30 minutes for feeding. If you offer a breast when your baby cries on demand, your baby will quickly learn that you are available to satisfy hunger and will actually cry less.

Looking after a new infant day and night is demanding and you should try to ensure you get as much rest as you can rather than trying to catch up with other tasks.

Make sure that you eat well and drink plenty of water. This is very important while breastfeeding to replace fluids. Be advised by your health professional about establishing a feeding routine, but have faith in your own instincts. Learn to enjoy being close to the baby, rather than becoming concerned. Cuddling and gentle stroking will relax you both. Accept that when the baby is hungry, he or she will almost certainly eat.

If your breasts become engorged, express some milk to be used later. A variety of breast pumps is available to do this comfortably, even when you go back to work. This will enable your partner to feed the baby, too. Some women develop cracked nipples. Lanolin cream or even expressed milk allowed to air dry will help heal them. Mastitis is a breast infection in which redness, a firm area on the breast, and sometimes fever occur. Should this occur, see your doctor promptly, who may treat the condition using antibiotics. You may continue breastfeeding.

Bottle feeding

You may choose to bottle feed, either because you don't want to, or can't, breastfeed. This can have the advantage of allowing your partner to become involved in feeding the baby right from the start. You can consult your doctor about how to prevent your breasts producing milk. Ask for guidance so that you know the right formula for the size of your baby, and follow instructions exactly.

Complications During Pregnancy

Many complications may occur during pregnancy, ranging from high blood pressure to miscarriage. Your health care team, consisting of your obstetrician and midwife, will monitor you carefully throughout your pregnancy so that they can detect and treat any problems early in the process.

MISCARRIAGE

The loss of a baby through miscarriage is more common than many people realize. Most occur within the first two months of pregnancy and many women may be aware of it.

Miscarriage is much less likely after 12-16 weeks. Warning signs are vaginal bleeding, cramps and backache similar to those of a period, and absence of pregnancy signs such as tender breasts and morning sickness. Once it starts, little can be done to halt a miscarriage.

What are the causes?

Evaluation of repeated miscarriages or one that occurred late in pregnancy should be done to exclude a treatable cause, but often the evaluation is negative. Most couples who lose a pregnancy do so for no clear reason and go on to have a healthy baby later. An evaluation may include referral to a genetic counsellor and blood testing for antiphospholipid syndrome, diabetes and various infections, as well as uterine or cervical abnormalities such as a cervix that prematurely dilates rather than remaining closed during pregnancy.

Testing risks

Certain prenatal tests carry a risk of miscarriage–these include chorionic villus sampling (CVS) (1 in 200) and amniocentesis (1 in 2,000).

CVS is carried out between 10 and 12 weeks using a fine needle inserted through the cervix or abdomen to remove uterine tissue that eventually becomes the placenta. This sample contains genetic information and may reveal whether the fetus has developed a chromosomal disorder, such as Down's syndrome.

Amniocentesis is normally carried out at 16-18 weeks. The procedure involves a needle being inserted through the abdomen into the uterus and amniotic sac to obtain a cell sample.

PREGNANCY COMPLICATIONS

Complications that may prevent a full-term pregnancy or live birth:

- Preeclampsia (a combination of high blood pressure, protein in the urine and swelling in late pregnancy. Can become very serious and include seizures if not treated early see box, next page).
- Rhesus factor (a type of antigen that may be present on the red blood cells. If absent in the mother and present in the fetus, it may result in severe fetal anemia and other problems. All mothers are tested for this antigen. If negative, they are given immunoglobulins to prevent it).
- Prenatal haemorrhage (bleeding from the placenta or other part of the reproductive tract of a pregnant woman).
- Too much or too little amniotic fluid (too much may be a complication of conditions such as diabetes and may result in early delivery; too little may be an early sign of poor fetal growth or fetal kidney problems).
- Retroversion of the uterus (a normal variant in the position of the uterus, so called "tipped uterus").
- Stillbirth (when the fetus dies inside the uterus prior to birth).

HIGH BLOOD PRESSURE IN PREGNANCY

Having your blood pressure (BP) checked regularly is essential during pregnancy. This identifies the woman who has an elevated blood pressure that puts her at risk for a complication of pregnancy called pre-eclampsia.

When it causes her to retain fluid and excrete proteins in her urine, she may need urgent treatment to reduce her BP, or labor may need to be induced to prevent the progression to eclampsia— which is defined as all the above signs of preeclampsia plus seizure. Eclampsia can have very serious consequences for both mother and baby. A woman is at higher risk if she is at either extreme of reproductive age, carries more than one baby, is pregnant with her first baby, has existing hypertension, diabetes mellitus, autoimmune disorders or kidney disease. Tests carried out in early pregnancy may identify women at risk.

Amniocentesis may reveal genetic or developmental disorders later in pregnancy. The test is also used to assess rhesus incompatibility and the fetus's lung maturity. These invasive procedures are generally carried out after an abnormal blood test in the first trimester screen or triple (quad) screen. The first trimester screen tests maternal blood for the blood markers HCG and pappA and includes an ultrasound measurement of the baby's neck fold thickness. The triple screen tests for the markers alpha fetoprotein, human chorionic gonadotropin and inhibin A. These markers may be abnormal in certain conditions, including neural tube defects, Down's syndrome or trisomy 18. The results will read as a ratio, not as a "yes" or "no" answer. For example, the ratio "1 in 350" means that for every 350 pregnancies with the same result, 349 are likely to be normal.

You should discuss the risks as well as the implications of such tests with your doctor. They can cause anxiety, and the wait for results can be difficult. While most come back normal, you need to consider how you would handle an abnormal result.

A problem with the placenta

Severe vaginal bleeding in the second or third trimester may indicate placenta praevia or placental abruption (placenta abruptio): both require urgent attention.

Danger signs

A serious problem of early pregnancy is an ectopic pregnancy, where the fetus develops outside the uterus (*see* box below). Symptoms include:
- Sudden, sharp or persistent pain in one side of the lower abdomen.
- Pain under one of the shoulder blades.
- Vaginal bleeding.

If an ectopic pregnancy is diagnosed, a laparoscopy is often used to remove the pregnancy and, sometimes, part of the fallopian tube. Alternatively, a chemotherapy drug methotrexate may be given to hasten the absorption of an early ectopic pregnancy. Women who have had one ectopic pregnancy are at greater risk of a subsequent one, but many women succeed in conceiving and achieving a normal pregnancy and delivery after an ectopic pregnancy.

Ectopic pregnancy

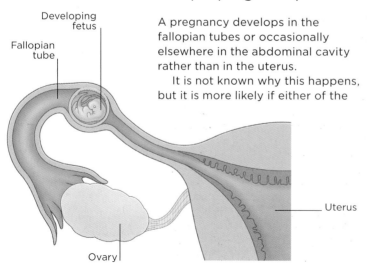

A pregnancy develops in the fallopian tubes or occasionally elsewhere in the abdominal cavity rather than in the uterus.

It is not known why this happens, but it is more likely if either of the fallopian tubes has been damaged by endometriosis, pelvic inflammatory disease (caused by chlamydia, gonorrhoea, and other sexually transmitted infections), pelvic adhesions, tubal surgery or by a previous ectopic pregnancy. Ectopic pregnancy is a potentially fatal condition that requires emergency attention. The symptoms include severe abdominal pain and vaginal bleeding in the presence of a positive pregnancy test. An ectopic pregnancy needs to be differentiated from other causes such as appendicitis or threatened spontaneous abortion.

Developing fetus

Fallopian tube

Uterus

Ovary

The Unintended Pregnancy

Nobody sets out to become pregnant in order to have an abortion. Yet many women, married and unmarried, find themselves in the position of having to make a choice about abortion that may affect them for many years to come. Remember that, if you are in any doubt, there is the option of giving birth to the baby and having it adopted.

HAVING AN ABORTION

Many pregnancies–about one in three in unmarried women and one in four in married ones–end in abortion, which is the voluntary termination of pregnancy before the fetus can live independently. There may be many reasons for a pregnancy to be terminated. Conception may have been unintentional, the woman may have a health condition that makes pregnancy risky, there may be an abnormality in the fetus or many other possible reasons.

Whatever the reason, the more thought and care that goes into the decision, the better the psychological outcome will be. Reliable advice and information should be sought on the methods used and what, if any, side effects they may have. Many women facing an unintended pregnancy benefit from counselling.

Make the decision

Some women know immediately that they want to terminate their pregnancy and will be comfortable with their decision; others are not sure. Most will want to discuss it with people closest to them, especially with their male partner, if appropriate. Having a supportive male partner can make a great deal of difference at such a time, but for many women this may not be an option. How a woman feels about the prospect of abortion will depend on why she wants one. A woman who definitely does not want to have a child is in a different position from a woman who would ideally like one, but for financial or other reasons is unable to cope with one at present. If abortion is against her ethical and social values, this can cause even more conflict. If there is any uncertainty, it is important not to feel pressured into having an abortion. You may wish to consider the alternative of continuing with the pregnancy and having the baby adopted.

Talk it through

Because it is much easier physically and psychologically to have an abortion as early in a pregnancy as possible, time may be an added stressor in the decision making. To help you place the experience in perspective, you need to talk to non-judgmental people familiar with the emotional issues involved. Having the opportunity to talk through your decision will help you to feel more reconciled to it later.

Meet with a counsellor

Having to make the decision to abort a wanted baby may be very traumatic and cause an incredible amount of anguish.

UNPROTECTED SEX?

Your first consideration after unprotected sex should be some kind of morning-after treatment, which may be effective in blocking pregnancy for several days after having unprotected intercourse.

THE TRAUMA OF SEXUAL ASSAULT

Sexual assault is one of the most traumatic things that can happen to a woman. The experience of being forced, coerced or manipulated into unwanted sex may remain with you for life. The humiliation you feel can prevent you from trusting men, affect close relationships and leave serious psychological sequelae.

The number of reported sexual assaults is increasing faster than other crimes of violence and includes penetration of the vagina, anus or mouth with a penis, finger or object. Most sexual assaults are carried out by a man known to the woman. So-called date rape, in which a woman is raped by a man with whom she has become friendly, has been a subject of controversy.

Contacting a Rape Crisis Centre, emergency department or counsellor will provide you with emotional and physical support after this terrible event. You may wish to discuss informing the police and what this might entail. Your first reaction may be to take a shower, but before you wash, you should have a medical check-up. This is best done by a doctor or at a hospital where there are staff experienced in examining sexual assault victims. A complete physical examination will be carried out, you will be given tests for STIs and, if there is a chance you could become pregnant, emergency contraception.

You should make an appointment to see your doctor two weeks after the incident for follow-up care. You may need ongoing counselling to deal with your emotions.

You may feel it is the only option because prenatal tests show the fetus to have chromosomal or physical problems such as Down's syndrome or spina bifida. These tests (blood, ultrasound scan and amniocentesis) are offered and carried out routinely; some are done at about 16 weeks of pregnancy and there may be a wait for the results. Your doctor, counsellor or support group can help you come to terms with the decision and to understand the implications for future pregnancies.

Abortion procedures

Termination of a pregnancy (under 24 weeks) can be done on request by a doctor at a family planning or abortion clinic or at a hospital. The needs and welfare of the woman are of prime importance, particularly if there are health problems, such as heart disease, blood clotting disorders or mental health conditions.

Abortion is a commonly performed surgical procedure, mostly done between 7 and 12 weeks. You may have a pelvic examination or an ultrasound scan. Tests may be done to see if you are anaemic and if you have a rhesus-negative blood type, and also for infection (STI). The doctor will want to know whether you have had a child or a previous abortion or miscarriage. This first appointment can be emotional, and a partner or friend can be a great support.

The termination is done by vacuum aspiration, a surgical procedure with local anaesthetic administered to the cervix and intravenous sedation. You may feel nauseated and have cramps,

similar to painful periods, after the procedure, which takes 10-15 minutes. You will probably be in the clinic for several hours afterwards. You will have bleeding as in a normal period, and you may receive medication to help the uterus to shrink and to lessen bleeding. You should ask your doctor when you can return to work (a few days' rest is usually advisable). Antibiotics are often prescribed to prevent infection.

Abortion after 12 weeks

At this later stage–the second trimester (12-24 weeks)–the health risks for the woman are much greater.

The first stage of the procedure is a D&E (dilation and evacuation) in which prostaglandin or laminaria (seaweed) sticks are used to gently dilate the cervix over several hours or overnight. Later on or the next day, vacuum aspiration under local anaesthetic/sedation is carried out in a similar fashion as in the earlier abortion procedure. In addition, the larger fetal parts are removed.

The risks

Having an abortion in the early stages of pregnancy is considered safe, but there are a few risks. Sometimes tissue is retained in the uterus that may have to be removed by D&C (dilation and curettage) later. You will be advised not to place anything in the vagina, including tampons, and to avoid douching and sex for two weeks to reduce risk of infection. Indications of infection are a high temperature, very heavy bleeding, foul-smelling discharge or severe abdominal pain; if you have any of these symptoms, go back to your doctor promptly for treatment. You should also see your doctor about contraception if a pregnancy is not desired in the near future.

Be kind

Loss and sadness are perfectly normal reactions after a termination, even when you are sure you have made the right decision. It is important that you show compassion to yourself at this time. Accept that it may take some time to recover fully, but if you feel you need help with your emotions, seek a support group or counselling.

THE ADOPTION OPTION

Abortion is not the only answer for a woman with an unwanted pregnancy. She may decide to carry the baby to term and then have it adopted. In this instance it is essential that she seeks reliable information and advice on what may be involved, including help with her own physical and emotional welfare during pregnancy and after giving birth.

Once the pregnancy has been confirmed by the doctor and the normal tests done, you should ask about your options, including adoption. The doctor or member of staff should be able to provide nonjudgmental counselling– whether a family member could possibly keep the child, for example, or if there are strong feelings about who the adoptive family should be.

If you decide to have the baby adopted, it is generally advised that the process begin immediately, under the direction of a social worker in an adoption agency. A case record of the history of the child, its parents and their state of health and religious or cultural preferences will be made. Sometimes, a birth mother deals directly with the people who wish to adopt her child (open adoption), but an independent agency may offer support during the pregnancy for this purpose.

If the birth mother is married, her husband automatically shares parental responsibility and his consent must be sought before the child can be adopted. If the woman is unmarried but puts the name of the father on the birth certificate (must be registered within six weeks after the birth), he may wish to be involved in the adoption process. You should seek legal advice about your particular situation. The adoption agency may be able to assist you in contacting an experienced legal counsel.

Care for yourself

A pregnant woman giving her child up for adoption should seek counselling to help her deal with the experience both physically and emotionally. Your doctor may have staff experienced in these matters. You will not be expected to provide care for your child. However,

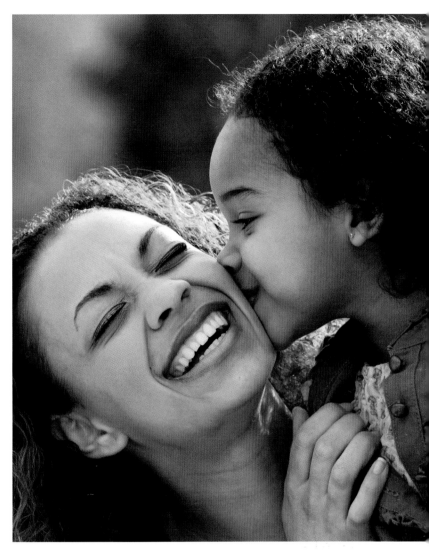

you may decide to look after the child and share the care under the guidance of the social worker. Issues such as whether to breastfeed or not should be part of any discussion.

Finding the right person to talk freely to about the reasons for giving up the child is important. You may not agree with termination or, if conception occurred after rape or violent assault, you may not feel able to care for a child conceived in this way. Perhaps you are not prepared to be a parent at this stage. Whatever your reasons, you need to address them, to allow yourself time to grieve so that you recover fully. Physically you need to see your doctor for a check-up six weeks after the birth to ensure you are healing well.

A WANTED CHILD
There are thousands of prospective parents seeking to adopt children. After a woman who chooses to have her child placed for adoption gives her consent, the process can begin quickly, and the adoptive parents can become involved soon after.

205

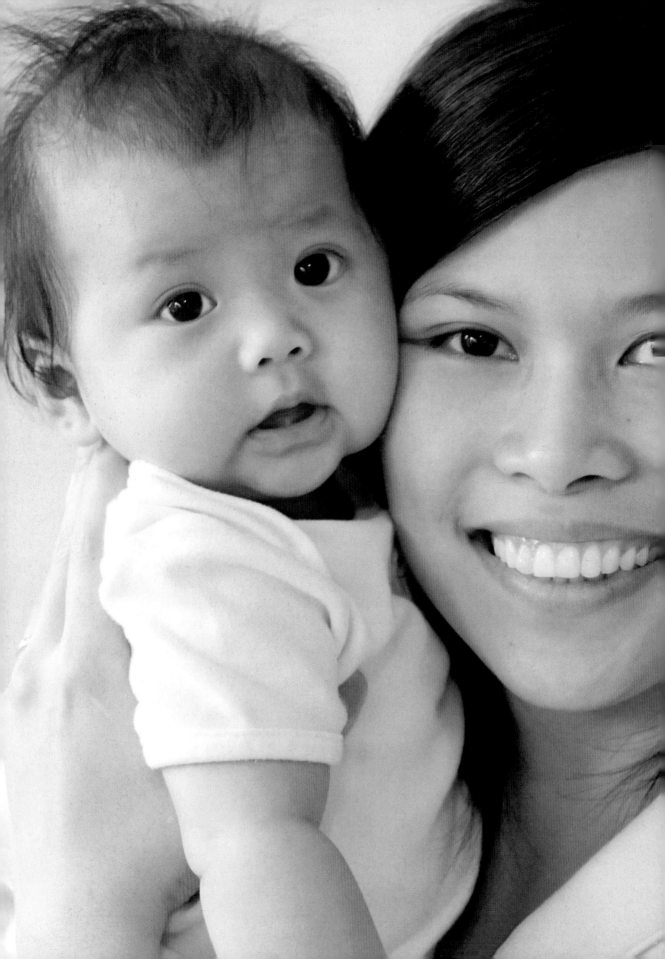

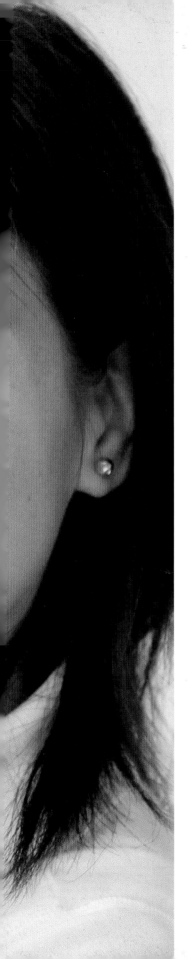

REPRODUCTIVE SYSTEM HEALTH

Along with the exciting ability to create new life, a woman's reproductive system also demands careful vigilance and maintenance. This chapter will help you screen for evolving problems in the system's key organs, understand what can go wrong–and know what to do when it does.

Breast Care

Your breasts play a crucial role in your sexual identity and in your nurturing role as a mother. They also tend to change size and shape as you progress from puberty to old age. Here's how to work out what these changes mean—and when you need to be checked by your doctor.

BENIGN BREAST CHANGES

There is an almost infinite variety in the shape and size of women's breasts. One can be bigger or higher or lower than the other. They can be rounded and full, or rounded and small. They may stand away from the chest wall or hang down. Some nipples are prominent, others may be inverted, and some women have extra nipples on the chest wall. And breast tissue may even extend into the armpit.

All of these describe "normal" breasts, which develop from puberty under the influence of the female hormone oestrogen, their shape depending on fatty and fibrous tissue surrounding the network of milk-secreting glands. Usually fully formed by the age of 20, breasts have no muscles, but they are suspended by ligaments.

Only a minority of women go through life without experiencing any breast discomfort at all, whether it is pain that starts before a period begins or the tenderness that heralds the onset of a pregnancy.

Some women regularly find lumps and bumps in their breasts. In women under 25 these are most often growths of harmless fibrous tissue. Between 30 and 40 a woman is more likely to develop cysts, which are full of fluid and can be painful (see p. 210).

Becoming familiar with the normal changes of your breasts will help you detect any new lump, thickening, or pain—and motivate you to see your doctor for an evaluation.

Breast pain

Medically known as mastalgia, breast pain is common and rarely a sign of serious disease. It is often described as cyclical, noncyclical or extramammary. Cyclical breast pain occurs in premenopausal women. It is usually worse just before a period when the breasts also tend to be lumpy; it subsides with menstruation. Although hormone therapy during the menopause years can trigger cyclical breast pain, most women find that breast pain disappears completely after menopause.

Noncyclical pain may be due to the weight of the breasts, muscle strain, a cyst or infection, pregnancy, prior breast surgery, oestrogen use and ill-fitting bras. It may be constant or intermittent, and typically occurs in the 40s or 50s.

If you have new onset breast pain, see your doctor. A breast examination and mammography or ultrasound may be done, and your doctor may suggest you keep a pain diary: it will help you judge whether your pain is cyclical and if anything makes it better or worse.

Potential causes of extramammary pain include referred pain from the chest wall and inflammation of the rib cage.

Persistent pain requires mammography and/or ultrasound to exclude a malignancy and a doctor's evaluation.

TAKE ACTION NOW!

Breast pain can often be effectively dealt with by some simple changes. Here are some things you can do:
- Have bras fitted by a professional
- Wear a sports bra during any vigorous exercise you do
- Reduce your intake of salt
- Ditch caffeinated drinks
- Switch to a lower-fat diet

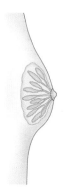 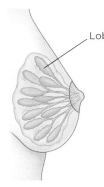 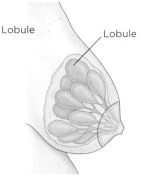 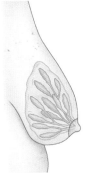

Lobule — Lobule

At puberty   **At maturity**   **When breastfeeding**   **After the menopause**

BREASTS AS YOU AGE
Mature breasts are composed of glandular tissue made up of 15–20 lobules. Milk-producing tissue becomes active in the days before a period, and some women have tenderness and lumpiness. In pregnancy the breasts enlarge, the milk-duct system expands and more lobules are formed. After the menopause, the glandular part shrinks as the proportion of fat increases, making the breasts less dense.

For persistent pain, your doctor may prescribe danazol, a hormonal drug that reduces oestrogen levels. However, this drug may have troublesome side effects, such as weight gain and acne. An alternative treatment is gamolenic acid (also known as evening primrose oil), which has no anti-oestrogenic side effects.

The elimination or dose reduction of hormone therapy may also alleviate breast pain.

NIPPLE PROBLEMS

Some women are born with inverted nipples. However, if a nipple suddenly becomes inverted, see your doctor since it could signal an underlying problem.

Nipple discharge is common and often due to benign causes. A green, grey, blue, brown or clear discharge is typically benign and associated with fibrocystic changes. Milky discharge may occur during pregnancy or persist for months after breastfeeding. Excess prolactin secretion may be caused by a prolactinoma, a benign tumour in the pituitary gland. Yellow or bloodstained discharge, or, rarely, a watery discharge may be due to a noncancerous tumour in a milk duct. The most common causes of a bloody nipple discharge are: first, an intraductal papilloma; next, duct dilation with or without inflammation; and third, cancer. Discharge containing pus usually indicates an infection for which antibiotics are needed.

The work-up of nipple discharge includes diagnostic mammography and/or ultrasound. Spontaneous, persistent bloody discharge or watery discharge from a single duct requires surgical duct excision to exclude malignancy, even if the breast imaging tests are normal.

Breast infections

A breast abscess is a collection of pus that forms a firm, painful lump. It develops if mastitis, or inflammation of the breast, caused by bacterial infection is not treated promptly with antibiotics. Mastitis most commonly occurs during breastfeeding, when bacteria in the baby's mouth can enter the breast through a crack in the nipple. It is characterized by redness and tenderness, a raised temperature and flu-like symptoms. Your doctor may prescribe antibiotics. If an abscess does develop, it should be drained, either with a fine needle or through a small incision made in the skin.

Mastitis is uncommon in a non-nursing woman. When such symptoms occur in this group, antibiotics are recommended as well as short-term monitoring by your doctor. If there is no improvement, a biopsy is advised to look for an underlying malignancy. A breast infection can be confused with inflammatory breast cancer.

Lumps in the breast

Many women have lumpy breasts; the lumps may become more obvious and tender just before a menstrual period. These are known as fibrocystic breast changes and are a normal response to the hormonal changes of the menstrual cycle. Women with fibrocystic changes are not at increased risk of breast cancer, although the condition may make it more difficult for new lumps to be noticed. Regular self-examinations (*see* box next page) will make you familiar with the usual texture of your breasts, so you are more likely to pick up new changes if they occur.

SEE YOUR DOCTOR

Even if you do have fibrous tissue or cysts on a regular basis you should never ignore new lumps or any other changes to your breasts because there is always the possibility that a cancerous growth is present. It is important to remember that the earlier breast cancer is diagnosed, the greater the possibility that it can be prevented from spreading.

Cysts are filled with fluid and may often be felt as smooth lumps. They are sometimes painful, but fluid can be aspirated to relieve any breast pain. Cysts do not necessarily need treatment, but ask your doctor to check them.

Fibroadenomas are another common cause of a benign breast tumour in a woman between the ages of 15 and 30. They often present as a single, firm mass and tend to move freely in the breast. They occur as a result of an overgrowth of the glands and fibrous tissue and rarely are associated with malignancy.

Fibroadenomas may enlarge with hormonal stimulation. Most tend to decrease in size with the menopause. The diagnosis of a fibroadenoma is done by breast imaging and possibly a breast biopsy. Some women have them surgically removed if they increase in size.

How lumps are investigated

If you notice a new lump or area of thickening in your breast, you should see your doctor immediately. Imaging tests such as diagnostic mammography or ultrasound scanning may be arranged. Fine needle aspiration, in which a small syringe needle is inserted into the lump to withdraw cells, may be performed. If the lump is solid or does not decrease in size after the aspiration, the cell samples will be sent for laboratory analysis. Further diagnostic mammography and/or ultrasound may also be needed.

Know your own breasts

Breasts are influenced by hormonal variation, which can make them sensitive, engorged, tender or lumpy. Every woman should become familiar with how her breasts look and feel at different times of the month, so that she is confident about knowing what is normal for her. Beginning at age 20, self-examination is encouraged once a month about one week after the beginning ends. Menopausal women should examine their breasts at the same time each month.

First, raise your arms over your head and look at your breasts in a mirror. Notice any changes such as dimpling, puckering, or rash involving the skin, whether the nipples appear as they usually do, without any sign of discharge, bleeding or a rash. To see how your breasts feel, lie down or examine yourself while in the shower. Place one arm behind your head and with the flat of your fingers of the opposite hand, feel all over the breast and armpit. Be careful not to prod or squeeze. Remember that most women do not develop breast cancer, and that if you do find a lump, nine out of ten that are discovered are benign.

- Stand in front of a mirror, raise your arms above your head and lean forwards so you can see the shape of your breasts and how they move from side to side.
- Put your hands on your hips so that your chest muscles tense. Look again, then turn sideways so that you can see the contours of your breasts from every angle.
- Lie down, put one arm behind your head, and use the flat of the fingers of your other hand to feel for any lump or thickening in the breast.
- Begin at the collar bone and use the three middle fingers to work your way around your breast with gentle sweeping strokes toward the nipple, like the spokes of a wheel.

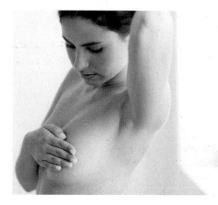

The presence of straw-coloured fluid with collapse of the lump determines that the problem is a cyst. A fluid sample will be sent for analysis only if it is bloody.

If you do find something during self-examination, you are bound to be anxious. Keep reminding yourself that nine out of every ten lumps are benign–in other words, they are noncancerous.

Your doctor may be able to reassure you that there is nothing to worry about but if there is the slightest doubt, you may be given an appointment at a breast clinic, where the problem can be fully investigated. You may undergo tests and procedures such as a mammogram or a biopsy–which involves taking a sample of cells for microscopic examination.

Mammography

The national screening programme offers women between the ages of 50 and 70 a mammogram–a breast X-ray–every three years. A woman who has a strong family history of breast cancer may be advised to begin screening 10 years before the age of the youngest affected first-degree relative in her family. Screening mammography performed before age 50 may be challenging because the breasts are denser, making the mammograms harder to "read".

The aim of mammography is to detect cancer at a very early stage, before it has a chance to spread. Because the incidence of breast cancer increases with age (1 in 14 by age 70, 1 in 10 at age 80), women may consider annual mammograms a worthwhile investment.

Mammography picks up most, but not all, cancerous tumours, and although you can feel reassured by a normal result, you should check your breasts regularly. An annual MRI (magnetic resonance imaging) scan may also be recommended for women who fall into a high risk group (see box, right).

How mammography is done

On the day of your examination, do not use deodorant or powder in the underarm or breast area. The radiology technician will ask you to undress to the waist and will then position each breast in turn between a clear plastic plate and the X-ray plate, so that the breast tissue is compressed. Two pictures of each breast will be taken.

The test may cause mild discomfort due to the need for breast compression, but it lasts only a few minutes. If your breasts have been augmented with an implant, inform the radiology technician since you will require special views to assess the tissue.

You will be asked to wait after the mammogram, while the film is processed to ensure the image is sufficiently clear, although the wait should usually not be longer than about 10 to 15 minutes. The X-rays will be analysed by a radiologist, who will normally give the result to your doctor. He or she may contact you directly if the image was not clear or an abnormality is detected that requires further views. Mammograms are now being performed in many medical centres using digital technology.

WHO IS AT RISK?

Between 5 and 10 per cent of women have an increased risk of developing breast cancer at an early age due to a genetic link. A woman with one first-degree relative—mother or sister—with breast cancer has a slightly higher risk than other women, especially if the first-degree relative was diagnosed with breast cancer before age 50.

Women who have had both breast and ovarian cancer, multiple cases of breast cancer, a male relative with breast cancer, a relative with ovarian cancer, are of Ashkenazi Jewish heritage or have had bilateral breast cancer may also fall into a high risk category. Women who fall into this category may wish to talk to a genetic counsellor to learn more about the risks, limitations and benefits of genetic testing based on their family history. Having a breast cancer gene does not necessarily mean that you will develop the cancer. Women who test positive for the gene mutation BRCA1 or BRCA2 have up to a 40 to 80 per cent lifetime risk of developing breast cancer.

In the Women's Health Initiative study that took place in the United States between 1993 and 2005, postmenopausal combination hormonal replacement therapy (HRT, oestrogen plus synthetic progesterone) was found to increase the risk of developing breast cancer. The risk was associated with long-term use of greater than three years. The increase in risk also falls after HRT is stopped.

The Women's Health Initiative study also looked at women who have had a hysterectomy and were threated with oestrogen-only hormonal therapy. No increased risk of breast cancer was found. It is important to understand that this risk level may not apply to women who have a significant risk for breast cancer due to a family history or other personal risk factors.

Age is the most common risk factor. Other risk factors include older age at birth of first child (35+ years), postmenopausal obesity, early menarche, late menopause and a history of prior breast biopsy that reveals a high rate of cellular proliferation in ducts or lobes.

BREAST CANCER

There is no doubt that finding a breast lump provokes anxiety and some women may be reluctant to go to a doctor. But time is very important because many forms of cancer, if caught early enough, have treatment options that will result in saving the breast, as well as improved recurrence and survival rates.

Treatment is likely to be more effective when it is provided by doctors who are experienced in dealing with a particular form of cancer. In recent years, the management of breast cancer has become complex. Seeking care or even a second opinion at a breast centre or a hospital that has a multidisciplinary team of breast experts is recommended. Talk to your doctor about the various options available.

What are the risk factors?

Some women may be more susceptible to developing breast cancer than others as a result of their genetic inheritance or lifestyle, although many individuals who have several or even all of the risk factors listed below will never do so.

Being over the age of 50   Younger women may be diagnosed with breast cancer, but 75 per cent of breast cancers are diagnosed in women over age 50.

A family history of breast cancer This is especially relevant if it developed at a relatively early age. Having one first-degree relative (mother or sister) with breast cancer doubles the risk; having two multiplies it five-fold.

Having no children, or a first pregnancy after the age of 35   These women have about double the risk of a woman who has her first child before the age of 20. Breastfeeding has been associated with a decreased risk of breast cancer.

Beginning your periods before the age of 12 and having late menopause (after the age of 50)   The longer the time between menarche and the menopause, the greater the risk. Improved nutrition and increased dietary fat intake, which are notable in developed countries, may result in early menarche. The result is long-term, uninterrupted cyclical hormonal stimulation of the breast.

In China, where there is a low incidence of breast cancer, the average age for a girl to begin her periods is 17 years, compared with 12.5 years in the UK and Australia.

Inheriting one of the genes known as BRCA1 and BRCA2   These genes are associated with a 40-80 per cent lifetime risk of developing breast cancer. However, only 5-10 per cent of all breast cancer is thought to be genetic in origin.

Lifestyle   Regular high alcohol consumption, obesity and an inactive lifestyle all contribute to a higher risk of developing breast cancer. In countries where a sedentary lifestyle and fatty food predominate, the incidence of breast cancer has increased drastically.

When cancer is detected

Breast cancer is identified by biopsy–taking a sample of tissue for analysis or surgical excision of a breast mass. A core needle breast biopsy provides tissue for a pathologist to examine and diagnose. The procedure can be performed by a radiologist using ultrasound guidance or by a surgeon as a day surgery procedure under local anaesthetic. The results are usually available in two or three days. The pathological analysis of the core needle biopsy will be able to tell whether the cancer is invasive or not. Invasive disease means cancer that has a tendency to spread outside the breast. Invasive ductal carcinoma is the most common type of breast cancer.

Non-invasive disease describes cancer that grows in just one place or is contained within the inside of the duct–it is called ductal carcinoma in situ. Non-cancerous abnormal cell growth, or atypical hyperplasia, is a marker for increased risk for breast cancer.

Other rarer types of cancer include: Paget's disease, in which a slow-growing cancer produces changes in the nipple and areolar region; intra-cystic carcinoma, a cancer growing within a cyst; and inflammatory cancer that causes changes on the skin such as redness, swelling and pain. This type often spreads quickly and often produces no evident lump.

Two crucial questions have to be answered before treatment is decided.

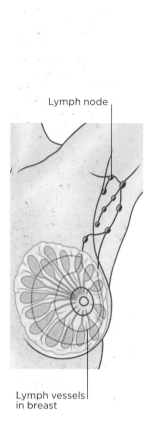

Lymph node

Lymph vessels in breast

SENTINEL NODE MAPPING
The technique of sentinel node mapping is used to detect whether cancer has spread to the lymph nodes. The "sentinel" node is the first lymph node draining a tumour. It is identified by injecting the tumour with a radioactive dye or methylene blue dye. The first node found to contain dye is dissected at the time of the breast cancer surgery. If there are no cancerous cells found, there is a 98 per cent certainty that the cancer has not spread to the lymph node in the armpit. If the sentinel lymph node is positive for cancer, then additional auxiliary lymph node dissection is required.

Is the chance of spread to other parts of the body high or low? And what can be done to reduce that chance? Doctors want to know whether the tumour has spread to the lymph nodes and, if so, how many are involved. They also look at the tumour size. Two tests are also extremely helpful in determining prognosis and the role of hormonal therapy or chemotherapy: these are known as the hormone receptor status and HER2 (human epidermal growth factor receptor 2) status.

The aims of treatment

Treating breast cancer has three aims: to remove the primary tumour, to reduce the chance of the cancer returning in the breast or armpit and to reduce the chance of the cancer establishing secondary tumours in the body (known as metastasis, or distant spread). The medical team's recommendations take into account all the factors that might affect you and consider the emotional, social, spiritual and financial aspects of treatment, as well as the physical. It is important that you are an active participant in the discussion and understand as much as possible about the proposed treatment. If you have a genetic susceptibility, you may also be asked to meet a genetic counsellor to discuss the role of genetic testing and its impact in evaluating surgical management options.

Surgery as treatment

The aim of breast cancer surgery is to achieve local control of the disease, prevent complications such as skin ulceration, determine the existence and extent of lymph node involvement and provide information regarding treatment and prognosis. The surgical options are:

Total or simple mastectomy This involves removal of the entire breast, but none of the chest muscle.

Lumpectomy This is a wide local excision of the lump and includes some surrounding normal breast tissue. This procedure is followed by breast irradiation treacment.

Modified radical mastectomy This procedure involves removal of the entire breast and axillary lymph nodes.

Subcutaneous mastectomy High-risk precancerous conditions are sometimes treated using subcutaneous mastectomy. Most of the breast tissue is removed, leaving skin and nipple intact. The breast can be reconstructed with an implant or your own tissue.

Sentinel lymph node surgery Surgical dissection of the sentinel lymph nodes is performed if the nodes test negative for cancer.

Lymph gland (axillary nodes) removal This procedure may follow the initial sentinel lymph node biopsy if the nodes test positive for cancer.

Breast reconstruction This is carried out either at the same time as a mastectomy or much later (*see* box p. 214).

Adjuvant therapies

Two types of therapy may be used, either before or after surgery, depending on where the cancer is.

Radiotherapy Normally given following lumpectomy, radiation aims to destroy any cancer cells that were not removed surgically. It may be delivered externally through the skin or internally by inserting radioactive material into the affected tissues under a general anaesthetic. The average course of treatment is five days a week for five or six weeks, starting three to six weeks after surgery.

Chemotherapy Chemotherapy is sometimes given in pill form, but it more often involves giving cytotoxic (cell-killing) drugs intravenously at intervals over four to six months. This type of treatment is usually suggested for premenopausal women and those with invasive tumours that are greater than 1 cm (2/5 in) in size, or if cancer cells are detected in the lymph nodes. It is usually done following surgery but may be given to shrink a large tumour before an operation to remove it.

Accelerated partial breast irradiation This therapy is a new investigational treatment carried out after lumpectomy. Delivered by radioactive implants or external-beam treatment, partial breast irradiation consists of a short course of therapy– usually 10 treatments over five days– and treats only the tumour region.

GETTING A SECOND OPINION

It is important not to rush into making a decision about treatment until you are sure that you have as much information as possible. While breast cancer treatment can be very successful, there is no such thing as the ideal treatment for all women. Much research is being done to develop new treatments and refine and improve existing ones. It is important that you build up a clear picture of the pros and cons. Questions that you might ask your doctor include:

- How long has this treatment been in use?
- What is the success rate for your patients?
- Are there any side effects and how common are they?
- How long does the treatment take?
- How much time should I take off from work?

Hormone therapy

Many breast cancers grow faster in the presence of the hormone oestrogen, so hormonal treatments are designed to reduce or block oestrogen from stimulating breast tissue. Tamoxifen, an anti-oestrogen, is given to premenopausal or postmenopausal women who have hormone-sensitive tumors. It may cause menopausal symptoms and an increased risk of blood clots and uterine cancer. A newer family of drugs, called aromatase inhibitors, works to reduce oestrogen levels and is used to treat hormone-sensitive tumours in postmenopausal women. It may cause menopausal symptoms, muscle and joint aches and increased risk of osteoporosis. These medications are often taken for five years either as initial therapy or in sequence. The decision about taking them is individualized and takes account of tumour stage and the medical history.

Ovarian function

Surgery to remove the ovaries or radiation to destroy them may be carried out to alter the levels of hormones in the body. Another option is an injection of the ovary-suppressing drug goserelin, which induces a reversible menopause in younger women. The additional benefit of these procedures when combined with standard therapy is still under investigation. The disadvantage of this treatment is that it causes an immediate menopause. Women at very high risk of recurrence may choose to give up their ability to have children in order to improve their chances of a cure.

Coping strategies

Having a serious illness is stressful and you may find that even the most caring doctors and nurses may not be able to help you think straight about the choice you make and what lies ahead. It is common to feel uncertain and alone.

It is important to remember that decisions rarely have to be made immediately. Seek the assistance of a psychologist or mind/body counsellor, who can help you develop the skills to cope and get through this critical time. Your partner, children and parents may be scared too and may also need reassurance and support.

Mind and body medicine is not a cure but provides you with tools for managing anxiety and discomfort. These include relaxation techniques, guided imagery, cognitive restructuring and training in assertiveness. Find out whether there is a group you can join where you can meet other breast cancer patients.

As with any disease, you should avoid any complementary therapy or practitioner claiming to offer you a cure. There is absolutely no evidence that such a possibility exists. However, wise use of complementary approaches, such as visualization, massage, aromatherapy and yoga, may make you feel better during cancer treatment. You should also think very carefully before deciding to discontinue any orthodox treatment while it still has something to offer you.

After the operation

You will be encouraged to get out of bed as soon as possible after surgery. There is no need to be in any pain; you can ask for painkillers if necessary. Your arm movement will be restricted at first, but exercise will help restore it. Stitches are usually taken out within two weeks and

Breast reconstruction

Women who have to have a breast removed may be offered a breast reconstruction, either at the time of the mastectomy or later. This can be done using an implant or with tissue taken from a muscle in the back or from the abdomen. If you are considering this option, discuss it with your breast surgeon and a plastic surgeon. While a reconstructed breast may never look exactly the same as before surgery, many women are happy with the results, but this type of surgery is not right for everyone. A prosthesis (artificial breast) worn inside a bra or swimsuit can look natural under clothes. There are also selections of beach, swim and sportswear available for women who have had mastectomies.

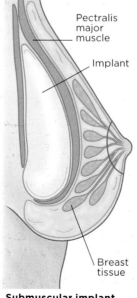

Pectralis major muscle

Implant

Breast tissue

Submuscular implant

the scar will heal in two to four weeks. Following radiation therapy or surgery to the lymph nodes, there may be problems with the flow of lymph that can cause the arm to swell (known as lymphoedema). Tubular compression garments can be made to help reduce the swelling. The usual treatment is massage to encourage lymph drainage, use of a mechanical pump to reduce swelling and exercises that involve raising the arm. Discuss the problem with your doctor if the lymphoedema continues or worries you.

Help your body heal
Once your treatment is finished, maintain a healthy weight and a diet of fresh fruit, vegetables, whole grains and fish. Begin to build an active exercise routine. Finding an exercise partner may help you stick to a regular workout routine and make your workout more enjoyable. Consider complementary therapies, such as yoga, massage or aromatherapy. Look for cancer survivor support groups in your area to help you meet others and learn more ways to speed your healing.

Postoperative exercise

You should start exercising to regain arm movement as soon as you feel able to do so, usually the day after the operation. Do exercises 1 and 2 only for the first 5 days, then add in exercises 3–6 and continue them until you can move both arms equally well. Try to use your affected arm as normally as possible; use it when brushing your hair or doing light housework. Build up gradually to heavier activities, but stop if it causes pain or strain. There may be discomfort at first and it may help if you take painkillers 30 minutes before you exercise.

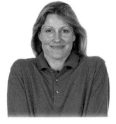

1 While sitting, hold your hands relaxed in your lap. Shrug your shoulders up to your ears, then push them down. Pull your shoulders forwards, then brace them back. Repeat 5 times, twice a day.

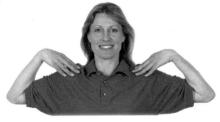

2 Stand with your arms by your sides. Keeping both arms straight, raise them to shoulder level. With your hands on your shoulders circle both shoulders back, then forwards. Repeat 5 times twice a day.

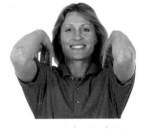

3 You can choose to do this either standing or sitting. Rest your hands lightly on your shoulders. Slowly lift your bent arms up in front of you, then lower them. Repeat 10 times, 3 times a day.

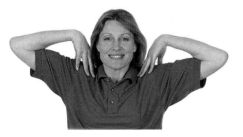

4 Keep your hands gently resting on your shoulders. Instead of having your elbows in front, move them out to the side. Slowly lower your arms to your waist then raise them up to shoulder level. Repeat 10 times, 3 times a day.

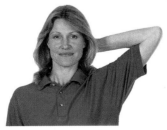

5 Raise your affected arm to shoulder level, then slowly lift your hand to behind your neck. Stretch the arm out again, then reach behind your back, with your hand at bra level. Repeat 10 times, 3 times a day.

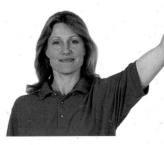

6 Stand with your affected arm stretched out to shoulder level. Gradually lift it above your head, then lower it slowly to where it was. Repeat the exercise with your arm straight out in front. Repeat 10 times, 3 times a day.

Menstrual Problems

From adolescence on, a woman's reproductive system has a major impact on her life. Her complex hormonal balance may at times be disrupted as she progresses from onset of periods to childbearing to the menopause. A woman needs to be able to recognize the warning signs so that she can seek medical help as early as possible.

MENSTRUAL DISORDERS

The majority of women will experience a menstrual cycle disorder of some kind at least once in their lives.

UNDERSTANDING THE MENSTRUAL CYCLE
Menstruation, when bleeding occurs, is the actual period and signals the fact that a fertilized egg has not implanted in the uterus. Blood flow that is absent, scanty, infrequent or too frequent, heavy or accompanied by pain, should be evaluated.

The normal menstrual cycle
Unless pregnant, a woman's menstrual cycle takes place about every month, from menarche (the first period, occurring between the ages of about 10 and 17) to menopause (the last period, occurring in the late 40s or early 50s). The average cycle length is from 28 to 32 days, but 24 to 35 days may be considered a normal range. The purpose of the menstrual cycle is to prepare the uterus for a possible pregnancy. The cycle is controlled by the complex interaction between hormones, starting with gonadotrophin-releasing hormone (GnRH) secreted by the hypothalamus in the brain that stimulates the endocrine system's master gland, the pituitary.

The first phase of the menstrual cycle is known as the proliferative or follicular phase. At this stage, several eggs, called ova, begin to ripen in follicles in the ovaries. This process is governed by two hormones secreted by the pituitary gland, follicle-stimulating hormone (FSH) and by the female sex hormone, oestrogen, produced by the ovaries.

As the oestrogen level rises, it inhibits further production of FSH and stimulates the release of LH (luteinizing hormone),

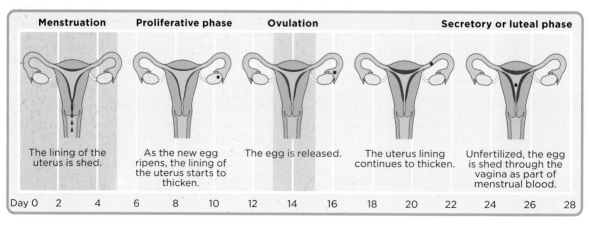

Menstruation	Proliferative phase	Ovulation	Secretory or luteal phase	
The lining of the uterus is shed.	As the new egg ripens, the lining of the uterus starts to thicken.	The egg is released.	The uterus lining continues to thicken.	Unfertilized, the egg is shed through the vagina as part of menstrual blood.

Day 0   2   4   6   8   10   12   14   16   18   20   22   24   26   28

IRREGULAR PERIODS

At various times in your life, your periods may change their usual pattern. If menstrual irregularities are bothersome or are accompanied by pain, you should discuss the problem with your doctor.

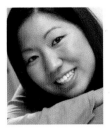

POST PUBERTY

Periods may be irregular during the first couple of years following the onset of puberty. Some women must wait until they are over 20 years old before their hormonal cycles become fully established and regular.

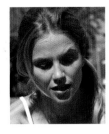

ATHLETE

Excessive exercise with a marked decrease in body fat may cause your periods to stop or become irregular. This is a reversible effect, but it may later result in osteoporosis caused by low oestrogen levels.

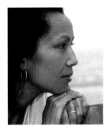

AFTER PREGNANCY

Normal periods usually resume about two months after giving birth if the mother is not breastfeeding. If she is, it may take longer or she may not resume periods at all until she stops breastfeeding.

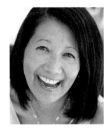

PERIMENOPAUSE

Irregular bleeding is one of the symptoms that indicates secretion of oestrogen and progesterone hormones are becoming more sporadic and inconsistent. This stage can last for several years.

also produced in the pituitary. This in turn causes the release of just one mature egg around the middle of the menstrual cycle, bringing this phase to an end. At this point, the body temperature rises slightly. After ovulation, upon LH stimulation, the ovaries secrete the other female sex hormone, progesterone, to complete the preparation of the endometrium, which is thickened for a possible pregnancy. The medical term for this is the secretory or luteal phase. If the released egg is not fertilized by sperm, the levels of oestrogen and progesterone begin to drop and approximately 14 days after ovulation the unfertilized egg is shed through the vagina, together with the endometrium, as a menstrual period.

The loss of blood is described as menses. It may last from 3 to 7 days with a varying amount of blood excreted–the average loss is about 60 ml (2 ½ fl oz). It may be less if you are taking oral contraceptives. When menstruation begins, for many young women it takes a couple of years for periods to settle into a regular cycle. Minor fluctuations are normal at every age, and the cycles may actually shorten in women over the age of 35 years prior to lengthening again around the climacteric (the time just prior to the last menses).

Absent periods

If menstruation doesn't start by the age of 16 years, or stops in a woman who is not pregnant or approaching menopause, she has amenorrhoea. If your periods become irregular (oligomenorrhoea)– that is, they arrive less often than once every 35 days or stop altogether–it is important that you see your doctor. A persistent lack of menstruation may affect your ability to become pregnant and weaken your bones, leading to osteoporosis later in life.

Late puberty is the most common cause of primary amenorrhoea, where periods do not start by about age 16 years. This may be because of poor nutrition (girls must reach a certain body weight before menstruation can start), hormonal disorders or a genetic disorder such as Turner's syndrome in which one of the female sex chromosomes is absent. Secondary amenorrhoea, where periods stop after they have started, can have several causes, such as stress, weight loss and diet. Often periods stop temporarily with excessive exercising and dieting (lowering the body fat to below 15 per cent)–common in athletes, dancers, models and anorexic women. Illnesses, such as the bowel disorder, Crohn's disease, or thyroid problems, may all affect menstruation.

SEE YOUR DOCTOR

The menstrual cycle is especially sensitive to external upsets, such as lifestyle changes (for example, prolonged travel) or an illness. However, you should see your doctor if:

- Your periods become unusually heavy.
- Your periods become irregular, are infrequent or stop altogether.
- You have bleeding between periods or after intercourse.
- You experience severe pain or heavy bleeding that interferes with your normal life.
- You start bleeding any time after menopause (usually defined as when you have been without periods for a whole year).

Another common cause of secondary amenorrhoea is polycystic ovary syndrome (PCOS). In this disease, irregular ovulation is linked to an excess of male hormones produced by the ovaries or the adrenal glands, or by premature menopause.

If your periods have not started at all, or if they have started and subsequently stopped, the doctor will want to do a careful medical history. A test to ensure that you are not pregnant will be done since pregnancy is the most common reason for amenorrhoea during the reproductive years.

The doctor will want to know whether you are taking any prescribed drugs that may be affecting your menstrual cycle. Blood tests will evaluate your hormone levels to determine whether your pituitary and thyroid glands are functioning as they should. If none is found to be a cause, the doctor may refer you to a gynaecologist to check that your ovaries are functioning as they should, and whether there are any other underlying factors. In cases where the cause is not obvious, no specific treatment may be given. Your doctor may suggest waiting a few months to see if your periods become reestablished. If blood tests find that there is an underlying hormonal imbalance, the doctor may prescribe drugs to correct the problem or to induce ovulation if you want to conceive.

Painful periods

Abdominal pain or cramping–medically called dysmenorrhoea–is common during a period. The pain, which can vary from mild to severe, is generally in the lower abdomen and may spread to the lower back and thighs. Severe pain may be accompanied by bowel disturbances such as constipation or diarrhoea, as well as nausea, dizziness and vomiting.

Most women experience a painful menstruation at some point. The mild cramp-like abdominal pains typical of primary dysmenorrhoea rarely begin after the age of 20. The pains are actually caused by muscular contractions of the uterus which are similar to–but not as intense as–labour pains. Natural, hormone-like substances called prostaglandins are involved in uterine contractions. They are produced by the cervix and also help to seal blood vessels in order to prevent excess blood loss as the endometrium is shed.

More severe pain caused by various conditions may occur at any age. The pain is usually recurring and may be a symptom of: endometriosis, in which fragments of the endometrium are found in other parts of the pelvic cavity and bleed cyclically; an infection of the fallopian tubes or of the ovaries; the presence of fibroids, which are benign tumours that tend to grow within the uterine wall, especially in women over the age of 30; and ovarian cysts.

The type of dysmenorrhoea dictates the treatment. The doctor compiles a history of the symptoms, when they began and occur and how long they last. A pelvic exam may also be carried out.

Primary dysmenorrhoea can usually be treated by a simple pain reliever such as ibuprofen or naproxen (types of NSAIDs), and by rest and relaxation techniques, as well as doing gentle exercise. Hormonal treatment such as the oral contraceptive pill may also be suggested.

Ease the pain

- Moderate physical exercise can be beneficial, but do not attempt it if the pain is severe. Gentle yoga-type stretches done through the day may help. Deep-breathing exercises will also help to alleviate the pain.

- Hugging your knees or lying on your back with your knees elevated may provide more comfort from menstrual pains.

- Heat can have a soothing effect—have a warm bath or shower or place a hot water bottle over your abdomen.

- Well-balanced meals containing plenty of fruit and vegetables can improve matters.

- Essential fatty acids (EFAs), especially from fish oils, have an anti-inflammatory effect which may ease pain.

- Aromatherapy, massage, acupuncture and acupressure have all been reported as techniques that can help some women.

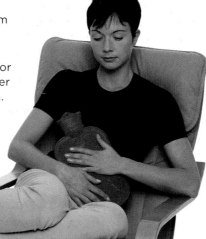

Mid-cycle pain

Pain that occurs in the mid-cycle–known as mittelschmerz–occurs in ovulatory cycles (during which an egg is released) and not in anovulatory ones (when no egg is released). It can be severe but usually does not last long and resolves without treatment.

Heavy periods

About 1 in 10 women of reproductive age suffer with heavy periods–called menorrhagia–in which the total blood loss exceeds 80 ml (3 fl oz) during one cycle. It is impossible in practice to measure how much blood you lose but, if you are menorrhagic, you may experience flooding, which soaks your underwear or bedclothes, may pass large blood clots, have to change pads or tampons frequently (more than every two hours) or have to wear extra absorbent tampons or double protection. Your periods may be so heavy that they limit your activities.

Some women always have heavy periods. If they are not anaemic and are comfortable with managing their periods, there may be no need for treatment. Periods can be heavier if you have recently given birth or have just stopped taking the oral contraceptive pill. Periods may also become heavier due to the development of a thicker endometrium as the menopause approaches. Irregularity that is caused by changes in the body's hormonal balance is also common at this time.

Other causes of heavy periods include fibroid tumours, polyps, endometriosis, pelvic inflammatory disease (PID), as well as a thyroid or blood-clotting disorder. Sometimes an isolated heavy period may be an early miscarriage that occurred before the woman knew she was pregnant. In other cases, the problem is caused by changes in the blood-clotting mechanism in the uterus, changes in the concentration of prostaglandins or by changes in the body's hormonal control of periods. However, quite often no cause can be detected at all. The doctor will perform a pelvic examination to check for fibroid tumours, polyps or other abnormalities of the uterus. A cervical smear may be

ENDOMETRIAL ABLATION AND RESECTION

In endometrial ablation, your doctor uses one of several techniques to permanently destroy the lining of your uterus. Endometrial resection involves your doctor using a wire loop to remove the lining of the uterus. Both of these procedures reduce blood loss in around half to three-quarters of women who experience heavy periods. These treatments are not suitable for women who have a very large uterus or those who may want to become pregnant in the future.

carried out, and if other symptoms include fatigue and breathlessness, a blood sample may be taken to test for anaemia.

The usual drugs prescribed include ibuprofen or naproxen, which can help reduce flow and provide pain relief. Other options for medical management are the oral contraceptive pill, patch or ring, or progestin preparations such as the contraceptive injection or oral progestin. A progestin-secreting IUD is very effective at controlling heavy bleeding and provides contraception at the same time.

Your doctor may recommend an ultrasound scan to check for abnormalities in the uterus, or perform a hysteroscopy and uterine biopsy in which a special telescopic instrument is used to examine the uterus and to obtain endometrial tissue for laboratory examination by a pathologist.

Breakthrough bleeding

Bleeding from the uterus between periods, which is called metrorrhagia, can be experienced for a variety of reasons. It is normal in some women throughout their reproductive life. It may be due to the presence of an IUD, contraceptive implant or occur while using hormonal contraceptives. It can also be a symptom of many vaginal or uterine disorders, such as fibroid tumours or polyps and may be a side effect of postmenopausal hormone therapy (HT). If you have breakthrough bleeding, you should discuss it with your doctor.

Cervical Problems

From the time a woman becomes sexually active, staying well and ensuring good reproductive health requires regular examinations of the genital area. Many changes that occur in the cervix, vagina and vulva can be detected by simple testing, and appropriately treated or carefully monitored.

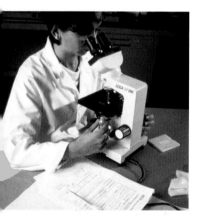

HOW CERVICAL SMEARS ARE ANALYSED

In the laboratory, the cervical cells are examined through a microscope by a cytologist—a specialist in cells of the body—or analysed by computer. There is a routine for checking the cells for changes in shape or colour.

CERVICAL SCREENING

By the time a woman turns 21 or within 3 years of becoming sexually active (whichever comes first), she should have a regular cervical cytology, also known as a Pap smear. In this, a collection of cervical cells is examined by a trained technician and a pathologist for any signs of cervical cancer or precancer (also called dysplasia). This is usually done in conjunction with a pelvic examination. Both tests should be done yearly until age 30 or longer if you have more than one partner or a new partner. Thereafter, testing intervals may be increased to every other year if all remains normal. If you are not sexually active, or are in a monogamous ongoing relationship, your doctor or nurse may consider stopping cervical cytology testing after three negative tests if this is appropriate for your situation.

There is increasing incidence of cervical cancer and dysplasia in younger women who smoke, have nutritional deficiencies or a sexually transmitted infection (STI). The Pap smear is the most efficient method of detecting the human papillomavirus (HPV), a common STI responsible for the vast majority of cervical cancer. The test is carried out in the doctor's surgery and can be done virtually any time during the menstrual cycle with the exception of very heavy bleeding days. Changes in the cervix–

the lowest portion of the uterus (womb)– or the surrounding tissue can range from the mildest degrees affecting only the surface of the cervix (dysplasia) to actual cancer, which involves the deeper layers of cervical tissue. If the diagnosis of dysplasia is made during a microscopic examination of the cervix in your doctor's surgery (called colposcopy) and a cervical biopsy in the lab, treatment can be a simple office procedure (if at the precancerous stage). If cervical cancer is found, it can be treated by surgical excision of the cervix (conization) or a radical hysterectomy (removal of the uterus and surrounding tissues where cancer is likely to spread). After these procedures, your doctor will suggest a close follow-up plan for your situation.

Cervical cytology and pelvic exam

To improve testing accuracy, you should avoid vaginal creams, foams or suppositories, douche, tampons and sex for 2-3 days prior to your examination.

The doctor or nurse will ask you to remove clothes and underwear below the waist and to lie on your back on an examination table. An instrument called a speculum will be inserted to part the walls of the vagina so that the cervix can be seen and checked for any sign of irritation or disease. Relaxing your thigh and buttock muscles will make the examination much more comfortable.

The doctor will collect cells from the cervix and the cervical canal with a special spatula and a small brush that will be smeared onto a slide or collected into a vial of special fluid, and sent to a laboratory for microscopic analysis.

The speculum will be removed and the doctor will inspect the vulva and vagina, then use two gloved fingers to examine your ovaries, uterus and fallopian tubes. Your doctor may also check the wall separating the rectum and the vagina, using a gloved and lubricated finger in the vagina and rectum, especially if you are over 40.

Women over 50 may be advised to have a yearly pelvic examination to help detect ovarian cancer, although this is very difficult to pick up. Ultrasound and blood testing can be used if an abnormality is found on examination.

What do the results mean?

If cervical cytology results are abnormal, further investigations and treatment will be required.

Abnormal dysplastic cells are classified as atypical (ASCUS), low-grade or mildly abnormal (LOSIL) or high-grade or very abnormal (HGSIL). Following a colposcopic examination and targeted biopsy, tissue is sent to the pathologist for definitive diagnosis. The degree of abnormality is then classified as CIN 1, 2 or 3, depending on how deeply the changes have affected the covering (epithelial) cervical cell layer. CIN stands for cervical intraepithelial neoplasia.

CIN1 Mild; with only one-third of the epithelial thickness affected with dysplastic change.

CIN2 Moderate; dysplasia affects two-thirds of the epithelial thickness.

CIN3 Severe; dysplasia affects the inner third of the epithelial thickness.

CIS Carcinoma in situ; dysplasia affects the full epithelial thickness. Despite the name, it is not cervical cancer.

Invasive carcinoma True cervical cancer that needs aggressive and prompt treatment by a gynecological oncology surgeon.

Milder changes (CIN1, CIN2) can be closely followed with repeat pap smear, HPV testing and/or colposcopy as indicated (*see* p. 222). In many healthy women, the HPV infection that causes these changes resolves spontaneously within 2 years. Boost your immune system by eating healthily, getting adequate rest and not smoking. It is very important to see your doctor at the recommended intervals to be sure that the dysplasia has not progressed to a point when treatment is necessary.

More severe changes (CIN3, CIS) are generally treated by cutting out (excision) the involved cervical tissue, by using laser or electrical current (loop electrosurgical excision procedure, LEEP) in the surgery or a conization in an operating theatre.

Warning signs

Early, precancerous changes rarely cause any symptoms and one stage can move to the other over years. It is known that dysplasia is most common between the ages of 25 and 35, carcinoma in situ between 30 and 40 and invasive cancer between 40 and 60. The symptoms of cervical cancer, such as bleeding between periods or after sex, are often ignored because women may regard them as a normal part of life.

See your doctor if you experience vaginal discharge that doesn't go away, especially if it smells unpleasant or shows traces of blood, pain or discomfort during sex or bleeding after sex.

Common cervical conditions

There are many possible causes for vaginal discharge or pain:

Cervicitis Inflammation of the cervix associated with STDs (chlamydia, gonorrhoea, trichomoniasis and genital herpes) or common vaginal infections caused by bacteria or yeast. An procedure called wet-prep is used to rapidly diagnose and treat some of the common infections by a microscopic examination of the vaginal discharge.

Cervical cyst (also called Nabothian cysts) Caused by a blocked mucus gland in the cervix. They require no treatment and clear up by themselves.

Cervical polyps Benign growths that may cause irregular bleeding, bleeding after sex and discharge. They are easily removed in the surgery.

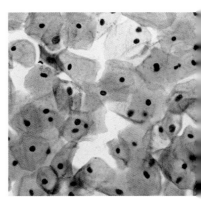

CELLS OF THE CERVIX
For close examination, cells are seen at a greatly enlarged size through a microscope. The cytologist will look for the presence of STIs and in particular HPV, which can cause cervical cancer. HPV incidence is highest in women aged from 18 to 28.

TAKE CARE

After cervical treatment, it's advisable to wash or shower every day and use sanitary pads or liners rather than tampons. You should not have long, hot, soapy baths, use soap inside the vagina or use "feminine hygiene" products such as sprays. Avoid wearing synthetic, tight-fitting clothes (such as tight jeans). Choose cotton underwear and clothing in preference to other types of fabric. You should not have sexual intercourse for the amount of time recommended by your doctor so as to prevent excessive bleeding at the treatment sites.

CERVICAL CANCER

When precancerous changes in cervical cells are found, tests will be carried out to find out how far they have spread.

The first test you undergo is likely to be a colposcopy, which involves examination of the cervix using a microscope. Tissue and cell samples will be taken from any area that looks abnormal for examination, a procedure known as a biopsy. A colposcopy usually takes about 15 minutes and should be only a little more uncomfortable than having a cervical smear.

If the colposcopy reveals a more serious abnormality, the next step may be an excision, in which a section of the central lining of the cervix is removed under local anaesthetic. This may get rid of all the abnormal cells and no further treatment will be needed. The tissue that was removed will be examined in a pathology lab, and you are likely to have to wait for a week or so for the results.

Possible treatments

There are three main types of surgical treatment to remove precancerous cells. Each of these can be carried out in an outpatient clinic using only local anaesthetic. They are:

Laser evaporation In this procedure, a concentrated beam of light of a specific wavelength "burns away" the cells.

Cryotherapy This technique uses a metal probe, cooled to about -160°C (-256°F), to freeze and destroy the abnormal cells.

Loop electrosurgical excision procedure (LEEP) In LEEP, a thin wire charged with electrical current is applied to the surface of the cervix to cut out the abnormal cells.

QUESTIONS YOU SHOULD ASK

If you're about to be treated for cervical dysplasia or cancer, here are some questions to ask your doctors:

- Will I experience any side effects from the treatment?
- Are there any complications I should expect?
- When is it safe to resume sexual relations?
- Are my periods likely to be affected?
- Should I be using sanitary pads rather than tampons?
- Can I become pregnant in the future?
- What is the likelihood of recurrence of the disease?
- When should I come back for my first check-up after treatment and for how many years should I return for regular check-ups?
- How often should I have a cervical smear?

GETTING GOOD ADVICE Use all the avenues you can to prepare yourself for eradicating the cancer. Find out from your doctor or medical team about what to expect during and after treatment. Counselling can help calm you.

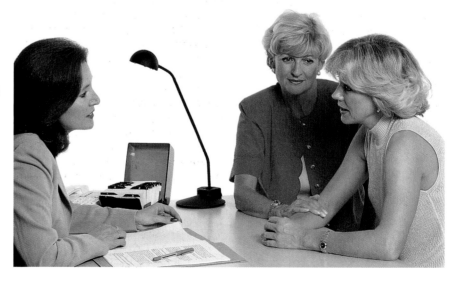

Treatments for invasive cancer

Invasive cancer is treated with surgery, radiotherapy and chemotherapy, in various combinations.

Surgery If tests indicate that the cancer is confined to the cervix or has only just begun to spread, it may be possible to get rid of it completely with surgery. This may mean removal of the uterus, cervix and possibly the nearby lymph nodes. Otherwise, a major operation known as a radical (or Wertheim) hysterectomy that involves removing the uterus, cervix, the upper part of the vagina and some adjacent tissues may be necessary.

An operation of this type can be a most upsetting prospect for a woman to face, and she may need help to come to terms with it. Many hospitals and cancer support groups offer counselling services that can also explain aspects of the surgery and the effects on your body. Though physical recovery takes only weeks, it may take a great deal longer to overcome the psychological consequences.

Radiotherapy This form of treatment is likely to be recommended if the cancer has spread any further than beyond the cervix itself, because it offers a greater chance of cure than an operation. It works by targeting the rapidly dividing cancer cells and destroying them.

Radiotherapy can be given externally–in much the same way as an X-ray is delivered–or internally, by feeding radioactive material through a tube leading directly into the affected area. Many women are treated with both in turn. Either way, the dose of radiation needs to be relatively high to be fully effective, and this means that there is a risk of side effects as a result of damage to healthy tissue during treatment. A premenopausal woman should be informed that the treatment will cause her to have instant artificial menopause because the ovaries stop working. There may also be other side effects at a later time, such as bowel and bladder problems, and it is essential to find out as much as possible about the potential risks from your medical team before treatment starts.

TYPE AND STAGE OF CANCER

Tests include blood tests, X-rays, pelvic ultrasound and body scans—CT (computer tomography) or MRI (magnetic resonance imaging). A pelvic examination under anaesthetic may be performed. Alternatively an intravenous urogram (IVU) is carried out, in which a dye is fed into your arm through an intravenous drip to enable the doctor to check for any abnormalities in the kidneys or urinary system. There are several stages of cancer of the cervix.

STAGE	WHAT IS HAPPENING
0	Carcinoma in situ, a very early cancer.
I	Cancer cells have penetrated the cervix but have remained confined to the uterus.
II	The cancerous cells have spread to other parts of the pelvis, such as the tissues around the cervix and the upper part of the vagina.
III	There is evidence of cancerous cells throughout the pelvic area, down to the lower part of the vagina and perhaps blocking the ureters that connect the kidneys to the bladder.
IV	The cancer has spread into the bladder or outside the pelvis.

The most common type of cervical cancer is known as squamous cell carcinoma and affects the covering of the cervix. A rarer form, called adenocarcinoma, may affect the glandular cells in the cervix. Only when all the tests have been completed will your doctor be in a position to discuss the most appropriate form of treatment.

Chemotherapy If a cancer has grown to the point where surgery or radiotherapy would be difficult, chemotherapy may be used to shrink the tumour first. It may also be needed after radiotherapy to reduce the chances of the cancer recurring.

Anticancer (or cytotoxic) drugs are given in liquid form as an intravenous drip or injection, or as a pill. The different doses and combinations of the drugs are unique to each person. Your doctor will explain how the treatment will be done and make you aware of possible side effects such as fatigue, increased susceptibility to infection and the effect on bone marrow. With modern treatment, the doctors will endeavour to reduce the nausea, sickness and hair loss that are toxic effects of chemotherapy.

Uterine Problems

The uterus is an adaptable, muscular organ at the core of the female reproductive system. It must be kept healthy so that it can provide the life support system for a growing fetus. However, the uterus is prone to a variety of treatable conditions.

The uterus lies behind the bladder and in a woman who is not pregnant is the shape and size of an upside-down pear: approximately 7.5 cm (3 in) long and 5 cm (2 in) at its widest point. The upper,

One in 20 women of childbearing age referred to a gynaecologist has endometriosis.

wide part of the uterus is known as the body and the lower, narrow neck that leads into the vagina is called the cervix. Before pregnancy, the cavity of the uterus is small and narrow. Its muscular walls have a thick middle layer known as the myometrium and an inner vascular lining called the endometrium.

The endometrium thickens every month under the influence of hormones in preparation for the implantation of a fertilized egg. If pregnancy does not occur, the endometrial cells degenerate and the uterus sheds them through the process of menstruation.

ENDOMETRIOSIS

In this disease cells similar to the type that normally line the uterus become established outside it. The cells may travel anywhere in the pelvic area– on to one or both ovaries, the fallopian tubes, the bladder, the uterus, the bowel, the peritoneum (the membrane lining the abdominal cavity) or on the pelvic wall. These cells then respond to the hormonal changes of the menstrual cycle –growing, breaking down and bleeding– in the same way as the uterine lining. Because these cells are trapped inside the pelvis, they irritate the tissue causing sticky bands (adhesions) between organs and/or the pelvic wall. Collections of endometriosis can fill with dark blood (known as chocolate cysts) causing

A TILTED UTERUS
About 20 per cent of women have a retroverted uterus. This is when the uterus tilts backwards rather than forwards. It is a harmless condition and is not associated with infertility as was previously believed. As the uterus enlarges during pregnancy, it naturally swings forwards.

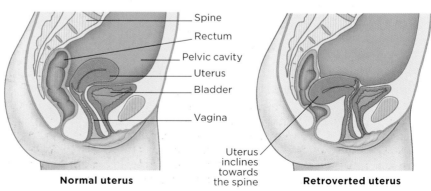

Spine
Rectum
Pelvic cavity
Uterus
Bladder
Vagina

Uterus inclines towards the spine

Normal uterus

Retroverted uterus

- Keep a pain diary: record your pain levels every day, three times a day (morning, noon and bedtime).
- Describe what you were doing at the time: eating, exercising, having sex, using the bathroom, etc.
- Rate the pain on a scale of 1 to 10: from not too bad to very painful.
- Look for anything that makes the pain better: relaxing, emptying bladder or bowels, lying down, etc.

painful masses that are diagnosed by examination or ultrasound.

Endometriosis is a complex disease, with symptoms such as abdominal pain, backache, cramps and sometimes nausea and dizziness. It often goes undetected, as women–and sometimes their doctors–attribute the symptoms simply to painful periods. However, it is a common condition and a leading cause of infertility. One in 20 women of childbearing age referred to gynaecologists has endometriosis.

The cause of endometriosis is unknown but one common theory links it to "reverse" menstruation where a small amount of the menstrual flow spills out of the fallopian tubes and the endometrial cells implant on the pelvic lining (peritoneum). Spread via the blood vessels or lymph channels is also thought possible and accounts for the rare instances of endometriosis found in the lungs, brain and nasal mucosa.

There is no known way of preventing endometriosis, although studies show that the oral contraceptive pill and pregnancy often improve its symptoms.

How is it diagnosed?

The most common symptoms are painful menstrual periods, pain with sex and difficulty becoming pregnant.

At present endometriosis may only be diagnosed by laparoscopic examination and biopsy–a minimally invasive surgical procedure in which a tube with a tiny camera at one end is inserted just below the navel into the pelvic area, and a tiny sample of suspicious tissue is removed

Polyps and fibroids

Polyps occur in the cervix or endometrium and are usually harmless overgrowths of uterine or cervical tissue. A cervical polyp may cause a watery, blood-streaked discharge between periods, after sex or after menopause. Polyps are removed surgically by hysteroscopy, in which a thin camera is inserted through the cervix into the uterus and an instrument is used to cut off the polyp.

Fibroids, made up of bundles of muscle fibres that grow in the wall of the uterus, can be smaller than a pea or larger than a full-term baby. They occur in 40 per cent of women over 40. Some have no symptoms; however, larger fibroids can result in heavy menstruation and anaemia, frequent urination, and a feeling of pelvic pressure. Diagnosis is made by a physical examination, ultrasound scan or a hysteroscopy.

Some fibroids can be removed through the hysteroscope. Outpatient surgery is an option with general or regional anaesthesia. Other treatments include drug therapy (to reduce oestrogen levels and temporarily shrink the fibroids), uterine artery ablation where the blood supply to the uterus and the fibroids is cut off, focused ultrasound ablation of the fibroid, myomectomy (p. 226) and hysterectomy (p. 227).

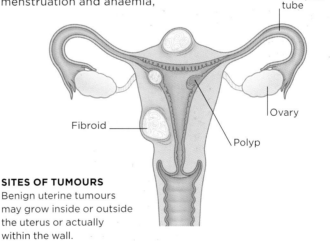

SITES OF TUMOURS
Benign uterine tumours may grow inside or outside the uterus or actually within the wall.

for pathological evaluation. It is performed under general anaesthetic.

Possible treatments

Treatment should be discussed with your doctor. Two main treatments are medical (hormones or temporary medical menopause) and surgery (either destruction of the endometriosis and adhesions by laser or cautery, or the removal of uterus and ovaries).

TREATMENT FOR UTERINE PROBLEMS

A number of disorders can affect the uterus ranging from structural problems to sexually transmitted diseases. Surgery and drugs are the most common types of treatment.

Pelvic inflammatory disease

Also known as PID, pelvic inflammatory disease involves inflammation of the reproductive organs, including the uterus, fallopian tubes and ovaries. Bacteria enter the body through the vagina and work their way up the cervix into the pelvic cavity. The bacteria responsible for gonorrhoea and

intercourse with an infected partner, but douching and procedures involving the uterus have also been linked to it.

PID can range from a mild condition with virtually no symptoms to a painful, even life-threatening, disorder requiring immediate medical attention.

Abdominal pain and fever are the most common symptoms. The pain evolves over a matter of hours and feels like a dull ache across the lower abdomen. It may be so severe that the woman cannot move and is only relieved by lying in the fetal position.

PID can cause infertility and increase a woman's risk of ectopic pregnancy seven-fold. The resulting scar tissue can cause pain during sex and chronic pelvic pain later in life.

PID is frequently the result of sex with an infected partner or douching.

chlamydia are thought to be the most common causes, although other bacteria–in particular some that normally exist harmlessly in the bowel or the vagina– may play a part, too. PID is generally a consequence of sexual

MYOMECTOMY

A myomectomy is the removal of uterine fibroids (leiomyomas), while leaving the uterus in place. Most commonly this is done when the fibroids are thought to interfere with carrying a pregnancy to term and can be quite successful. Under general anaesthetic an incision is made into the wall of the uterus, the fibroids shelled out and the uterus sewn up. There are, however, a number of possible complications with this procedure. Complications may include weakening of the uterine wall precluding future vaginal delivery, heavier intraoperative bleeding than with hysterectomy requiring transfusion, and postoperative adhesions. Some fibroids can be remove by hysteroscopy without needing to make incisions into the uterus. Many of these patients can have successful vaginal deliveries.

To diagnose PID, the doctor will do a physical examination, taking swabs of vaginal fluid for bacterial culture to confirm the source of the infection. Additional testing including blood tests, ultrasound or even laparoscopy may be recommended to evaluate the severity and treatment for this condition. Evidence of past PID is sometimes detected when a woman undergoes testing for infertility. The symptoms of PID can be similar to those of endometriosis and appendicitis, and accurate diagnosis is important for proper treatment.

PID is usually treated with antibiotics, given in the hospital intravenously or in oral form as an outpatient. Patients are advised not to douche (which may introduce bacteria into the cervix) and to practise safe sex.

Pelvic prolapse

The forward or downward displacement of an organ caused by weakness of the surrounding tissues is known as prolapse. The uterus and the vagina are the most common organs to be affected, particularly postmenopausally when the muscles and ligaments slacken as a result of past vaginal childbirth and hormonal changes. Some women have naturally weaker pelvic floor supports and are at greater risk of developing pelvic prolapse. All women should strengthen their pelvic muscles by doing pelvic floor exercises regularly. Your doctor can show you how to do them.

The most common symptoms include discomfort, a feeling of pelvic heaviness and something falling out. When the rectum and bladder are also displaced, women may experience constipation and difficulty evacuating bowel movements and urinary incontinence when she coughs, laughs or sneezes.

On examination, the cervix can be felt in the lower vagina especially if a woman stands or strains. The cervix may even come out of the vagina pulling the inverted vagina with it. Losing weight, and avoiding constipation, heavy lifting and coughing may help in minor cases, along with regular exercise. Pelvic floor muscle exercises may improve the symptoms, but in more serious cases a hysterectomy may be required to remove the uterus, with or without the ovaries, and repair the pelvic floor replacing the bladder and bowel back to their original position.

As with any elective surgery, the risks and benefits need to be thoroughly discussed with the patient. If she chooses not to have surgery, or is not a good candidate for it, a flexible device

called a pessary, may be inserted into the vagina to lift and hold the pelvic organs in place. Generally the patient needs to remove the pessary frequently for cleaning and to monitor the vaginal tissues for any signs of injury caused by the pessary.

Hysterectomy

The surgical removal of the uterus, because of uterine disorders or disease or menstrual problems, is known as a hysterectomy. It may be partial, total or radical and may also include the removal of the fallopian tubes and ovaries (*see* p. 228). As it involves major surgery, it is performed under general or regional anaesthetic. Hospitalization is required for several days after an abdominal hysterectomy, followed by a recuperation period of about six weeks when patients need to avoid sex, douching and heavy lifting. The recovery from a vaginal hysterectomy is generally faster and patients may go home as early as 24 hours postoperatively.

The most common reasons for a hysterectomy include severe, uncontrollable uterine bleeding (menorrhagia); pelvic infection or endometriosis that does not respond to medical treatment; cancer; pelvic prolapse; or fibroids.

The two consequences of a hysterectomy are that periods cease and the woman can no longer bear a child. The impact either of these have may vary according to the age of the woman and understanding the ramifications should be an essential part of gynaecological care. A woman should also be counselled as to whether it would be best to remove the ovaries (oophorectomy) along with the uterus and about the hormonal changes that inevitably result.

HOW A HYSTERECTOMY IS DONE

A hysterectomy can be performed through an incision in the abdomen—either a horizontal one just above the pubic bone (bikini cut) or a vertical midline cut as used in cases of large fibroids or cancer.

A vaginal hysterectomy leaves no visible scar. It is generally less painful, causes less bleeding and has lower risk of adhesions than other hysterectomy procedures. It may be assisted by a laparoscopy—keyhole or minimally invasive surgery through the navel and two small incisions. Your surgeon will discuss with you the safest and most appropriate approach for your situation.

Types of hysterectomy

There are different types of hysterectomies. The most commonly performed operation is known as a total (or simple) hysterectomy, in which the uterus and the cervix are removed. Sometimes the fallopian tubes and the ovaries are removed in addition to the uterus. This is known as a total (or simple) hysterectomy with bilateral salpingo-oophorectomy. A radical hysterectomy, in which the uterus, the cervix, part of the vagina and the pelvic lymph nodes are all removed, is used to treat early cervical cancer. This method is preferred over radiotherapy to treat cervical cancer, especially in young women, since the ovaries may be left in place. They will continue to produce hormones and premature menopause is avoided.

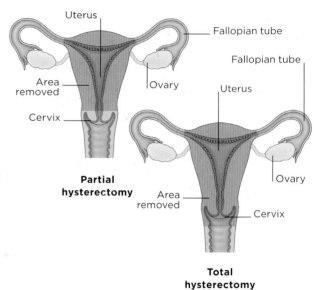

Partial hysterectomy

Total hysterectomy

UTERINE AND ENDOMETRIAL CANCER

Cancer of the uterus results from a hormonally supported overgrowth and cancerous transformation of the uterine lining. Women who started having periods relatively early and ended them late are at increased risk along with heavier women and those with diabetes, high blood pressure or a history of infrequent periods due to polycystic ovaries. The majority of women develop the condition after menopause.

How do I know what's wrong?

The hallmark of uterine cancer is unusual vaginal bleeding. This may include the resumption of vaginal bleeding after the menopause (by definition 12 months of absence of periods), bleeding that lasts longer than normal and bleeding between periods. Infrequent menstrual bleeding in some women increases the risk of developing uterine cancer. Any of the abnormalities described should be promptly reported to your doctor.

The doctor will evaluate the problem by taking a sample of your uterine lining either in a uterine biopsy (also called endometrial biopsy) or in a minor operation known as a D&C (dilation and curettage). This sample is examined under a microscope to make the diagnosis. Additional tests include transvaginal ultrasound to determine the thickness of the uterine lining or a biopsy taken by inserting a flexible instrument called a hysteroscope through the vagina and into the uterus. A cervical smear is not sufficient to diagnose uterine cancer.

The treatment

In the majority of cases, a hysterectomy in which the ovaries are also removed will offer a cure. If the cancer has spread or there is a suspicion that it might recur, you may also need radiotherapy. This can be done either externally or by inserting a radioactive tampon into the uterus for 24 to 48 hours, or both. Sometimes treatment with synthetic progestogen either in pill or injection form may be necessary if there is a risk of the cancer coming back or if it does so following surgery.

After the operation and treatment you may want to discuss with your doctor how often you will need to be checked and ways of maintaining good health. Whether you have passed the menopause or not, the doctor is unlikely to prescribe any drugs containing oestrogen because the hormone may be implicated in triggering the development of the cancer.

Ovarian Problems

The ovaries are under the influence of hormones, and their role in the menstrual and reproductive cycles is beyond your control. The ovaries are well protected inside the body, but they can be susceptible to various disorders.

CYSTS

The two ovaries, normally about walnut size, are responsible for producing eggs and oestrogen throughout a woman's reproductive life. Ovarian health can be affected by cysts, tissue sacs that form on or inside the ovary. These can be caused by the normal hormonal cyclic changes leading to ovulation and support of an early embryo (corpus luteum cysts) or they can be abnormal. A cyst is filled with fluid. If the growth is solid, it is known as a tumour and may be benign (harmless) or malignant (cancerous).

Some types grow large, causing swelling of the abdomen and placing pressure on other pelvic organs such as the bladder or bowel, making bathroom visits more frequent. Other symptoms are irregular periods, bleeding between periods, pelvic pain, growth of facial and body hair and deepening of the voice. Your

doctor will do a pelvic examination and possibly an ultrasound to assess the cyst.

Normal physiological cysts generally disappear within weeks. Resolution is generally confirmed with a repeat ultrasound in about 6 weeks. If the cyst remains or has a worrying appearance, surgical removal may be recommended.

Surgical options

Various operations can be carried out to remove ovarian tissue. It can be drained or removed entirely via a laparoscope. If the mass is large or possibly cancerous, it is best removed via an abdominal incision (with a thorough exploration of the abdominal organs). It is important that a pathologist evaluates the removed tissue for any abnormality including cancer. Options are oophorectomy (*see* box left), hysterectomy (*see* p. 227) or salpingectomy (in which both ovaries and fallopian tubes are removed).

OOPHORECTOMY

The removal of one ovary is called an oophorectomy; the removal of both is termed bilateral oophorectomy. If the uterus is removed as well, the operation is known as a hysterectomy. The removal of both ovaries will cause an abrupt premature menopause if the woman has not yet reached it. In this case, hormone replacement therapy (HRT) may prove beneficial and should be discussed with your gynaecologist.

POLYCYSTIC OVARIES

The word polycystic literally means many cysts. Medically speaking, a polycystic ovary is one that contains at least 10 cysts that lie just below the surface, causing the ovary to become enlarged. The covering of the ovary thickens, which makes ovulation–the release of an egg–increasingly difficult or can prevent it from happening at all.

The condition is brought about by a malfunction of the pituitary gland in the brain. In this case the pituitary gland produces too much luteinizing hormone (LH) and too little follicle-stimulating hormone (FSH). The ovaries are therefore subjected to excess stimulation and produce abnormal amounts of male hormones (androgens).

The cyclic production of oestrogen and progesterone by the ovaries is disrupted, and consequences include irregular or absent periods, infertility, miscarriage, excess body hair growth, acne and weight gain. Women with polycystic ovaries are also abnormally resistant to insulin and therefore may be at risk of developing diabetes.

How do you know what's wrong?

The first step to diagnosis is a physical examination, followed by blood tests to check hormone levels, and an ultrasound scan. Polycystic ovaries are a common cause of infertility and may be discovered during investigation for that disorder.

PREMATURE MENOPAUSE

In most women, the menopause occurs naturally over a period of about two years between the ages of 45 and 55. But a premature menopause can be caused by certain drugs—notably chemotherapy—radiotherapy and surgical procedures such as a hysterectomy. Common menopausal symptoms include hot flushes, night sweats, insomnia, mood changes, anxiety, irritability, poor memory and concentration, vaginal dryness and decreased interest in sex.

In order to deal with the symptoms you are experiencing in premature menopause, you should discuss matters with your doctor, who can talk to you about the increased likelihood of heart disease and osteoporosis and how to prevent them. He or she may, for example, recommend dietary changes. You should also discuss hormone replacement therapy (HRT) and the risks and benefits of its long-term use.

Treatment varies according to the symptoms and goals, which may include pregnancy, control of hair growth or acne, weight reduction or improvement of high blood sugar. Oral contraceptives may be given to correct hormone imbalance and help improve menstrual regularity, acne and hair growth. Ovulation can be induced with hormonal means to help achieve pregnancy. Weight loss may also help to correct polycystic ovaries.

A POLYCYSTIC OVARY
Tiny follicles or cysts proliferate on the surface of enlarged central tissue. The condition is associated with overproduction of androgen hormones.

Uterus

Fallopian tube

Polycystic ovary

OVARIAN CANCER

Most women who develop ovarian cancer are in their 50s and 60s. It is more common in Western countries than in places such as Japan, although relatives of Japanese women who move to the West seem to become susceptible, suggesting that environmental factors may play a role in triggering it.

In some cases genetic inheritance may be involved: a woman who has a close relative with ovarian cancer and others with breast or colon cancer diagnosed at an early age may be at increased risk. Interrupting long stretches of monthly ovulation–such as during pregnancy and breastfeeding, or taking the oral contraceptive pill–offer some protection. Women with risk factors should discuss screening with their doctor.

What are the symptoms?

Unfortunately, ovarian cancer may cause few ill-defined symptoms especially in the early more treatable stages.

Although they may be caused by other noncancerous conditions, it is worth making an appointment with your doctor if you experience persistent unexplained symptoms. For example, a change in your usual bowel habits, indigestion and nausea or feeling bloated or having a loss of appetite for more than a few days. You may have unexpected vaginal bleeding, although this is relatively uncommon.

Because the ovaries have plenty of space in which to enlarge, it may be a long time before symptoms are noticed. Generally, symptoms appear when the increasing size of the tumour exerts pressure on other organs. If you are in middle or later life, it may be worth questioning a new diagnosis of irritable bowel syndrome as the symptoms can be similar to those of ovarian cancer.

Check it out

After a thorough physical and pelvic examination by your doctor, you may be referred for blood tests, and a pelvic ultrasound scan. If the ovary is enlarged, additional testing or repeat testing in a few weeks or months may be recommended. A sample of abdominal fluid may be taken under local anaesthetic, and the doctor may also decide to look inside your abdomen under a general anaesthetic. The most common ovarian cancer–epithelial cancer of the ovary–starts in the covering (epithelium). Other types can start in other components of the ovary.

Pregnancy and breastfeeding may protect against ovarian cancer.

Cancers of ovarian tissue are known as sarcomas, and cancers that start in the ova-producing part of the ovary are known as germ-cell tumours.

Is it treatable?

Ovarian cancer is generally diagnosed at an advanced stage. The best treatment involves radical surgery with removal of as much tumour as possible, known as "optimal debulking". This is followed by chemotherapy with a combination of agents. A gynecological surgeon and an oncologist will discuss the best options.

How do you know?

Levels of a chemical marker in the blood, known as CA 125, may be raised in a woman with ovarian cancer, but this is not a screening test. False-positive elevations can be present in a woman having her period, with fibroids, endometriosis or other conditions irritating the abdominal lining (peritoneum). Likewise a Pap smear does not screen for uterine or ovarian cancer. The best strategy is to have a regular pelvic examination and to follow with ultrasound if an abnormality is found.

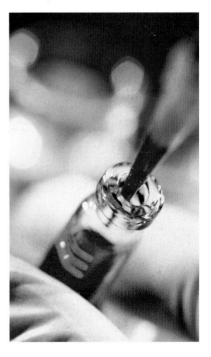

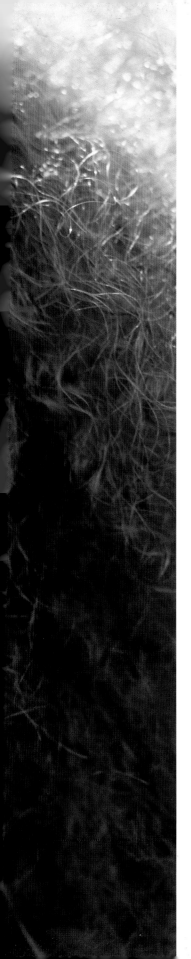

SEX AND SEXUALITY

Whether you're single or in a relationship, young or old, sexually active or sexually celibate, sexuality is an important aspect of your life. It's part of who you are. It's formed by your genetic makeup, your environment, the events of your childhood and your years of growing up. Helped by your own level of awareness and the parameters set by the society in which you live, how you feel about your sexuality frequently determines how you feel about yourself. And the way you feel about yourself can frequently determine the outcome of relationships.

Your Sexual Self

The essence of sexuality is the way a woman develops her sexual potential and becomes knowledgeable physically and emotionally. Many issues have a bearing on both, including past events and the way her feelings change through the years.

UNDERSTANDING SEXUALITY

The first step to having a happy and rewarding sexual relationship is to understand what sex and sexuality mean to you as a person. This means having clear knowledge of yourself and what makes you the way you are, knowing what influences came from your past and understanding their impact—good and bad—on you.

Becoming aware may be a long process, as the effects of some of those influences may have been subtle. They may now be so deep-rooted that they seem second nature, yet they may underpin the way you act in a relationship and be important to it. For example, do you depend on others to feel good about yourself? Do you fantasize about love and romance, about finding the lover of your dreams?

Where do you come from?

Like every woman, you have your individual history involving background, religion, cultural beliefs and personality. All combine to make you the sexual being you are today.

The way sexuality and relationships were viewed in your family will affect how you regard sex as an adult. This can be positive or negative. For instance, if your parents were loving to their children and to each other, the chances are that you will believe a close couple relationship will be rewarding for you. Not all people, however, experience such a positive background. If your parents argued a lot, for instance, you may find it hard to accept that loving relationships are in fact possible.

HOW FEELINGS MAY CHANGE

Many things can have an effect on your sexuality, and they may differ throughout your life. Your relationships, whether you become a parent and whether you choose to remain single will all have different degrees of significance for you at different ages.

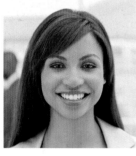

TWENTIES
You probably form relationships easily with both sexes, enjoying the mix of fun and pursuit of a career. You may vacillate between wanting commitment and preferring freedom.

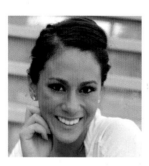

THIRTIES
You will know yourself better by now and may be in a relationship. You may have embarked on a life of sharing, balancing work and play. Marriage and having a child may be issues at this time.

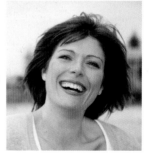

FORTIES+
At this stage your sexuality may be influenced by meeting the needs of your partner, your family and your own changing feelings about what the future may hold for you after the menopause.

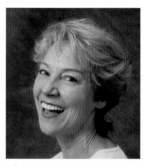

SIXTIES+
Sexuality does not stop as you get older. It continues to have an effect on your attitude to relationships. But with maturity you may have a different perspective on your priorities and wants.

DISCOVER YOUR SEXUALITY

You need to know your body well in order to have the best sex that you can. You should find out for yourself what brings you pleasure–and what doesn't. Women who rely on their partners to teach them what will bring them pleasure put the responsibility on someone else to control a sexual experience when it should be a joint endeavour–with equal pleasure for both.

When women describe their bodies, they often find fault with the way they look. However, you will never be able to relax fully if you find yourself worrying about your appearance or if you are not happy with your body for whatever reason. Being able to concentrate on the feelings you are experiencing and what is happening to your body during sex enhances your enjoyment.

Some partners may try to impose on you standards of beauty or hygiene that conflict with your own views. The pleasures of sex can be diminished if the expectations you have of each other are either unrealistic or cause you to have doubts about the other person. If you feel your physical self is not being valued as it is, your own self-respect should make you realize it is best to say "Thanks, but no thanks".

Explore your body

Discovering that sex can be joyous, wonderful and pleasurable, can come from a new partner or you can find it out by yourself. Getting to know your body and exploring the physical sensations that can be aroused can help you realize what you most appreciate and want from a sexual relationship.

One way to do this is to look at your body in a full-length mirror, noting the shapes of the different parts, the folds and creases. The purpose is not to be critical, but to reveal which of these parts could be a source of pleasure. Take a warm bath, dry yourself with a fluffy towel, then slowly rub your whole body with body lotion. Use a light massage movement, stroking your arms, legs, torso and breasts, drawing your fingers

and palms along the skin, teasing the nipples, moulding and pressing on muscle and tissue. Don't rush, relax into the feelings. Try different types of touch–firm or gentle, with fingertips or the whole hand–so you can feel your body responding all over.

Masturbation

A normal process, masturbation is an activity that many women discover by accident, usually during childhood when exploring their bodies. Not only does it feel great, it also helps you learn what

Masturbation allows you to learn what your body likes sexually.

kinds of touch you like and don't like when it comes to having sex with another person.

If embarrassment or lack of understanding about your genital area prevents you from masturbating, try becoming familiar with your genitals through reading a well-illustrated book about anatomy and sexual practice. On your own, gently touch and stroke the area to find the responses it invokes.

YOUR SENSUAL SELF
Your body will provide the clues to your sensuality. However, you must make time to discover what gives you pleasure. Delight in the sensuousness of touch and warmth in a scented bath.

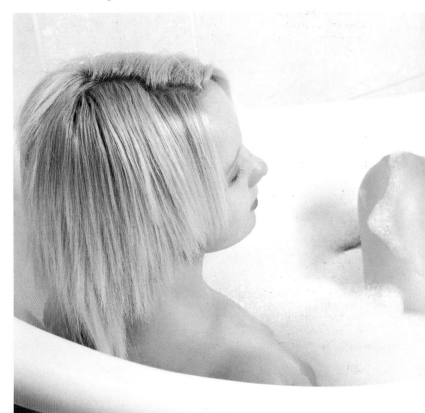

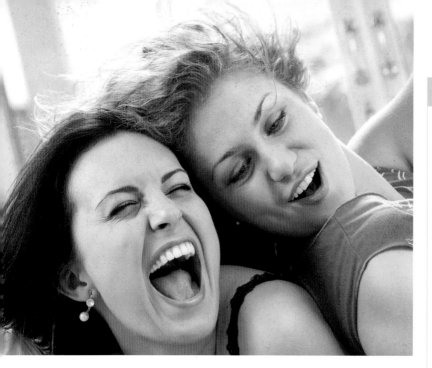

SEXUAL IDENTITY
A close, loving and sexual relationship between women can begin at any age.

Now imagine an unknown lover is pleasuring you; bring into your mind's eye the fantasy person you would like to have sex with. Take as much time as you want, touching and stroking your clitoris and vagina, feeling the area swelling and lubricating until you are thinking only of the pleasure.

Masturbation trains your body to react sexually, so you know your own arousal levels and how close you are to orgasm. Women who may have trouble having an orgasm with a partner can often do so when they are alone, using their hand or a vibrator.

No sex?

Many women choose to spend some time in their lives without being in a sexual relationship. They choose celibacy so they can concentrate on other things, or have a period of reflection, perhaps after the ending of a long-term relationship. Others may be celibate because they cannot find a suitable partner, or for religious reasons. It may also be forced upon some by a change of circumstances, such as the death of a partner and the loss of desire.

Celibacy does not stop you from having sexual feelings. You may not have the intimacy of a relationship–whether by choice or not–but you remain a sexual being. If sex is important to ensure self-esteem, masturbation and fantasy are valid options.

WOMEN WHO LOVE WOMEN

It is not unusual for girls and young women to be attracted to other women for a while, even hugging and kissing. Some women eventually find that they want a man as a sexual partner; others realize that they are lesbians, but may have to choose their time to reveal that to others. These women may have existing family who reject anything that differs from the heterosexual "norm", or they may be in a marriage they cannot leave, perhaps because of children or illness. Or perhaps they may not feel psychologically able to handle the emotions that might be triggered by this revelation and so go on denying their lesbianism to themselves.

In most cases women need to take time to come to terms with their feelings and to decide how open they want to be about their newly found identity. One of the first stages of coming out may be to contact helplines that provide understanding and advice, offer friendship and put a less antagonistic perspective on lesbian and bisexual women. You may learn, from those who have already faced the problem, of ways to broach the subject with your friends and your family. You will also want to talk through with them the risks involved in coming out.

There is in both heterosexual and lesbian society an assumption that someone is either "one of us" or not—and it is this attitude that can cause unhappiness. A woman who loves another woman can face opposition and oppression. Mothers who become lesbian may be challenged in regard to custody of their children. They may become targets of violence, and at work they may be discriminated against or receive unwelcome sexual attention from men or harassment from females. Being aware that any of these situations might happen is preparation in itself. There is now, however, greater awareness of sexual diversity and more people accept lesbians and bisexual women as simply part of a wider society.

Being honest with yourself about your feelings is the basis of finding happiness. As in any partnership, each of you needs to feel equal to make it work, and any problems have to be ironed out together. A relationship that is mutually beneficial and supportive is as prized by two people of the same sex as it is by a heterosexual couple.

WHAT A SEXUAL RELATIONSHIP MEANS

Sex within a relationship can bring a couple closer together, increase their sense of bonding with each other and give them a feeling that cannot be shared with anyone else.

There are different issues, joys and pleasures in a new relationship compared with a longstanding one. When you are first attracted to someone, the mere sight of that person may be enough to make you want sex. As soon as you touch, you are excited. With the development of your relationship, you learn more about each other, mentally and physically, and a new approach may replace that earlier excitement. It is not unusual for a woman to need more stimulation before she is ready for sex, and her partner may indicate preferences to make penetration more enjoyable for both. Most couples find that sex improves over time, as they get to know each other's bodies and learn to trust each other implicitly. The potential for giving each other profound, deep pleasure becomes greater with time.

In a longstanding relationship, sex can be many things depending on your mood—fun, comforting or deeply, intensely loving. During the course of such a relationship, you may make love many thousands of times, but if it becomes routine, you risk sexual boredom, which may break the bond you have established. If you don't always do exactly the same things, in the same order, in the same place, a relationship stays fresh. On the other hand, as time goes by, such familiarity may be appreciated by both of you.

Sex reflects your relationship

How sex is between the two of you often reflects how things are in the rest of your relationship. For instance, a man who is successful in his career may feel dominant over his partner who is at home with the children. At a later stage, she may be achieving in her career when he is facing a crisis in his own. Both changes are bound to have an effect on a couple's sex life—although the precise way depends on their affection for each other and their personalities.

Anger in a relationship may generate exciting sex for some. But this is not satisfactory long term, since the anger may too easily lead to physical violence. A partner who is physically stronger may hurt you even in play.

Misunderstandings or blocked feelings—particularly those that arouse resentment or jealousy—can influence

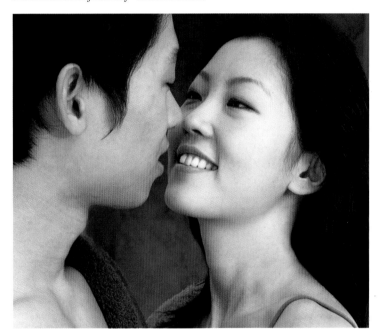

your attitude towards sex. You need to find out what is upsetting you, and try to work it out with your partner before it becomes a problem that divides you.

Good sex, bad sex

Nothing is abnormal if both partners are happy with it. So if both of you only want sex in the bath or shower, always want sex in bed in the dark or want to do something that would make everyone you know burst out laughing, that's entirely up to you—providing it does not damage your relationship or hurt anyone else.

Bad sex is anything you don't want to do or find boring, uncomfortable or painful. If your partner likes certain sexual practices and you don't, you have every right not to do them. If you give in when you don't want to, it may begin a pattern of pain and hurt.

ENJOYING SEX
For both of you to enjoy sex, you must be aroused. This is likely to happen more quickly for a male partner than for you so, if you are not ready, encourage your partner to stimulate you more to arouse you fully.

NEVER EXCUSE ABUSE

Domestic violence is a significant source of women's illnesses and injuries, which the victim may not be willing to talk about due to fear or embarrassment or pretence that it hadn't happened. Physical abuse can include anything from slapping, kicking, pinching and choking to forced sexual activity. Emotional abuse involves continuous criticism and undermining of self-worth, unpredictable responses, threats of violence, withholding of affection and manipulation through unreasonable demands. Certain factors have been identified that may indicate susceptibility to violence or battering when they are present in a relationship. So ask yourself, does your partner:

- Always want to know where you were and whom you were with?
- Limit, control or try to stop your contact with family or friends?
- Throw things or hit objects when angry?
- Show violence towards anyone else?
- Abuse alcohol or drugs and is violent when drunk or high?
- Put you down and belittle your opinions?
- Believe that he ought to be in charge?
- Have views about men and women that are very traditional?
- Imply that everything that goes wrong is your fault?
- Have violence or abuse in the family background?
- Seem to behave worse as your relationship develops?

If you experience any or several of these types of behaviours, or if you have been injured in any way by your partner, you should not assume the behaviour will change. It's more likely to escalate. You need to remove yourself from the dangers and get help: tell your doctor, the local hospital or the police. Call a domestic abuse helpline.

It can also too easily become physical abuse if you don't pay attention to your sense of fear. Be warned if after hurting you, your partner sends roses or makes some other "romantic" gesture and promises never to hurt you again. In a relationship such as this, you must put your physical safety foremost and try to find a way out, bearing in mind that attempting to leave an abusive relationship is known to prompt further violence. You should seek help.

Fantasy sex

The mind plays as great a part as the body in bringing about sexual enjoyment. Learning to fantasize and sharing the experience can make a relationship stronger and enhance lovemaking. The best sex is not static; it changes and grows as you discover what you like and what satisfies you. You may have fantasies that help you reach orgasm, but you may choose to share them only when you are sure of your partnership and know that your thoughts won't offend.

Fantasies come in many guises, from those that take you away from reality to those that add something extra to it. The one that works for you may encompass play acting (for instance, pretending that you have never met before). It may be something that in theory you could do, but which has an element of danger (such as having someone else in bed with you). It may be an outlandish dream (such as having sex on a raft at sea). Using some form of harmless bondage may add to the fantasy as long as you both want it.

LOVING MOMENTS
Affection, warmth, respect and humour bring the closeness that a sexual relationship needs to develop. Being able to express your thoughts and feelings without worrying about your partner's response is key to an emotionally and physically mature partnership.

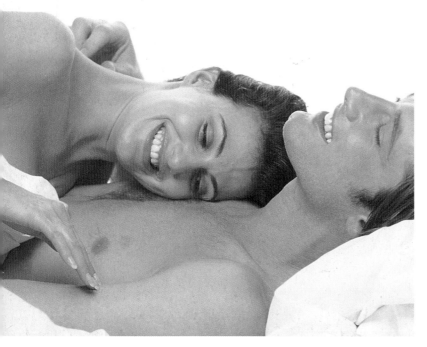

INTIMACY

The basis of happy sexual relationships is intimacy. This means knowing someone as they are, rather than as they appear to be or as you would like to see them–and accepting it.

Intimacy takes time to develop and it does not happen automatically. You need to remain emotionally open to your partner and make an effort to keep getting to know him, as he needs to do with you. Wanting to find out more about your partner's responses and feelings is the best way to keep your passion healthy and thriving.

Many couples believe they are communicating because they talk to each other all the time. But talking about the practical things–such as taking the children to school, paying the bills–is only part of the communication that leads to real, deep closeness. For that, you need to be talking about yourselves and your thoughts, sharing ideas and attitudes whether they are positive or negative. Relationship counsellors find that most couples who come to them seeking their help have problems communicating on a personal level. Talking is the first step, but you need to listen, too. And you need to accept what your partner feels and thinks, even though it may be different from what you think and feel. Some subjects can be difficult to talk about honestly, but ultimately this is what leads to trust.

It is essential to spend time together as a couple, making space and taking time for yourselves as two people together. If you see each other only as parents, you may not be sexually aroused. Equally, if you are both totally involved in your individual careers, you may neglect your partnership. You need intimacy and closeness for an abiding sexual relationship.

Men do not always find it as easy to discuss or verbalize their feelings as women do. They may not have been encouraged to do this by their own families and may not see any point to it if, on the surface, everything appears to be going well. However, if your partner's restraint affects the development of your relationship, you may need to encourage him to open up more. It may take time and patience. Quizzing him gently and affectionately when you are getting along well may help him turn his thoughts into words and communicate them to you.

Stroking and touching, without necessarily leading to intercourse, can be helpful in bringing a couple together.

Touch

The skin of the hands is extremely sensitive and the feeling of skin on skin is both sensual and comforting. Through touch you attune yourselves to each other. All sorts of touch–ranging from friendly cuddling and stroking, body massage to more intimate caressing–can relieve the stresses and strains of daily life, making you feel relaxed and close. Being touched can take you back to the warm security of childhood, while cuddling someone can make you feel nurturing and loving. Touch arouses both of you and relieves tension.

CHANGING PATTERNS
Inevitably the life of a couple will change when they become parents. You may not want sexual intercourse for a while after the birth, but your sexual intimacy can move to a new level through touch. Caressing and stroking can be loving and comforting at the same time, just as it is for the baby you have created together.

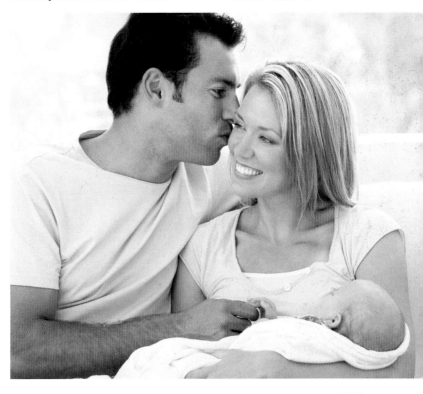

Stroking and touching that does not necessarily lead to intercourse can be helpful in bringing a couple together. Using the principles of sensate focusing, you can take all the time you need to work out what you like. By exploring your sexuality together, you will discover things about yourselves both as a couple and as individuals, helping to develop an excitement and trust that will help to carry you through the adverse times in your relationship.

Try to set apart a time of the day when you can lie in each other's arms, being quiet and peaceful. This will add to the closeness and affection that is essential to intimacy.

Ask for what you want

Skilful negotiation is important in many parts of life and essential to your most intimate relationships. You will both have the best sex you can if you are able to ask for what you want in bed.

The thought of talking about what you want and being honest about what does and does not work for you raises a lot of fears for both women and men.

You may think, for instance, that you run the risk of rejection. Or you may find the prospect of talking about sex embarrassing. You may also fear hurting the partner you love deeply if you tell him that he is not doing what you like. At other times you may not even know what it is that you want—for instance, after the birth of a baby when tiredness and getting enough sleep become more of a concern than having sex.

The real point about relationships is that you should not expect your partner to read your mind, whether the subject is sex or the household chores. Explanation and making requests are part and parcel of a relationship between equals. You need to give some thought to what pleases you and to realize that you have a right to ask for it, as does your partner. For instance, a man may want to start penetration before the woman is ready. Asking lovingly—yet assertively—for more foreplay will add to your pleasure. Similarly, if you don't like the way he rubs your clitoris, gently redirect his hand to indicate this. You can use body language to reveal your preferences, too,

to show your partner what you like by doing it to yourself. There may be other times when you have an increase in desire which your partner cannot meet—he's too tired, falls asleep or is away from home. In this case masturbation may be the best resolution.

Negotiation is part of all relationships, heterosexual and homosexual. While a woman may feel she knows instinctively what another wants, all women do not necessarily like the same thing—and if the process of finding this out is enjoyable, it makes for a better relationship. Intimacy relies on your being honest both with your partner and with yourself.

All relationships have troughs and peaks; by its very nature, sex can't or won't be perfect or satisfying every time. If you know this, and you and your partner have learned to be confident with each other, you can laugh about it together when the unexpected happens. Such warmth and humour are as much elements of intimacy as touch, and are to be prized in a loving relationship.

THE LIMITS OF TOUCH

As a relationship develops, it is important to take a lead from your partner as to which parts of the body it is good to touch and also to convey your preferences to your partner. Although touch will be arousing in a sexual sense, it can also be worrying or alarming.

- With an established partner, if you do not like a particular touch, say so, even if you liked it in the past.

- If you are with a new partner and feel at all uncomfortable about anything, let that person know as soon as possible. If you continue to be uncomfortable and he does not change, you should leave the situation.

- If you are single, always be clear about sexual limits right at the start of a date.

- If you find yourself in an abusive relationship, be aware of the risks at all times (see p. 238), and take action to protect yourself from physical subjugation. Seek help from a domestic helpline or women's shelter or from the police.

Sexual Problems

Decreased libido is the most common complaint. Not being able to make love because your body won't do what you want it to can be frightening and frustrating. It happens to men and women and can cause worry and anxiety. Talking to your doctor is important and may help to relieve the problem.

WHEN LOVE HURTS

Sex should be pleasurable, not painful. If something is hurting you, the first thing you should do is stop–or ask your partner to stop. Painful intercourse can be caused simply by a man thrusting too hard or too deeply. It may also happen if you have a chronic medical condition, in which case all that may be necessary is to find a more comfortable position.

If intercourse continues to be painful, there may be other reasons. Infections such as yeast vaginitis, cystitis or pelvic inflammatory disease (PID) can be the cause of discomfort. If you have an infection, you will need to see your doctor for antibiotic treatment; until the infection is gone, you should not have sex. Inflammation of the vagina can also be the result of an allergy to perfume in soap and body lotion; the pain should disappear when you stop using them. If you bleed after intercourse, you should report this to your doctor who may arrange tests.

Lack of lubrication

Some women find that intercourse is uncomfortable because their vagina is not lubricated sufficiently. This may occur because sex is infrequent or you are not yet sexually aroused, in which case more foreplay may help. Other women may not produce enough lubrication no matter how excited they are. This can apply particularly at the menopause and after, when the vaginal walls thin and shrink from lack of oestrogen. Using a lubricant can overcome the problem, as can topical oestrogen therapies, which make the tissues more like they were before the menopause.

A woman's first sexual experience may cause pain–either because there is not enough lubrication or the hymen may be unbroken. Take things very slowly, make sure your vagina is moist, and your partner stretches the opening with his fingers first.

After childbirth the memory of physical pain can reduce desire for sex and cause anxiety. Overcoming this requires a gentle partner, much reassurance and the use of a lubricant so intercourse can be enjoyed once more.

Tight muscles

Vaginismus is a condition in which the vaginal muscles tighten so much that penetration is painful and sometimes impossible (an internal examination or cervical smear cannot be done). Vaginismus is usually caused by anxiety about sex and is not permanent. The best way of treating it is to try to establish a relaxation ritual during which, at your own speed, you find out for yourself how to relax the vagina. Then, with your partner, have lots of foreplay so your vagina is well-lubricated before any penetration. If you have tried these suggestions and are still having pain, stop attempting penetration. Do not force yourself to have intercourse because you think you should. Your body may start associating sex with pain, affecting desire and leading to a bigger problem. A trained sex therapist and pelvic muscle training can be helpful.

ERECTION PROBLEMS

Some men cannot achieve an erection from time to time, and this is quite normal. Other men may ejaculate far too quickly, becoming limp and leaving their partners frustrated. It helps to know that some causes of erectile dysfunction and premature ejaculation are psychological and can be alleviated by simple exercises a couple can learn with the help of a therapist trained in sex therapy. Remember that if you and your partner are having penetration quickly to avoid loss of an erection, you may be compounding the problem, causing discomfort and anxiety for both of you.

When a man is unable to get an erection at all, or cannot maintain one for long, there may be a physical factor involved; encourage your partner to get medical advice.

SEX AND RELATIONSHIPS

When sex is going well, it is just one part of a loving relationship. When it goes wrong, it can feel as if it is taking over not just your relationship, but every element of your life.

The most common sexual complaints women have fall into four categories: decreased libido, difficulty with arousal, dissatisfaction with frequency of orgasm or the type of stimulation required to reach orgasm, and painful or uncomfortable sexual activity (*see* p. 241). Factors that can affect these include depression, anxiety, fatigue, alcohol consumption, low hormone levels and drug use–either prescription or illegal–including antidepressants and treatment for high blood pressure and fluid retention. Your lack of sexual response should be discussed with your doctor, particularly if there is any type of illness involved.

Both men and women can have sexual problems, and if one partner has a problem, the other is invariably affected by it. A sexual problem that has always existed is called a primary problem and may have either a physical or a deep-seated psychological cause. When problems start during a previously happy relationship, it is essential to consider the reasons rather than ignoring them.

Many couples remember a time in their relationship when sex was good. Those memories and their fondness for each other should reassure them that, whatever is causing the present upset, it can be overcome.

No interest?

Between 50 and 70 per cent of women report loss of desire at some time in their lives. Men who complain of impotence may well be masking a lack of desire. People can feel bewildered and upset when desire deserts them, but it is only a problem when one or both of you think it is.

It is not uncommon to find you want to have sex less frequently the longer you know each other. If you remain close and intimate, you will be satisfied by quality rather than quantity. If on the other hand, you have no interest in making love, you may have relationship difficulties. This is the most common cause of decreased libido and also arousal and orgasm problems.

The reasons can be complex. What you were taught in childhood about what sexual expression should and should not be may have predisposed you to certain emotional traits that do not sit well with your current relationship–often without your realizing it.

Each new relationship brings different pleasures and problems, but people do tend to bring their sexual habits and assumptions with them. In the early days, you are likely to have a lot of fantasies about your sexual partner, because there are always new things to discover. There can be an air of secretiveness to add to the excitement. Once a relationship is established, sexual arousal can depend on different factors.

When dissatisfaction strikes

The most obvious cause of many sexual problems is to be found in the pressures of day-to-day living. Work demands, little time to relax, even good events such as the birth of a child or a new job, can stop you from wanting sex. You may not be feeling well or on top of things, and other parts of your life take priority.

It helps to know in any relationship that this is inevitable and will happen from time to time. However, if sex loses its importance to both of you, you will lose intimacy, too. In this situation it is essential that you make time for sex and for each other. Organize it so that the two of you can be alone without other distractions. Plan a date together, doing something you enjoy, spend some time hugging, hand holding, give each other a massage or a foot rub, and see where it takes you. You may not solve all your problems, but you will be closer.

Let go

Sex-related anxiety is not uncommon in both men and women and can prevent you from reaching orgasm or even allowing yourself to be stimulated. If you know your lovemaking is likely to be interrupted, perhaps by children, it can be difficult to relax and enjoy yourselves. Or you may worry about becoming pregnant. Such concerns should be resolved before the anxiety becomes disabling to your relationship.

Changes in your lifestyle–giving up work, having a baby, changing jobs or neighbourhoods–can cause you to look anew at your sexual relationship. If you can't reach orgasm now, was it always this way, or were you once able to be satisfied? Have you become stuck in certain sexual patterns or habits? Perhaps there are other reasons why you can't relax. Your desire may be inhibited by a plethora of deep feelings–other problems within the relationship can leave you with blocked anger, repressed emotions and no way of talking about them. These emotional issues can be resolved by increased communication.

If you find that you can't talk to each other or there is too much anger felt, it may be worth seeing a counsellor who is trained as a sex therapist who can facilitate communication, look at the emotions and may guide you through a series of sensual exercises to connect with your sexual self and each other.

The purpose of sex therapy

When normally loving people have problems in their sex lives, a sex therapist may help them find the answers they seek. Sex therapy can be based on behaviour therapy or insight-oriented, psychodynamic psychotherapy, or preferably both. A therapist who is also trained in sex therapy will alternate between these as needed during the treatment with a couple or individual depending on the issues revealed.

A therapist can show you how to change the way you approach or have sex in order to overcome specific and solvable problems, such as premature ejaculation or insufficient arousal.

In the 1960s, sex therapists Masters and Johnson developed a programme called sensate focusing, which is still used today to help couples discover more about their feelings and sensations. You are given a set of exercises to do at home in your own time. You take turns pleasuring each other through massage, touching and stroking parts of the body, but not the genitals. As you progress in your understanding of each other's reactions and have confidence in saying yes to what you like–and you both find your excitement increasing–non-intercourse-related genital activity is encouraged. Finally your sex life is restored to normal, or better, so that your relationship should benefit from a return to shared values–and prosper.

FOCUS ON SENSATIONS
When a couple starts therapy for sexual problems, the first stage will encourage them to discover more about their feelings and sensations. Pleasuring each other through the gentlest massage and stroking brings new understanding of what arouses them.

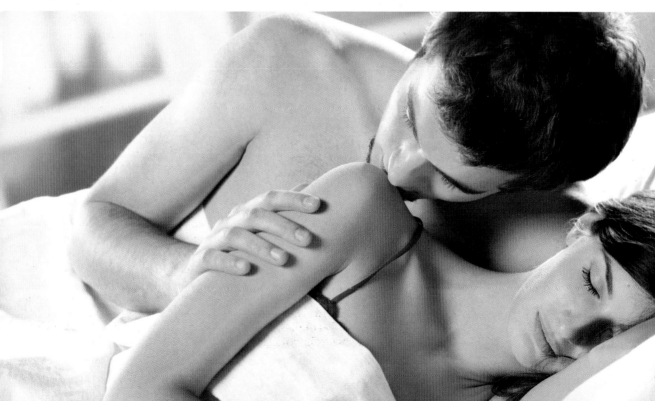

Sexual Infections

Once called venereal diseases, sexually transmitted infections—or STIs—are infections spread from one person to another by sexual contact. They are a worldwide problem and can have particularly serious consequences for women.

THE DANGERS OF SEX

Women are at greater risk from sexually transmitted infections than men—a woman is, for example, more likely than a man to catch an STI from a single sexual encounter. There are about 25 different infections classified as STIs. The best known is HIV—the virus that leads to AIDS. A woman is 17 times more likely to catch HIV from a man than a man is from a woman. Viral STIs, such as HIV and herpes, cannot be cured; bacterial STIs can be cured if they are treated promptly.

If there is any chance that you have contracted an STI, even if you have no symptoms at present—and women often have fewer noticeable symptoms than do men—you have a responsibility to yourself as well as to your sexual partners to be diagnosed and treated and to inform any partners about the situation.

If you have caught an STI, it will not clear up on its own. If left untreated, some STIs, such as chlamydia and syphilis, may have further consequences for your health and fertility in the long term. An STI infection during pregnancy may also lead to complications and illness for the baby.

STOP!

If it is possible that you have an STI or if you have any of the following symptoms, do not have sex until you've seen your doctor:

- unpleasant vaginal discharge
- pain during intercourse
- pelvic pain
- pain on passing urine
- swelling in the groin
- sores in the genital area
- flu-like symptoms

How do you catch them?

STIs are usually caught by having sex–vaginal, anal or oral–with an infected person and exchanging bodily fluids, such as semen, blood and vaginal fluids. Very rarely, an STI is passed on through blood transfusion. STIs cannot be caught from toilet seats or swimming pools, although some, such as pubic lice, can be picked up in close, nonsexual contact. Other infections, such as cystitis and thrush, may be passed on or worsened by sex; these may also develop without sexual contact.

Who's at risk?

Almost anyone who is sexually active is at risk of catching an STI. There are only two totally risk-free choices: abstinence and life-long monogamy. If you and your partner have only ever had sex with each other, then you are not at risk. However, it is very uncommon today for a person to have only one sexual partner in a lifetime. You may be in a trusting and long-standing relationship but, because some STIs do not present obvious symptoms, it is possible that one of you may be infected with something caught many years previously. The more partners you have, the greater your risk.

Be honest

It may be difficult to tell your partner or partners that you have an STI–although this depends on the circumstances in which you contracted it. A longstanding but recently diagnosed STI, such as chlamydia, may be seen as a health issue, rather than a relationship crisis. Professionals at the clinic can inform casual partners if you feel unable to.

Being told that your partner has an STI can be as hard as breaking the news yourself, although it does not necessarily mean that the infected partner has contracted the disease while in the relationship. However, you must be examined and treated as necessary if your partner is infected. Feelings of hurt, betrayal and anger–on either side–will need to be discussed, and you and your partner may find counselling helpful.

HPV VACCINE

The first vaccine to offer protection against the human papilloma virus (HPV) is now available in Europe and Australia. It is a three-dose vaccine that has the trade name Gardasil. HPV is associated with the development of cervical cancer and genital warts (see also p. 247). Although the vaccine does not guarantee prevention from cervical cancer or warts, it does protect against the most common viral types that cause 70 per cent of cervical cancers and 90 per cent of warts. It is recommended that girls receive this vaccination before becoming sexually active. Ongoing studies are looking at how long the levels of antibody will last and whether women who receive the vaccine may need to have booster shots in the future. The vaccine is tolerated well, although it is common for there to be some pain at the injection site. A rare disorder that causes muscle weakness, known as Guillane-Barre Syndrome, has been reported in some women after vaccination.

SEXUALLY TRANSMITTED INFECTIONS

Symptoms may develop weeks, months or years after the initial exposure to the infection. A sexually active woman should ensure that she has regular pelvic examinations and cervical smears, as these may reveal problems. If you have had unprotected sex with a person who you think may have an STI, see your own doctor or go to an STI clinic. Don't be embarrassed. Nobody knows why you are there.

Disease	Symptoms	Detection	Treatment
HIV			
The human immunodeficiency virus (HIV) is a leading cause of death of young people in many countries. After contracting HIV, people may have no symptoms for years, but over time the virus attacks the body's immune system, leaving it susceptible to acquired immune deficiency syndrome (AIDS). This is a collection of symptoms that prevents the body from fighting a range of infections and conditions.	Mild flu, which comes and goes, then vulnerability to infections such as thrush, shingles and herpes; loss of appetite and weight	The virus becomes apparent in blood tests typically within three months after the infection has been contracted.	Focus is on achieving the maximum suppression of symptoms for as long as possible. This aggressive approach is known as highly active anti-retroviral therapy (HAART). The aim of HAART is to reduce the amount of virus in the blood to very low or even nondetectable levels, though this doesn't mean the virus is gone. This is usually accomplished with therapy that combines three or more drugs.
HEPATITIS B			
A liver infection caused by a virus 100 times more infectious than HIV. Symptoms appear 2–6 weeks after infection caused by sexual contact or through infected blood or other body fluids (saliva or faecal matter). Most people recover, others become carriers and may pass it on to sexual partners as well as remaining at risk of serious liver disease later. Family and sexual partners of those with hepatitis B can be vaccinated.	Jaundice, loss of appetite, nausea, headaches	Blood tests; in rare cases, a liver biopsy	Includes rest and restricted physical activity. For chronic hepatitis, the drug interferon may be given.

(continued)

Disease (continued)	Symptoms	Detection	Treatment
TRICHOMONIASIS			
This is caused by a microscopic protozoan single-celled animal. It is uncommon but is associated with other STIs such as gonorrhoea, chlamydia and genital warts. It is spread through sexual contact and may be passed on by syringes or shared devices used anally or vaginally. Trichomoniasis does not usually produce serious disorders and only rarely reaches the upper genital tract.	Vaginal discharge is smelly and may be green and frothy. Soreness of the vulva and pain on passing urine are common, as is discomfort on penetration.	Testing vaginal secretions	Antibiotics: metronidazole, tinidazole Pessaries
SYPHILIS			
A bacterial infection, which, if untreated, can develop over several years into serious illness and possible death. In modern times, syphilis is usually diagnosed and treated before it gets to the tertiary, or final, stage for which there is no treatment. Syphilis is passed on through sexual contact. If anything leads you to think that you have been exposed to the infection, you must contact a doctor immediately. Syphilis screening is carried out as part of prenatal care and for giving blood.	First stage of infection is a painless sore on the genitals, which may come and go unnoticed. Second stage, up to three months after infection, has flu-like symptoms and a bodyrash lasting 2–10 weeks.	A blood test may not be effective if infection occurred less than 10 days before. If there is a genital sore, a smear of cells is examined microscopically. A blood test is then done to confirm diagnosis.	Antibiotics, usually injected penicillin; azithromycin or doxycycline are used for those with a penicillin allergy. Partner should also be treated. This may be ongoing, depending on the results of three monthly tests.
GONORRHOEA			
Gonorrhoea is caused by bacteria that spread around the vagina and urethra. It is highly contagious. Sufferers may have no symptoms, but if untreated, it can lead to serious problems—chronic stomach pain, infertility and other STIs. It can infect a fetus in the womb via the birth canal, causing blindness. It is spread by sexual contact, including oral sex.	Unpleasant vaginal discharge, an urgent need to pass urine, pain on urination, bleeding between periods	Testing of a sample of cervical fluid	Often resistant to some antibiotics. Ceftriaxone, ciprofloxacin, doxycycline and cefixime (not available in Australia) can be used. Both partners must be treated.
CHLAMYDIA			
The most common STI, caused by a bacterium, chlamydia often has no symptoms and is particularly common in young people. It has been recommended that all young women be screened annually. Left untreated in women, the infection can lead to pelvic inflammatory disease (PID), which in turn can cause infertility. Men who contract chlamydia can be made sterile. After one bout of PID, the disease tends to be recurrent.	Pain during intercourse, thin vaginal discharge, burning when passing urine	Swab of the cervical fluid is tested	Antibiotics of the doxycycline or tetracycline type, such as azithromycin

Disease	Symptoms	Detection	Treatment
GENITAL HERPES			
The most common viral STI caused by the herpes simplex virus HSV-2, which is similar to the cold sore virus HSV-1 and the Epstein-Barr virus of glandular fever. Genital herpes is contagious, incurable, but not fatal. The virus remains in your body, although it may not show symptoms, and can be triggered by stress and tight-fitting undergarments and clothing. It is spread by sexual contact, which can include kissing or touching infected areas. Babies born vaginally during an active herpes infection may, rarely, become infected.	A few days after infection, flu-like symptoms, pain on passing urine, burning in genital area, lower back pain. There may be vaginal discharge, swollen glands and small red bumps in or near the vagina that blister.	A doctor takes a sample of fluid from a blister and sends it away for testing. If no blisters are present, herpes can be hard to diagnose.	Antiviral drugs help healing during attacks and can be taken long term to reduce the frequency. Bathe sores in tepid salty water; use a topical painkilling cream. Wash hands after touching sores. Reduce stress.
NONSPECIFIC URETHRITIS			
This bacterial infection of the urethra can be caused by chlamydia, ureaplasma or trichomonas. In a man, one sign is a cloudy discharge from the penis. Early treatment prevents spread of infection into the pelvic cavity. There is no firm evidence that irritants such as perfumed soaps can cause urethritis.	Pain or burning when urinating; frequent urination	Testing of urine and urethral discharge	Antibiotics: doxycycline, azithromycin or erythromycin
PUBIC LICE AND SCABIES			
Two types of tiny, irritating parasites that live on the skin but can't be seen. Pubic lice, often called crabs, are pinhead-sized insects that lay their eggs in hairy parts of the body, particularly the groin. Scabies is an itchy rash caused by a mite burrowing under the skin to lay its eggs. They are passed on by sexual or other close contact with an infected person.	Pubic lice: intense itching or rash in the pubic/groin area

Scabies: generalized itching | By sight | Your doctor or clinic will suggest relevant shampoos or creams. It is not necessary to wash clothing and bedding in very hot water, as previously assumed. |
| **GENITAL WARTS** | | | |
| These contagious warts are caused by the human papilloma virus (HPV). HPV types can also cause cervical cancer and other less common cancers, such as cancers of the vulva, vagina, anus and penis. As the virus may be involved in precancerous changes, it is important to have regular smears. Genital warts are passed on through sex with an infected person. | There are no obvious symptoms of infection. Warts can grow in or outside the vagina or around the anus and may be puffy and pink or hard and grey. | Small, painless lumps that may itch appear around genitals or anus 3 weeks to 6 months after infection. Associated with cervical dysplasia (precancerous changes), caused by HPV. | Visible warts can be burned off, frozen off or treated with laser surgery, but virus remains in the body. May be self-treated with drugs such as podophyllotoxin cream at home. If given to girls before they become sexually active, a vaccine can protect from the four types of HPV that cause most cervical cancers and genital warts. |

HIV AND AIDS

HIV, the human immunodeficiency virus, is passed on when an infected person's bodily fluids, such as blood or semen, enter another person's bloodstream. This is most likely to happen during sexual intercourse, both heterosexual and homosexual. Women generally acquire the virus from men rather than passing the virus to their male partners.

Other methods of transmission are through the use of hypodermic needles shared with someone who is HIV-positive, or when the infection is passed on by a woman in childbirth or to a baby from its mother's breast milk.

In the past, some people were infected through treatment with blood or blood constituents contaminated with the virus, but these substances are now screened before use. Although the virus is present in the saliva of infected people, there is no evidence that it can be passed on by activities such as kissing or sharing a drinking glass. However, bleeding gums can be an entry point. Anal intercourse is risky because the tissues in the rectum tear easily. Women who have open sores on their genitals from herpes, for example, are also at risk during sexual intercourse.

Once in the bloodstream, the HIV virus attacks T-cells in the immune system (known as CD4 lymphocytes) that are taken over and begin the task of reproducing the virus instead of performing their normal function of defending the body against infection. If these T-cells are destroyed in sufficient numbers, the infected person develops acquired immunodeficiency syndrome (AIDS), although it may take many years– even as long as a decade–before this stage is reached.

What are the symptoms?

Blood is tested for antibodies that the body produces against the HIV virus. However, the antibodies may not appear in measurable quantities until at least 3 months after infection and in some cases up to a year later.

A positive result has profound implications for the person concerned,

INFECTIONS KILL

When the immune system is not functioning properly, the individual is vulnerable to infections that would be easily controlled by a healthy person. These are called opportunistic infections and affect the most susceptible—the very young, old, frail and people who are HIV-positive. Common infections for HIV-positive men are a type of pneumonia called *Pneumocystis* pneumonia (PCP) and infection from an organism called *Cryptosporidium*, which is found in water. These infections can be treated, and prophylactic medication to prevent them may be recommended for people when blood tests show their immune system is weak. For women, the most dangerous infection is bacterial pneumonia.

The diagnosis of AIDS is usually made after a person has contracted one or more life-threatening infections. For a woman these may be invasive cervical cancer and serious ulcerative genital lesions, both of which are difficult to treat. A CD4 count of less than 200 is another sign; CD4 cells are the most important white blood cells involved in immunity. Women and men with AIDS can develop tuberculosis, non-Hodgkin's lymphoma, and a herpes infection called CMV (cytomegalovirus) that leads to blindness, colitis and oesophagitis (inflammation of the oesophagus).

PROTECT THE CHILDREN

Most children with HIV acquire it from their mothers. The infection is passed on either in the uterus or during breastfeeding. If a woman who is HIV-positive has a baby and breastfeeds, there is a 25–35 per cent risk of the baby becoming infected, unless preventive measures are taken. Antiviral drugs are now available that can reduce this factor to as little as 2 per cent. In developed countries, antiviral drugs such as zidovudine can be given in cocktails to pregnant women and can reduce their viral load so that the risk of transmission is much reduced. If the mother has not been treated, small amounts of antiviral drugs can also be given to infants that significantly reduces their risk of infection.

as well as for those close to him or her and for anyone with whom they have had unprotected sex. It is therefore important to prepare for the test by discussing the possible outcome with a counsellor; this will normally be offered at clinics specializing in HIV concerns as well as through national support organizations. A counsellor will also be able to discuss the various treatment options that are now available and advise who should be told about the diagnosis. In addition, decisions about employment and insurance may have to be made. The counsellor may have advice on making lifestyle changes, including practising safer sex.

Supportive medication

There is as yet no cure for HIV or AIDS, but modern treatments can often temporarily halt or retard the progression from HIV infection to the development of the syndrome. Since a person who is HIV-positive may continue to feel well, the CD4 cell count and viral load are monitored closely. When the CD4 cell level goes down and the viral load up, treatment is started. Doctors usually recommend prophylactic medication before the immune system is irreversibly damaged. Issues that need to be considered include the fact that the drug therapy for HIV is costly, complex, disruptive and has psychological as well as physical side effects.

Slow viral growth

The first objective of treatment is to stem the proliferation of the virus in the body, the second is to prevent and treat so-called opportunistic infections (*see* box, left) and the third is to boost and maintain immune system function.

Anti-HIV drugs are usually taken in combination. While they cannot eradicate HIV infection, they can often slow viral replication and maintain the protective T-cells at near-normal levels. It is essential to take such medications exactly as prescribed (which may involve waking up at night to do so), despite experiencing unpleasant side effects. Although early symptoms, such as aches and pains, fever, diarrhoea, breathing difficulties, swollen glands, weight loss and persistent dry cough, will be the same in women as in men, women may also have menstrual problems. Abnormal cervical smear results may occur, and recurrent yeast infections may not clear.

Strengthen your immunity

The advice usually given when someone has been found to be HIV-positive is to pay careful attention to a healthy diet and food hygiene.

With a weakened immune system, you should be scrupulous when handling uncooked meat that may harbour infectious organisms such as *Campylobacter* and *Salmonella*. You should avoid raw or lightly cooked eggs for the same reason and drink boiled tap water or bottled mineral water because of the risk of *Cryptosporidium* infection (*see* box left). A consultation with a nutritionist or dietitian can be useful to devise a healthy and affordable diet.

Keeping up to date with information on the constant new developments in treatment is important. Counselling and support from various organizations offer help to HIV-positive people, their partners, friends and families.

Fight back

Controlling the infections, which are inevitable with AIDS, with antibiotics or blocking the reproduction of the virus

with a drug such as zidovudine (AZT) can improve the survival rates for AIDs sufferers. AZT may be given while a woman is pregnant since it appears not to affect the mother or child adversely and reduces the chances of transmitting the virus to the child. It has been found that combination therapy (that is, using a number of drugs) is more effective than monotherapy (using one drug only).

Immunizations against contagious and life-threatening illnesses such as diphtheria, mumps, measles, rubella, tetanus, hepatitis B and influenza should be administered. Women should have a cervical smear every 6 months. Blood tests are performed every 3-6 months so that the levels of CD4 cells and viral load can be measured. There is no vaccine to prevent AIDS at present, although there continues to be extensive research into the development of one.

TAKE ACTION NOW!

Male or female condoms can substantially reduce the risk of infecting the partners of HIV-positive people. HIV-positive people who have sexual intercourse with a person who is also HIV-positive should take precautions as well, because there may be a potential risk of infection from a different or drug-resistant strain of the virus.

Most children with HIV acquire it from their mothers.

TALKING CAN HELP

One of the chief problems if you have HIV may be that you feel you can't talk about your condition. Ask your doctor for a referral to a trained counsellor who can guide you through the everyday problems of living with the virus.

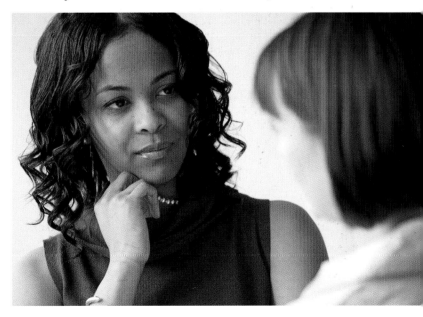

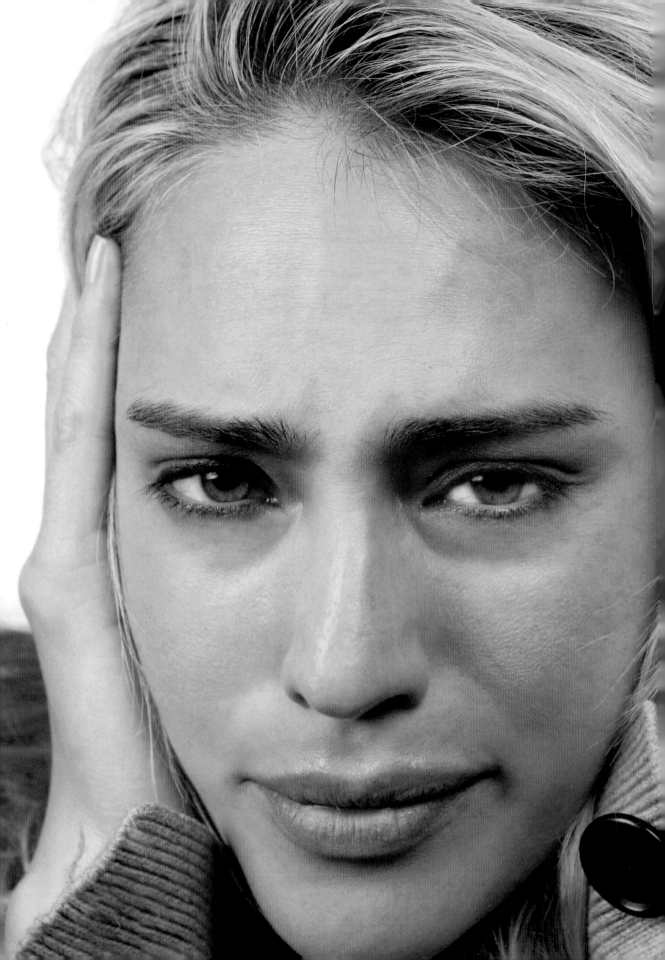

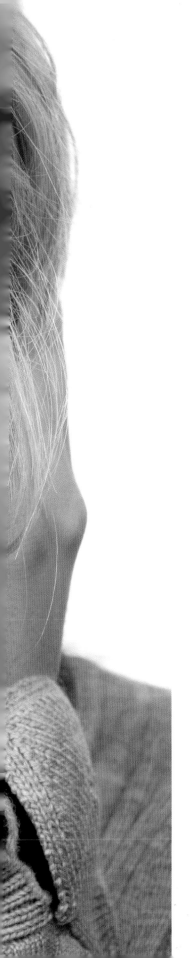

URGENT
ILLNESSES

Handling a sudden illness in the middle of the night or being called upon to deal with an emergency in the neighbourhood–choking, bee stings, dog bites, nosebleeds, broken bones, heart attacks and pizza burns–is a part of every woman's life. This chapter will help you learn how to handle an urgent or emergency situation until a doctor is available to help.

Acute Infections

If you get an infection that strikes suddenly, you should make sure to see your doctor as soon as possible. Such infections require prompt medical treatment to prevent them from spreading. Without medical attention, acute infections may rapidly worsen and become chronic.

PELVIC INFECTION AND INFLAMMATION

The entrances and exits to your reproductive and urinary systems are so close to each other that infections can affect both systems. Some infections are more common in your 20s and 30s but may also occur at and after the menopause.

TAKE ACTION NOW!

Cystitis can be prevented by:
- Drinking water or cranberry juice
- Cutting down tea, coffee and alcohol
- Emptying your bladder regularly
- Wiping from vulva to anus
- Not using perfumed soaps
- Avoiding vaginal deodorants
- Wearing cotton underwear
- Avoiding tight jeans
- Wearing thongs only occasionally

Cystitis

Women are more susceptible than men to cystitis–inflammation of the bladder–which can lead to kidney damage if not treated promptly. Cystitis is usually caused by *E. coli* bacteria that live harmlessly in the bowel until they are transferred to the bladder or urethra.

Triggers of cystitis include poor hygiene, pregnancy, sexual intercourse, putting off urination and some forms of contraception. Some women experience recurrent attacks around the time of their period. The usual symptoms are an urgent need to urinate, with only a little amount of urine passed, a burning sensation during urination, and cloudy or sometimes bloody urine. If the inflammation has spread up the ureters to the kidneys, there may be fever, backache, nausea and vomiting.

At the first sign of cystitis, take a painkiller and flush out the bacteria by drinking 275 ml (1/2 pt) of water immediately and then every 20 minutes for 2 hours. Over-the-counter cystitis remedies, taken at certain times over 48 hours, can be used to reduce the urine's acidity. If the symptoms persist or if you have signs of a kidney infection, see your doctor. If a test of a urine sample shows bacteria, a short course of antibiotics may be prescribed.

Urethral syndrome

This is the medical name for chronic inflammation of the urethra. It is much more common in women than in men and has cystitis-like symptoms. The cause of the inflammation is often unknown, since usually there are no bacteria present in the urine, and kidney function and urinary tract anatomy are normal. Urethral syndrome may occur in women at or around the time of the

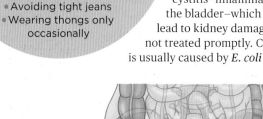
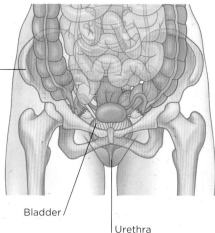

Pelvic bone

Bladder

Urethra

PELVIC AREA
The bladder is lower down the pelvis in a woman than in a man, and the urethra—through which urine is passed—is only one-fifth as long. As a result, women tend to have more urinary tract infections.

menopause and may be due to lack of oestrogen. This causes the tissues of the vulva to become thinner, which is combined with less vaginal moisture. The vulva and urethra (which lies close by) become vulnerable to trauma and irritation. The vulva may also be sore, making intercourse painful.

There is no specific treatment, although urethral syndrome may be eased with the same self-help measures as cystitis. You should also use a vaginal lubricant during sex and avoid any foods causing irritants, such as chocolate, spicy or acidic foods, mature cheese, tomatoes, alcohol, caffeine, nicotine and carbonated drinks. Your doctor may prescribe oestrogen or steroid creams to soothe the inflammation.

What colour is your urine?

In a healthy body, urine is normally pale in colour and has little odour. It can be discoloured by foods such as rhubarb, beetroot or blackberries, but returns to normal within 24 hours. However, you should see your doctor if you experience dark-coloured or red urine (which may be a side effect of a drug or viral infection) or dark yellow urine (which indicates overconcentration and a lack of fluids).

You should also consult your doctor if you have cloudy, smelly urine (which is usually caused by a urinary tract infection) or blood in the urine (which may be caused by a kidney or bladder infection). Low levels of urine may indicate kidney problems, a kidney stone or severe dehydration, while high levels of urine could be a symptom of diabetes. In either case, it is important that you arrange to see a doctor.

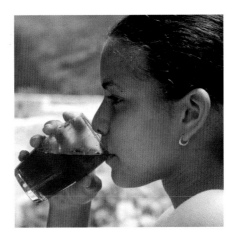

CRANBERRY JUICE
As well as having a number of substances that stop the growth of bacteria, cranberry juice can raise the acidity of urine, helping to kill bacteria in the kidneys and urinary tract.

Kidney stones

Medically termed renal calculi, kidney stones are crystals formed by chemicals in the urine. They can vary in size from a grain of salt to a marble. Some people seem to be more prone to stones than others, although it is not known why. Stones are much more common in men. Kidney stone formation is associated with hot climates, drinking too little fluid and frequent urinary tract infections.

Small stones may be excreted in the urine and in fact most stones pass naturally if large quantities of water are drunk. Larger stones can cause serious problems.

You may experience a severe, sudden pain in the small of the back that spreads down and round the front of the abdomen to the groin when a kidney stone develops. The pain may come and go for minutes or hours (most stones pass in the urine within a few hours). There may also be nausea, blood in the urine and frequent, painful urination. If stones become lodged in the bladder, you may experience loss of control of urine (incontinence).

Diagnosis is by ultrasound or X-ray. If the stones are large or if there is an infection, surgical treatment may be necessary to prevent damage to the kidney. A non-invasive technique called extra-corporeal shock wave lithotripsy (ESWL) may be used to shatter the stones into small fragments that can be passed in the urine.

WHEN A KIDNEY IS IN TROUBLE

Swelling of tissues, listlessness, nausea, rapid breathing, diarrhoea and difficulty urinating are all symptoms of kidney failure. It can be caused by diabetes, scleroderma, lupus, high blood pressure, by traumatic injury or congestive heart failure. Rarely it is a complication of pregnancy. Whatever the cause, it needs prompt medical attention in order to prevent damage to the organ.

HOW TO PREVENT STONES
To prevent stones from recurring, as they do in 50 per cent of cases, you should drink at least eight large glasses of water a day, avoid large doses of vitamin D and dairy products and cut down on protein foods.

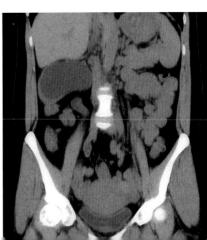

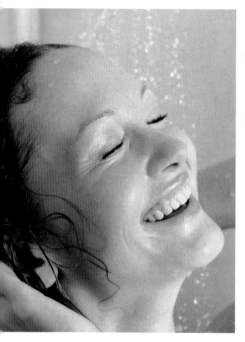

YEAST INFECTION

This condition–also known as candidiasis, thrush or monilia–is caused by a yeast-like fungus called *Candida albicans*, which is normally present in the vagina and in the mouth in small quantities. Usually it is kept in check by the naturally occurring bacteria, but this delicate balance is easily upset, and the fungus then grows out of control. Candida most commonly infects the vagina, but the infection may also be found in the mouth or on the skin. It is a very common and irritating condition with severe itching as the primary symptom.

Broad-spectrum antibiotics are a common cause, since they may destroy friendly bacteria, allowing the yeast to grow. Steroids or immunosuppressive drugs may also allow the yeast to proliferate. Candida feeds on sugar, so untreated diabetes (which causes high blood-sugar levels) and hormonal changes during a menstrual period, pregnancy or the menopause (which affect the sugar levels in vaginal tissues) increase the risk of candida infection.

What does it look like?

In the mouth candida infection produces sore, yellowish patches; on the skin it may infect damp folds and form an itchy rash. Vaginal yeast infection causes a thick, white discharge resembling cottage cheese, and with an unpleasantly sweet and "bready" smell. The vagina and vulva feel sore and itchy and urination is painful.

What to do

Applying natural live yogurt to the vaginal area may relieve the symptoms, perhaps by increasing the acidity of the vaginal area. Over-the-counter remedies, such as antifungal creams, vaginal tablets or suppositories kill off the yeast. Even so the infection can take up to a week to clear up. You should not use local anaesthetic creams formulated for itching as these can cause sensitivity and make the condition worse.

If an over-the-counter treatment does not work, make an appointment to see your doctor. A yeast infection should be properly diagnosed because it can be similar to other vaginal infections. The doctor will do an internal examination and take swabs of the discharge for laboratory analysis. Once the diagnosis is confirmed, your doctor may prescribe an antifungal treatment in the form of pills or cream. Candidiasis is not strictly a sexually transmitted disease, but it can be passed on to sexual partners. Men rarely experience symptoms, but if you have recurrent attacks, it is possible that your partner may need to be treated, too.

PREVENT RECURRENCE
To prevent the recurrence of candida infection, take cool baths or showers in hot weather. Avoid using perfumed soaps, bubble baths, vaginal deodorants or bath oils. Wear cotton underwear and loose clothes (especially on warm days) that allow air to circulate. You may find it helpful to reduce your intake of foods containng sugar and yeast (bread, for example).

STIS

STIs—or sexually transmitted infections as they are more formally called—can be difficult to detect in women, since many have nonspecific symptoms, such as vaginal discharge, pelvic pain, genital itching and pain on intercourse. However, they can cause long-term damage. For example, chlamydia can lead to infertility, while hepatitis and genital warts (fleshy lumps occurring around the genitals) can increase the risk of cervical cancer.

There are over 25 different types of STIs. Women most at risk are young adults, people from ethnic minorities and the socially and economically disadvantaged. If you suspect you may have an infection, you should act promptly and visit your doctor or gynaecologist. You will have a physical examination, and blood and urine tests. Many STIs can be treated with antibiotics or antiviral drugs if they are caught early enough. You should notify your sexual partner(s) so that they can be tested—and possibly treated—too. (The clinic may offer to do this for you.) You should avoid any further sexual contact until you are sure the infection has cleared.

Applying natural live yogurt to the vaginal area may relieve the symptoms.

EYE INFECTIONS

Infections of the eye can cause anything from mild discomfort to a serious threat to your eyesight. Eye infections are easily passed on through touch–at schools, colleges or day care centres, for example.

Conjunctivitis

The conjunctiva is the transparent membrane covering the white of the eye and inside of the eyelids. Inflammation of the conjunctiva is called conjunctivitis or pink eye. It can be caused by a bacterial or viral infection or an allergy (to cosmetics or pollen, for example). The eyes are red, sore and itchy, with a gritty tight feeling. With an allergy or viral infection there is a watery discharge; with a bacterial infection there may be a thick, sticky, yellowish discharge that dries at night, making the eyelids difficult to open. This crust can be removed with a moistened cloth or a cotton wool ball (in warm water).

Viral conjunctivitis may last several weeks but usually gets better on its own. Antibiotic eyedrops or ointment can clear up a bacterial infection, while antihistamine or anti-inflammatory eyedrops relieve allergic symptoms.

Sty or chalazion

If an eyelash hair follicle becomes infected, a painful, inflamed abscess, or sty, appears at the base. It develops a white head of pus that bursts within a few days, relieving the pain. The eyelash then falls out. A warm compress applied three times daily can help relieve pain and the infection may be treated with an antibiotic ointment if the sty is persistent or recurs. Never squeeze a sty: this can spread the infection to other hair follicles. Sties usually subside within a week but tend to recur in diabetics or in teenagers or women under stress.

A chalazion develops on the eyelid and is often painless. Warm compresses and antibiotic creams help with healing and the problem usually resolves in a month.

Blepharitis

Blepharitis (seborrhoeic dermatitis) or inflammation of the eyelid, is often associated with dandruff. The eyes may be sore, itchy and have flaky lids. The flakes of skin can cause conjunctivitis. If the eyelids become infected, they develop small blisters that cause the lashes to fall out. The eyelids should be cleaned with a cotton bud dipped in cooled, boiled water. Medicated shampoos will help treat the dandruff. Your doctor may prescribe an antibiotic eye ointment. If the eyelid becomes ulcerated, the infection may spread to the cornea, which must be treated immediately.

Corneal ulcer

The cornea (outer part of the eyeball) may be infected and develop ulcers. Some of these infections clear up quite easily, but if the infection is with the herpes virus and leads to an ulcer, the virus may enter the eyeball. You should contact your doctor immediately.

Acute iritis or uveitis

In rare cases, the iris (the coloured part of the eye) may be infected, often due to other conditions, such as tuberculosis or syphilis. This condition can also be associated with autoimmune joint diseases. Symptoms include one pupil becoming smaller than the other, red eyes, blurred vision and pain. Early treatment is vital, since it may cause long-term visual problems, such as corneal ulcers, glaucoma and cataracts.

A doctor can prescribe steroid ointment or eyedrops to reduce inflammation. Persistent inflammation of the uvea can cause visual loss.

Healthy eyes

You can keep your eyes sparkling with health by following a few simple precautions:

- Bathe irritated eyes in cool, boiled water. Never rub them.
- Never share towels or washcloths.
- Get plenty of sleep.
- Do not wear eye make-up when you have an infection.
- Use eyedrops to flush out minute particles.

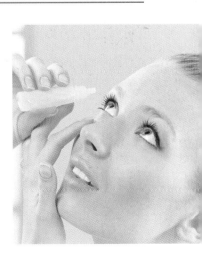

UPPER RESPIRATORY TRACT INFECTIONS

Infections that commonly affect the upper respiratory tract are known collectively as URTIs. Your ears, nose and throat are generally involved. Most URTIs make you feel miserable, but they tend to be short-lived and harmless. However, they can easily become more serious if you are run down or your immunity is impaired for any reason. Some are contagious, so you should take care not to spread any infection.

Cause	Symptoms	Treatment	Duration
COMMON COLD			
Over 200 different viruses	Feeling under the weather with a sore throat, a congested or runny nose, a cough and headache	Ease symptoms with pharmacy remedies: paracetamol for fever, lozenges for sore throat, decongestant for stuffy nose and cough syrup.	Most colds last a week at the most.
COLD SORES			
Caused by the herpes simplex virus, which lies dormant between attacks. They can be triggered by a cold, sun or stress; some women experience outbreaks around their period; highly contagious.	Sores that appear around your mouth or nose. The first sign is a tautness and a tingling feeling on the skin, which develops into a small painful blister. The blister turns into a weeping sore, which dries to form a scab.	Antiviral treatments at the tingling stage can prevent the sore from developing. One self-help measure for pain relief is to try over-the-counter anaesthetic gel or ice. Avoid eating nuts, chocolate and seeds.	Five to 10 days. Don't touch a cold sore, as you can spread the virus to your eyes or genitals.
SINUSITIS			
Excessive buildup of mucus following a cold, which settles in the air-filled spaces in your cheekbones, forehead and near the bridge of your nose. Persistent sinusitis may be due to allergic rhinitis, which can be triggered by pollen, dust and pollutants.	Pain in the face, nose and forehead, and in severe cases laryngitis or an ear infection	Should be treated with decongestants and antibiotics; otherwise, it may become a chronic problem and may require surgery to improve drainage of the sinuses. You can ease congestion by inhaling steam over a bowl of hot water with a towel over your head.	Up to 10 days. Don't use decongestants—either pills or sprays—for longer than one week, since they may make the congestion worse.
EAR INFECTIONS			
After a cold or allergic reaction, catarrh or inflamed mucus may block the eustachian tube, which connects the middle ear to the nasal cavity.	Loss of balance, dull throbbing pain and fever indicate an infection of the middle ear (otitis media). If untreated, the ear drum can rupture and cause hearing loss.	Decongestants and paracetamol can help to ease discomfort, but severe pain needs medical advice. A middle ear infection can be treated with antibiotic or steroid ear drops.	One week

Cause	Symptoms	Treatment	Duration
PHARYNGITIS			
Throat infection triggered by a virus or streptococcus bacteria (known as a "strep throat"). If it is recurring, it may be caused by smoking or an allergy, such as hay fever.	Back of the throat hurts when swallowing, voice becomes hoarse, and glands under the jaw become enlarged; headache.	Drink plenty of fluids, gargle with warm salt water, suck throat lozenges, use NSAIDs for pain. Antibiotics may be needed for the bacterial infection.	One week to 10 days
LARYNGITIS			
Usually follows a cold but can be caused by straining the voice box (from too much talking or shouting) or smoking. The swollen larynx restricts the airflow through your vocal cords, causing a temporary loss of voice.	Hoarse voice and an irritating cough	Should be treated like a mild attack of flu: stay in bed, take paracetamol and drink warm fluids. Rest your voice. Inhale steam from a hot shower.	If hoarseness or loss of voice lasts for more than a week, consult your doctor, since this can be a sign of cancer in rare cases.
INFECTIOUS MONONUCLEOSIS			
Very common viral infection of the white blood cells (lymphocytes or mononuclear cells), also known as glandular fever. It is passed on through close contact, mainly kissing, and is especially common in teenagers and young adults.	Fever, a sore throat, enlarged tonsils and swollen lymph glands in the neck, armpits and groin may develop over four to six weeks. General malaise and lethargy, and a measles-like rash may appear on the body, arms and legs.	No specific treatment. If a sufferer takes the antibiotics ampicillin or amoxicillin, a red, blotchy rash may appear. The infection can enlarge the spleen and spread to the liver, causing jaundice or hepatitis.	It can take six months to recover. Relapses are common and it is vital to have plenty of rest, since chronic fatigue syndrome can occur.
TONSILLITIS			
Can be caused by bacteria or a virus. Highly contagious infection. Tissue at the back of the throat is covered in tiny white pus-filled spots.	Severe sore throat, swollen neck glands, a cough, fever and fatigue	Stay in bed, drink plenty of fluids, gargle with warm salt water, eat soft foods. A bacterial infection needs antibiotics.	10 days. If a quinsy (tonsil abscess) forms, antibiotics will be necessary.

NOSE SENSE

If you have a congested nose, don't blow too hard or too often. This can make the congestion worse, force infected mucus back into your sinuses, or weaken the small blood vessels in your nose, causing nosebleeds. Applying too much pressure when blowing can sometimes rupture an ear drum.

MENINGITIS

Meningitis is an inflammation of the meninges, the delicate membranes surrounding the brain and spinal cord. The most usual cause is a virus, which is rarely severe. However, a bacterial infection can be dangerous and needs urgent diagnosis and treatment.

Types of meningitis

There are two types of meningitis–one that's life-threatening and one that's not.

Viral (aseptic) meningitis The most common form of meningitis is rarely life-threatening. It is caused by many viruses, such as mumps, polio, varicella zoster (related to chickenpox and shingles) and herpes simplex (which causes cold sores). The viruses are spread by coughing or sneezing or can be picked up in areas of poor hygiene from contaminated food or water. The symptoms vary from a mild flu-like illness with a bad headache to a more severe condition that resembles the bacterial form.

Bacterial meningitis This is a serious infection spread through close contact, such as kissing, sneezing and coughing. The most common symptom is a severe headache, usually associated with an intolerance of bright lights. The sufferer may also feel feverish, have a stiff neck, feel nauseous and vomit. Local outbreaks can occur among groups gathering in restricted space. One type of infection, meningococcal meningitis, tends to affect children and young adults, while another, pneumococcal meningitis, is found more often in people over 45 years of age. *Hemophilus influenzae* meningitis is less common today, since babies are now routinely immunized with the Hib vaccine.

One in 10 people has the meningococcal bacteria in their throat and nasal passages without realizing it. The infection, which mostly occurs in winter, develops if the bacteria overcome the body's immune defenses. There are three types of meningococcus bacteria–A, B and C–with B being the most common and most dangerous. Although the bacteria are highly contagious, they can survive for just a few minutes outside the body and therefore can only be spread by very close contact. Because the symptoms of meningococcal meningitis develop very rapidly, you need to be aware of the danger signs (*see* box opposite).

LUMBAR PUNCTURE
Also known as spinal tap, this procedure is done under a local anaesthetic. It involves inserting a needle between two lower spine bones so that a sample of spinal fluid can be taken for analysis.

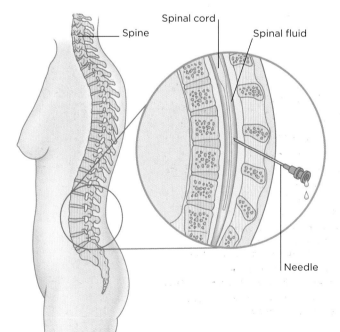

Spine

Spinal cord

Spinal fluid

Needle

WHEN DO YOU NEED AN ANTIBIOTIC?

When you get an infection, you need to know the cause so that treatment will be effective. Viral infections are common, are usually mild and clear up on their own over several days—you rarely need a doctor's help unless your immune system is challenged by chronic illness or older age. Antibiotics do not work against viruses. However, they are highly effective in treating bacterial infections, which have more severe symptoms. Antibiotics can cause side effects such as diarrhoea and skin rashes.

Because of the widespread use of antibiotics, bacterial resistance is occurring. It is probably also the result of people not finishing a prescribed course of treatment. In these cases the antibiotic kills off the weakest bacteria, but the toughest ones are left to breed, mutate and become stronger, creating a resistant "superbug". This means that some diseases may no longer respond to common antibiotics.

How do you know if you have it?

All cases of meningitis are regarded as potentially dangerous. The symptoms are so similar that it may not be immediately obvious whether the cause is viral or bacterial. For this reason, a person showing symptoms of meningitis may be given antibiotics before the infection is properly diagnosed to give the doctors time to complete various

How to prevent it

Meningococcal meningitis is a medical emergency that always requires rapid hospitalization and treatment–immediate injection of penicillin and drugs to reduce the swelling of the brain and the risk of an epileptic seizure. Because of the risk of passing on the infection, the patient may be treated in isolation and will stay there until the infection is eradicated. Preventive

One in 10 people has the meningococcal bacteria in their throat and nasal passages without realizing it.

tests. The usual method of diagnosis is a lumbar puncture (*see* opposite). Normal spinal fluid is clear, so meningitis is suspected if the fluid is cloudy and contains pus cells. Samples of blood and urine may also be tested. A chest or sinus X-ray may be done.

Two different treatments

In viral meningitis there is no need for antibiotics, although they may help prevent secondary infection (*see* box left). The usual treatment is bed rest, plenty of fluids to drink and anti-inflammatory drugs for headaches. Viral meningitis usually has no lasting effects. The symptoms are mild and resolve in 1-2 weeks.

With a diagnosis of bacterial meningitis, the patient will need antibiotics (intravenously initially and then by mouth), anticonvulsants to reduce the risk of epileptic seizures and antinausea drugs for sickness. If bacterial meningitis is diagnosed early enough, the patient may make a complete recovery. However, the infection can be fatal or lead to permanent damage, particularly in the very young or elderly. Babies are most susceptible and the bacteria may cause deafness, neurological damage, cerebral palsy or epilepsy. The bacteria may also cause the cerebrospinal fluid to accumulate in the brain and this fluid may need to be drained.

antibiotics may be given to all people who had intimate or direct contact with the patient within 7 days of the infection being diagnosed.

Vaccinations against *Streptococcus pneumoniae* and *Hemophilus influenzae* type b (Hib vaccine) are given around the age of 2 months. Meningococcal vaccine is recommended for university students–who are at risk because large groups of young people are in close proximity. Vaccination is also recommended for travellers to countries where meningitis is more likely.

DANGER SIGNS

Meningococcal meningitis develops quickly from minor flu-like symptoms to the severe disease. There are a number of symptoms, but all of them are quite easy to detect:

- A severe headache
- Neck pain and a dislike of bright light
- Vomiting and dizziness, accompanied by a very high temperature
- A purple rash that looks like pin pricks (which can indicate septicaemia—blood poisoning)
- Drowsiness, convulsions and, occasionally, a loss of consciousness

In such cases, you should call your doctor immediately.

Emergency First Aid

Knowing what to do and being able to help promptly when a child or an adult is injured can save lives. Staying calm will allow you to act sensibly and give you confidence to assist in the wide range of first-aid situations described in these pages.

IN AN EMERGENCY

- Make sure the help you give does not endanger your own life.
- Sum up the situation quickly and act fast.
- Call 999 if immediate medical assistance is needed.
- If you suspect a head, neck or back injury, do not move the person.
- Check the airway, breathing and circulation (ABC) first (*see* right) so the brain is not starved of oxygen.
- Place an unconscious person in the recovery position (*see* opposite) unless you suspect a spine or neck injury.
- Put pressure on an injury to stop any severe bleeding, but do not use a tourniquet.
- Treat the person for shock (*see* p. 262).

Check the unconscious person's airway, breathing and circulation (ABC, *see* below). If there is both breathing and a pulse, put the person in the recovery position (*see* opposite). Cover with a coat or blanket and talk reassuringly until help arrives. If there is a pulse but no breathing, begin mouth-to-mouth resuscitation (*see* p. 262). If there is no pulse and no breathing, begin CPR (*see* p. 262).

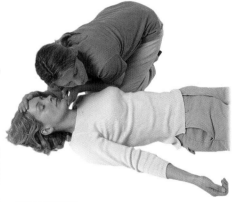

BREATHING
Listen for sounds around the mouth and nose, watch for movements of the chest and place your face close enough to feel the breath on your skin.

IF SOMEONE IS UNCONSCIOUS

This is a procedure to follow in any situation with an injured person:

- SPEAK, asking "Can you hear me? Are you all right"?
- SHAKE her shoulders gently without jerking the neck.
- LISTEN for breathing by placing your ear close to the mouth.
- LOOK along the chest to see if it is moving up and down.
- CHECK that there are no signs of fracture, neck or spinal injury.
- PLACE person in the recovery position if there are no signs of injury.

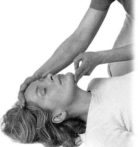

AIRWAY
The passage between the mouth, nose and throat must be clear. If the person is lying face up, press down on the forehead with one hand while lifting the back of the neck with the other. Move this hand to tilt chin up. Turn head to one side and use your first two fingers to sweep around inside mouth to remove any obstruction. Do not attempt this if a neck fracture is suspected.

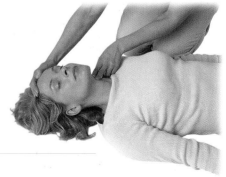

CIRCULATION
Place the tips of your first two fingers in the depression at the side of the Adam's apple and feel for a pulse.

THE RECOVERY POSITION

The aim is to turn the injured person so she can breathe without the danger of the airway being blocked by vomit or by the tongue falling back and cutting off the airway. Stay with the person until help arrives, monitoring breathing and pulse every 10 minutes.

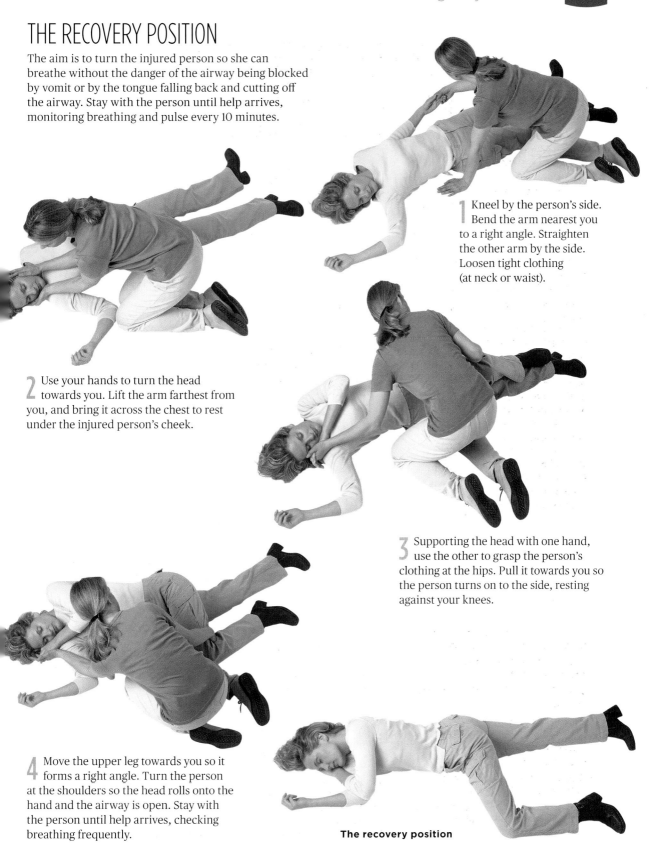

1 Kneel by the person's side. Bend the arm nearest you to a right angle. Straighten the other arm by the side. Loosen tight clothing (at neck or waist).

2 Use your hands to turn the head towards you. Lift the arm farthest from you, and bring it across the chest to rest under the injured person's cheek.

3 Supporting the head with one hand, use the other to grasp the person's clothing at the hips. Pull it towards you so the person turns on to the side, resting against your knees.

4 Move the upper leg towards you so it forms a right angle. Turn the person at the shoulders so the head rolls onto the hand and the airway is open. Stay with the person until help arrives, checking breathing frequently.

The recovery position

261

MOUTH-TO-MOUTH RESUSCITATION

(when there is a pulse but no breathing)

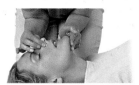 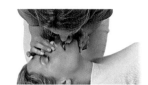 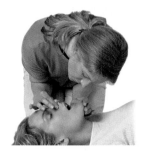

1 Tilt the head back using two fingers under the chin. Pinch the nose between index finger and thumb. Take a deep breath and place your lips around the person's mouth, making a seal.

2 Blow firmly and slowly for two seconds into the mouth until you see the person's chest rise. Remove your lips and release the nose. Count to four, take a deep breath and repeat.

3 If the chest does not rise and fall, check the airway for an obstruction. Sweep the mouth with a finger to remove anything there. Repeat the resuscitation procedure.

CHECK!

Always check to see if a person is wearing a MedicAlert bracelet or pendant. Both will give vital information in an emergency. People vulnerable to shock or coma (for example, through diabetes, epilepsy, heart problems and dangerous allergies, such as reactions to nuts or bee or wasp stings) wear them; some also carry a syringe filled with adrenaline for immediate use for allergic reactions. It should be injected into the middle part of the thigh.

CPR

Cardiopulmonary resuscitation is used to help someone whose breathing or heart has stopped. It combines mouth-to-mouth resuscitation, in which you blow your breath into the person's lungs, with compression of the chest in order to help the heart contract and keep the blood circulation going. Compression is hard work and it is usually recommended that

1 Place your middle finger where the breastbone meets ribs and your index finger above it. Slide the heel of your other hand down to fingers.

2 Lift first hand over second, interlock fingers. Count: on 1 lean forwards and press on breastbone; on 2 depress it up to 5 cm (2 in); on 3 release pressure. Repeat 15 times. Give mouth-to-mouth resuscitation twice, repeat compression.

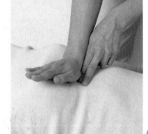

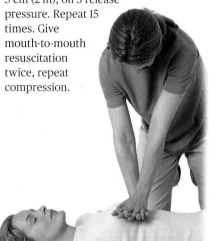

it be done only by a person who has been trained. Mouth-to-mouth resuscitation may help the person until the arrival of medical aid.

CPR is required for the following symptoms: skin tone pale or bluish, no sign of breathing in chest or from mouth, no heartbeat or pulse.

ANAPHYLACTIC SHOCK

Sudden collapse with swelling of the tongue, throat and mouth. Call 999. Check if person is wearing pendant or bracelet or carrying an adrenaline injection kit. Follow instructions given with the kit. Loosen clothing at neck, waist and wrists, take pulse and breathing rate. Cover with coat or blanket and be prepared to give mouth-to-mouth resuscitation.

TREATMENT FOR SHOCK

When giving any form of first aid, keep an eye on the injured person's face. Signs of shock are: skin becomes pale, grey looking, or is cold and moist with sweat. If pulse is weak and rapid and breathing is fast and shallow, don't give the person anything to eat or drink. Raise the feet and put a coat or cover across the trunk for warmth. Call 999 for immediate medical assistance.

HEART ATTACK

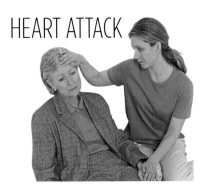

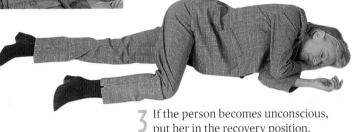

1 If the person is conscious, make her comfortable in a half-sitting position with good support to the head and shoulders. If there's no wall to lean against, the back of another person, sitting with knees bent, will substitute.

2 Loosen clothing around neck and waist. Call 999. Give reassurance and make a note of breathing and pulse rates. Ask if she carries any medication for heart problems; if so have her take it. If she is fully awake, give her an aspirin to chew.

3 If the person becomes unconscious, put her in the recovery position. If breathing stops, turn her on to her back and begin CPR (*see* opposite).

STROKE

Call 999. If the person is conscious lay her down, with head and shoulders raised and supported by rolled clothing. Turn her head to one side and loosen her clothing. If the person is unconscious, place her in the recovery position.

FAINT

Brief loss of consciousness. Place the person flat and lift the legs to help blood flow back to the heart and head. If the person is sitting, bring the head forwards between the knees. Call 999 if person doesn't recover quickly.

BE ALERT

If someone is unconscious:

- SPEAK, asking "Can you hear me? Are you all right"?
- SHAKE her shoulders gently without jerking the neck.
- LISTEN for breathing by placing your ear close to the mouth.
- LOOK along the chest to see if it is moving up and down.
- CHECK that there are no signs of fracture, neck or spinal injury.
- PLACE person in the recovery position if there are no signs of injury.

WHEN A CHOKING ADULT COLLAPSES

1 Turn the person on to the side and give five sharp blows with the flat of your hand between the shoulder blades. Turn the person on to the side and sweep inside mouth with fingers. If obstruction is not removed, slap the back again.

2 If that doesn't work, turn the person face upwards with head tilted back. Sit astride the person, placing the heel of one hand below the rib cage and the other hand on top. With straight arms press sharply inwards and upwards five times.

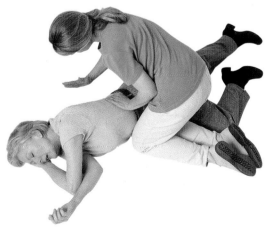

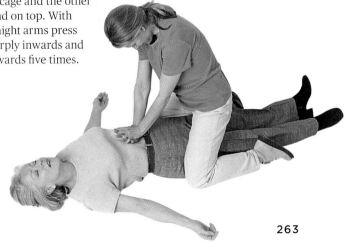

263

WHEN AN ADULT IS CHOKING

If something is stuck in the airway, breathing will be difficult. Act quickly.

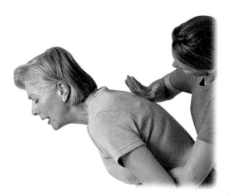 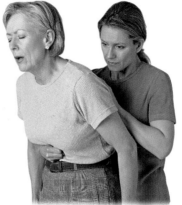 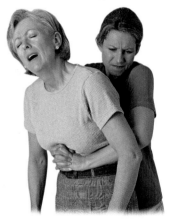

1 First get the person to breathe in deeply, then to cough forcefully. If that doesn't work, get the person to bend over from the waist and slap the back sharply between the shoulder blades.

2 If this doesn't work, do the Heimlich manoeuvre. Stand behind the person, make a fist with one hand and place it thumb inwards in the middle of the abdomen.

3 Grab the fist with your other hand and pull both sharply against the person's body, inwards and upwards. Repeat four times if necessary, but it should force the obstruction out of the throat like a cork out of a fizzy bottle.

IF A CHILD IS CHOKING

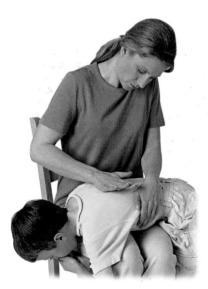 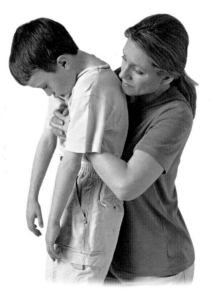 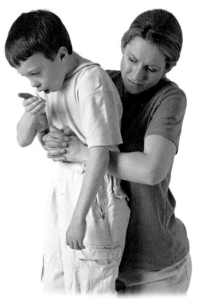

1 Sit on a chair and pull the child across your upper legs, with his head and face down. Give four quick but not too forceful slaps between the shoulder blades with the heel of your hand.

2 If the object is not dislodged, kneel behind the child, make a fist and grasp it with your other hand. Make five sharp inward thrusts against the lower breastbone.

3 If this doesn't work, move your arms down and make five thrusts between the rib cage and the navel.

IF A BABY IS CHOKING

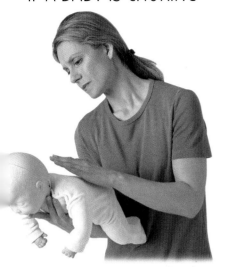 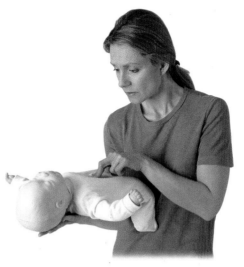

1 Place the baby, tummy down, along your arm so the head is below the chest and your hand supports the head and shoulders. With your other hand give five firm, but not hard, slaps between the shoulder blades.

2 Turn the baby over and check the airway. If the object was not dislodged and you can't hook it out with your finger, repeat the first step.

If a child becomes unconscious, call 999
Put into recovery position and watch ABC carefully until medical help arrives.

EPILEPTIC FIT OR SEIZURE

Do not move the person or put anything in the mouth or between the teeth. If possible loosen tight clothing (around neck or waist), but do not restrict his or her movements. Protect the person from harm (for example, against the edges of nearby furniture or railings), staying until he or she recovers fully, usually after several minutes. Place her in the recovery position.

FEBRILE CONVULSION

Sponge or bathe the baby or child with lukewarm water to try to lower the temperature. Call the doctor.

DROWNING/RESUSCITATION

1 Once out of the water lay the person flat and check ABC. Get someone to call 999. Turn the person's head to the side, sweep around inside the mouth with two fingers to clear it–this may also cause her to vomit water. Begin mouth-to-mouth resuscitation.

2 If the chest does not rise and fall, check the airway again for an obstruction. If the person is choking, push her on to the side and slap the back five times with the heel of your hand. Repeat resuscitation procedure. As soon as breathing is restored, put the person in the recovery position.

EMERGENCY WARMING

When someone has been immersed in water or been exposed to extreme cold, it is esssential to try to raise the body temperature. Remove wet clothes and replace with dry ones. Put person in recovery position and wrap well from head to toe with anything available. Shield from the wind. Stay with person until medical help arrives, carefully watching breathing.

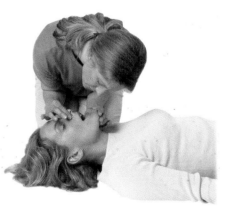

ELECTRIC SHOCK

The first objective is to break the connection between the person and the electricity without endangering yourself. Make sure your hands are dry. Switch off the current at the mains or electric point. If that's not possible, take a wooden broom handle or wooden stool, stand on paper of any sort and push the electric gadget well away from the person. Check ABC and begin mouth-to-mouth resuscitation if necessary. If unconscious but breathing, place in the recovery position. Call 999.

GENERAL BURNS

If the burn is extensive, cool the area as quickly as you can with clean water from a fine sprinkler of a hose or watering can.

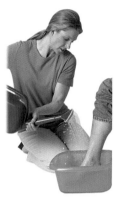

CHEMICAL BURNS OF THE EYE

If possible, place the person's face sideways to a sink under a tap so cold water runs gently into the eye for at least 10 minutes. Otherwise place the person down on his or her side, lift and turn the head and gently pour cold water into the eye for 10 minutes, making sure water doesn't run down the face or into the other eye. Seek immediate medical help.

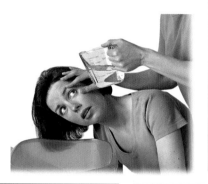

DO NOT TOUCH!

There is a high risk of infection when skin is damaged. Do not touch the injured area, do not try to burst any blisters and do not use lotions or ointments of any kind. Water is the best treatment for most injuries since it cools and cleans the area.

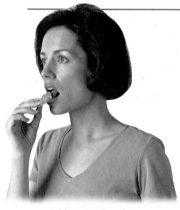

BURNS TO MOUTH

Call 999. Loosen clothing round the neck. Give small sips of cold water or an ice cube to suck. Do not try to make the person vomit; if a corrosive has been swallowed, vomiting will make matters worse. Watch for signs of shock or restricted breathing and take action until help arrives. Do not give mouth-to-mouth resuscitation since this may endanger you.

TIPS FOR SUCCESSFUL FIRST AID

- After cleaning a wound, exposure to the air will allow the blood to clot naturally. Holding a bleeding cut under running water will prevent clot formation and the blood will continue to flow.

- If a cut or wound is large, press the edges together with your (clean) fingers until a clot forms, then cover the cut with a dressing to allow healing to take place.

- If a wound is deep or has ragged edges, stitches may be needed to bring the skin together.

- Keep a magnifying glass in your first-aid box so you can see inside the wound clearly.

- Never put undiluted antiseptic on a wound.

- Don't use fluffy materials such as cotton wool as a dressing on small grazes and cuts. Fibres get caught in the scab that forms, and bleeding will start again if you try to remove them.

POISON

Common poisons include pills, household and other corrosive liquids, solvents, fumes, berries, fungi and alcohol. Call 999. Check the ABC.

If the person is breathing but unconscious, place in recovery position.

If there is an indication of burning in and around the mouth and the person is conscious, help her to drink a glass of water or milk, then put in the recovery position.

Monitor pulse and breathing until help arrives.

FRACTURE

If you suspect a bone is fractured, do not move the person until you have immobilized the injured area. Seek medical help.

BITES

If a bite is of animal or insect origin and the skin is broken, it should be taken seriously. Wash well, allowing blood to flow, then cover with a sterile pad or sticking plaster. Contact the doctor as tetanus injection or antibiotics may be needed.

Insect bites may be swollen and red, an allergic reaction to what the insect has left. Wash area well then cover with a sticking plaster.

Snakebites signs are pain, swelling and puncture wounds. Lay the person down, keeping injured leg or arm flat. Clean area, wiping away from the wound, then bandage firmly. Seek immediate medical help.

SKULL, NECK AND BACK INJURIES

Injuries to the skull, neck and back are serious and need expert help. Call 999. If you are alone, do not attempt to move the person. If someone can help, hold the head steady while he or she puts rolled-up clothing on either side to immobilize the neck and shoulders. If the person is turned on the side and resuscitation is needed, you will need help to ease her on to her back. At all times you should keep the head supported and aligned with the neck and back. Check ABC every 10 minutes.

THE FIRST-AID KIT

A first-aid kit should be kept in a safe place in your home, accessible to you but well out of the reach of children. It need not be large, but it should contain all you need if someone is injured. If you are in doubt about what to do, call 999. Keep in it: aspirin, paracetamol, magnifying glass, thermometer, a range of different types of bandages (roller, tubular), safety pins, sticking plasters or dressings, disposable gloves, antiseptic wipes for wound and skin cleansing, and tweezers.

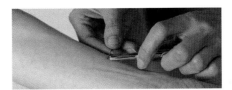

REMOVING SPLINTERS

Clean the area around the splinter with an antiseptic wipe. Press tweezers on to skin and catch protruding splinter. Gently ease it back out, in the direction it went in. If you can't see splinter end, sterilize a sewing needle in a flame. Try to get it under the splinter so you can grab it with the tweezers. Clean area with antiseptic wipe.

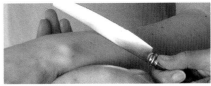

STINGS

Remove the insect's venom sac by scraping it from the skin, in one direction only, with the blunt edge of a knife or your fingernail. Don't use tweezers since these push the venom into the skin. Clean area with an antiseptic wipe and place an ice cube or wrapped pack of frozen peas on the site. Also *see* anaphylactic shock (p. 262).

NOSEBLEED

Use your thumb and index finger to pinch the soft part of the nose (the nostrils), lean forwards and breathe through the mouth. Hold this position for 10 minutes so that a clot forms. Do not touch or blow the nose for several hours, in order to prevent further bleeding.

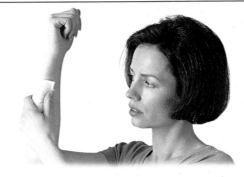

CUT THAT WON'T STOP BLEEDING

Place under cold running water for a few seconds, then raise the arm above chest height, cover the injury with a clean lint-free dressing or adhesive bandage and apply direct pressure with your other hand or fingers until the bleeding has stopped.

STOP THE BLEEDING!

Stopping the blood flow in an artery at pressure points in the upper arm or groin by pressing the artery against the bone needs strength and is only done as a final resort when indirect pressure on the wound itself fails. Do not use a tourniquet, and do not compress artery for more than 15 minutes. Both can stop blood flow entirely.

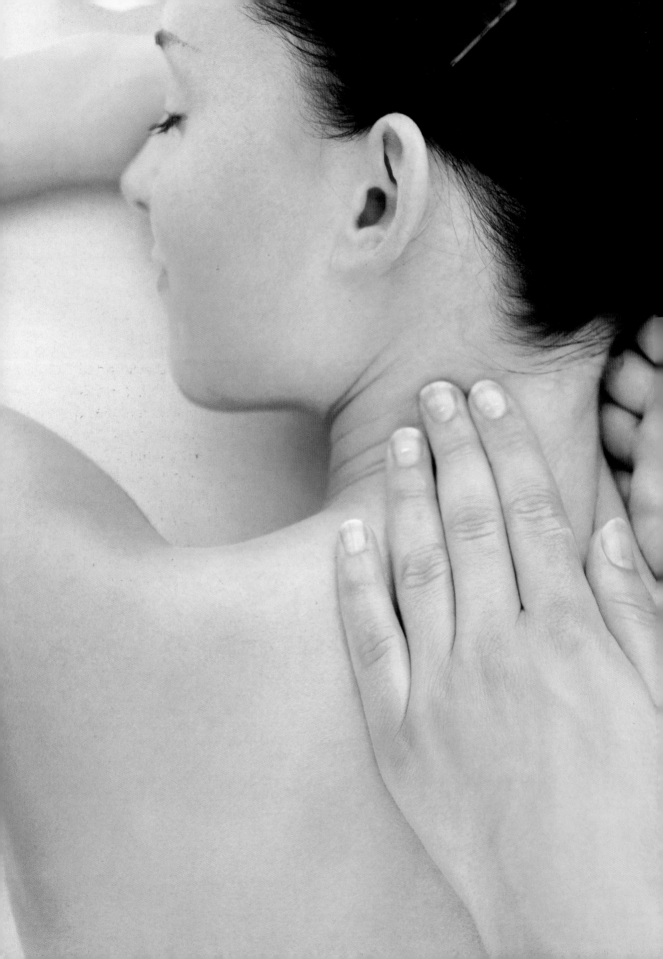

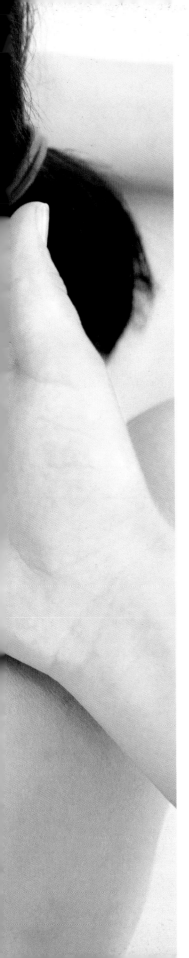

HEALING
THE BODY

Over the past decade, research has uncovered the molecular secrets of hundreds of diseases and conditions that strip us of health and energy. Tests have been developed to reveal their presence; specialists have been educated to treat them. What's more, an amazing number of therapies and treatments have been found to fix or manage whatever might be slowing us down. Exercise, diet, massage, relaxation, acupuncture, drugs, surgery—all are helping us live longer and live better. On the following pages, you'll find everything you need to do exactly that.

Treatment Plans

When you seek medical help, you benefit from having as much information relating to your condition as possible before you're called upon to make decisions.

FIND THE FACTS

Once you've made an appointment with the doctor to evaluate a new symptom or a medical concern, he or she will take a history, do a physical examination and then determine what diagnostic tests are needed to help make a diagnosis. Your provider will use all this information to find the best way to treat your condition. Whether you are pregnant or uncertain about a symptom or a collection of symptoms, you have every reason to expect that you will receive optimum care. It is helpful to know what potential tests may be obtained or what questions to ask your health care provider before the medical appointment. This chapter provides up-to-date information on a variety of treatment plans and diagnostic tests.

Understand your records

The relationship you have with your doctor is confidential, and what is shared between you and him or her should not be disclosed to a third party unless it is part of ongoing treatment. You have the right to access the records that your doctor keeps on you. These records may be shared with other medical personnel as part of your treatment. The data on the records may be written in medical language that is hard to understand. Ask for an explanation if you don't understand something. Take a friend or family member to your appointment–it may help if what the doctor has to say is complex and involves a range of investigations and specialists.

You will want to know possible risks of the proposed treatment as well as the benefits. It is important to understand the suggested plans and the scale of time of the treatment. Unless the situation is an emergency, you should not feel hurried into making decisions. You should feel comfortable asking for a second opinion if you feel you need more information to help you make a decision or understand the treatments or options.

Know your team

Your doctor will explain the diagnosis and discuss the tests, treatments and any medications that are required. In many conditions the expertise of a wide range of professionals will be required. Find out who your point of contact will be or who the coordinator of your care will be in case you need more information.

Get a clear explanation of anything you sign. Consent forms should indicate the exact medical or surgical treatment you agree to, particularly if it is going to take place under an anaesthetic. Make sure your family, partner or caregiver has your written instructions should you be unable to make decisions.

Get some backup

If you have difficulty coming to terms with the diagnosis and treatment, or have other concerns, find a service to help you. You may need psychological and social support to deal with your anxieties, fears or family issues.

INVESTIGATIVE TESTS

Doctors may carry out or arrange a wide variety of tests based on your presenting symptoms as part of the process of working through a differential diagnosis to either eliminate or confirm a diagnosis. Certain tests may be performed as part of regular check-ups while others may be part of the medical evaluation. Making sure you know what the test involves prepares you and makes the experience less stressful.

TYPE	PURPOSE	WHERE DONE/ANAESTHETIC
Amniocentesis	Antenatal screening	Clinic or hospital/mild tranquillizer
Arthroscopy	Joint problems	Hospital/general or local
Balloon angioplasty	Unblocking artery	Hospital/general
Barium enema	To check small and large intestines for abnormalities	Clinic or hospital/none
Biopsy	Laboratory examination: breast (needle), cervical (curette), endometrial, skin (scalpel), vulval	Clinic or hospital/local or none
Blood	Range of tests to diagnose or rule out disorders: complete blood count, coagulation, glucose, enzymes and electrolytes (for heart, liver or kidney damage), uric acid, cholesterol, triglycerides, albumin and globulin (abnormal protein levels), thyroid, prenatally (anaemia, rubella, rhesus factor, hepatitis, STIs), HIV, syphilis, bilirubin	Clinic or hospital
Blood pressure	To check that it is not above 140/90 (adults, pregnant women), and for those with a family history of high blood pressure	Clinic/none
Cervical smear	Simple method of obtaining cervical cells for laboratory analysis	Clinic/none
Colonoscopy	To get an inside view of large intestine using an endoscope (flexible fibre-optic tube); enema or laxatives given first to clean out colon	Hospital/light sedation
Colposcopy	Visual examination of the cervix if cervical smear shows an abnormality; may be combined with biopsy	Clinic or hospital/none
Computerized axial tomography (CT) scan	Evaluates soft tissue (after stroke or hemorrhage), for cysts, abscesses, tumours using X-ray to produce 3D image; contrast dye may be given intravenously to enhance detection of abnormalities	Hospital/none
Coronary angiography	Detects blockages in heart arteries; dye injected intravenously to visualize arteries	Hospital/general
Cystometric tests	To evaluate bladder volume and function	Clinic or hospital/none
Cystoscopy	Examination of the inside of the bladder using a thin fibre-optic scope passed along urethra; may be combined with biopsy or cautery treatment	Clinic or hospital/local or general

(continued)

271

TYPE (continued)	PURPOSE	WHERE DONE/ANAESTHETIC
ECG and stress ECG	Electrocardiogram traces activity pattern of heart at rest; a stress ECG is done while walking or jogging on a treadmill. Either may be done in conjunction with thallium scanning (nuclear medicine scan)	Hospital cardiac unit or surgery/none
Echocardiography	Ultrasound to assess heart function, heart valves and indirectly to detect blockage in heart vessels by assessing heart movement	Clinic or hospital/none
EEG	Records electrical activity in brain	Clinic or hospital/none
Endoscopy (oesophageal, gastric, duodenal)	Method of visually examining inside of the upper gastrointestinal organs using flexible fibre-optic instrument called an endoscope; may be combined with biopsy	Clinic or hospital/light sedation
Exercise stress test	Also called a stress ECG or exercise tolerance test; assesses blood available to heart during exercise	Clinic or hospital/none
Fluorescent angiography	Test for macular degeneration by evaluating blood vessel pattern in eye; special dye is injected into arm vein	Ophthalmologist's surgery/none
Hysterosalpingogram	Method of assessing shape of uterus and whether fallopian tubes are open; usually performed as part of an infertility workup	Clinic or hospital/light sedation
Hysteroscopy	Endoscope is inserted via vagina and cervix to assess the inside of the uterus; problems found during test may be treated by gynaecologist at the same time	Clinic or hospital/general
Immunoassay	Test for antibody concentration in immune system disorders	Clinic or hospital/none
Intravenous pyelogram (IVP)	X-ray of kidney and bladder; dye is injected into arm vein; may be done as part of a workup to assess disorders of the renal system	Clinic or hospital/light sedation
Laparoscopy	Minimally invasive surgery for evaluating gynaecological problems; involves a fibre-optic scope being inserted via the umbilicus through a small incision	Hospital/general
Laparotomy	Abdominal surgery to detect, diagnose or treat conditions; incision is 10–13 cm (4–5 in) long, above pubic region	Hospital/general
Lumbar puncture (also know as a spinal tap)	To obtain spinal fluid from the lower back for analysis as part of an evaluation of infections such as meningitis	Clinic or hospital/none
Lung function test	To check capacity of lungs, airflow and oxygen/gas exchange	Clinic or hospital/none
Magnetic resonance imaging (MRI)	Imaging study to view and photograph inside of body, using no radiation; may involve intravenous contrast dyes to enhance images	Clinic or hospital (Note: those who are claustrophobic and cannot tolerate small spaces can ask for short-acting anti-anxiety medication to take 45 minutes before the test)

TYPE	PURPOSE	WHERE DONE/ANAESTHETIC
Mammogram	X-ray of breast tissue for early detection of cancer or other breast symptoms (nipple discharge, breast pain, breast lump)	Clinic or hospital/none
Pelvic examination	Routine check-ups of external and internal reproductive organs performed to evaluate gynaecological symptoms; may combine external, internal (speculum), bimanual (gloved finger inside vagina, hand pressing outside) and rectovaginal (gloved fingers in vagina and rectum)	Clinic/none
Physical examination	Carried out as part of preventive health screening or to evaluate new symptoms or signs	Clinic/none
Postcoital test	Much like cervical smear; to obtain cervical mucus after intercourse as part of infertility workup	Clinic/none
Proctoscopy	Examination of anus and rectum to assess bowel conditions using a rigid scope	Clinic or hospital/none
Radionuclide scan	Technique to assess liver and to check for gallstones	Clinic or hospital/none
Sigmoidoscopy (also known as flexible sigmoidoscopy)	Uses flexible lighted tube to view lower part of large intestine known as the sigmoid colon	Clinic or hospital/none
SPECT (Single Photon Emission Computed Tomography)	A radiological test to look at blood flow in the brain	Hospital/none
Stool test	Examines stool sample for blood, mucus, bacteria, fat or bile	Clinic or hospital/none
Thallium scanning	Radioactive material is injected into a vein in conjunction with exercise ECG	Clinic or hospital/none
Tonometry	Measure of pressure of fluid in eye to diagnose glaucoma	Ophthalmologist's surgery/eyedrops containing anaesthesia
Ultrasound	Internal view of body using high-frequency sound waves recorded on screen to form a picture; wide range of uses	Clinic or hospital/none
Urine tests	Regular part of pregnancy or physical examination; also used to detect infection, glucose, acidity or alkalinity	Clinic/none
VER (visual evoked response)	Used to detect retina reactions under a range of different conditions (bright lights, flashes, etc.)	Ophthalmologist's surgery/none
X-rays	Radiation image of various organs, bones and soft tissue as part of the medical or surgical workup of symptoms or disorders. A woman who suspects she may be pregnant should inform the technician prior to undergoing the test because X-rays may be harmful to the growing fetus	Clinic or hospital/none

Healing the Body

WHO CAN HELP?

Medical care is a team effort and involves a range of qualified practitioners who work together in planning and carrying out tests and treatment. Consultation and other services may be available at a clinic, large group practice or hospital. A range of professional staff, who have had specialized training in a specific area of medicine or surgery, may be consulted by your health care provider to assist in your medical or surgical evaluation and needs. This chart lists some of the people you are likely to meet.

MEDICAL PROFESSIONAL	
Audiologist	Specializes in the study of impaired hearing that cannot be improved by surgical or medical treatment
Cardiologist	Physician skilled in the diagnosis and treatment of heart disease
Dermatologist	Physician skilled in the study of skin disorders and diseases
Embryologist	Specializes in the science of the development of the individual during the embryonic stage of life
Endocrinologist	Physician skilled in the study of disorders and diseases of the glands and hormones
Gastroenterologist	Physician skilled in the study of diseases and disorders of the stomach and other parts of the digestive tract
General practitioner	Physician skilled in providing primary health care and prevention of disease; someone who provides you with regular and ongoing health care
Geneticist	Specializes in the study of possible genetic factors influencing the occurrence of certain diseases
Immunologist	Specializes in the study of diseases of the immune system, including allergies and hypersensitivities
Nephrologist	Physician skilled in the study of disorders and diseases of the kidneys
Neurologist	Physician skilled in the study of diseases and disorders of the brain and other parts of the nervous system
Obstetrician/ gynaecologist	Specializes in the care and treatment of pregnant women and the delivery of babies and also treats diseases of the genital tract in women
Oncologist	Physician skilled in the study and treatment of cancer
Ophthalmologist	Physician skilled in the study of disorders and diseases of the eye
Otolaryngologist (ENT)	Physician skilled in the study of disorders of the ears, nose and throat
Paediatrician	Specializes in the diseases, disorders and development of children from birth to post-puberty; may specialize in paediatric endocrinology or immunology, or neonatal medicine
Psychiatrist	Physician skilled in the diagnoses and treatment of mental and emotional illness; a neuropsychiatrist specializes in the combined practice of neurology and psychiatry
Psychologist	Specializes in the study of the relationship between physiological processes and behaviour; provides counselling as part of the management of mental disorders

MEDICAL PROFESSIONAL *(continued)*

Pulmonologist	Physician skilled in the disorders and diseases of the lungs and chest
Radiologist	Physician skilled in the interpretation of X-rays, ultrasound, MRI and CT scans, mammograms and other diagnostic imaging tests
Rheumatologist	Physician skilled in the study of disorders and diseases of the joints and rheumatic disorders in particular
Urogynaecologist (women)	Physician skilled in the combined practice of urology and gynaecology
Urologist (men)	Physician skilled in the study of disorders and diseases of the bladder and urinary tract in men

SURGICAL SPECIALISTS

Anaesthetist	Physician skilled in the study of anaesthesia and anaesthetics, provides anaesthetics before an operation and monitors a patient's condition during surgery; anaesthetists may also run clinics for pain management
Cardiothoracic surgeon	Surgeon skilled in the surgery of the heart and the great vessels around it
Cardiovascular surgeon	Surgeon who specializes in the surgery of the heart and blood vessels, aneurysms and coronary artery disease, for example (also known as a cardiothoracic surgeon)
Cosmetic surgeon	*See* Plastic surgeon
ENT (ear, nose and throat) surgeon	*See* Otolaryngology surgeon
General surgeon	Surgeon skilled in the surgery of the abdomen; may also operate on other surgical emergencies such as an inflamed appendix, hernia or intestinal problems
Neurosurgeon	Surgeon skilled in the surgery of disease or trauma to the brain, spinal cord and other parts of the nervous system
Oral and maxillofacial surgeon	Surgeon skilled in the surgery of diseases and problems of the mouth, teeth and jaw; oral surgeons are trained both in medicine and dentistry
Orthopaedic surgeon	Surgeon skilled in the surgery of bone diseases and disorders, including surgical repair of bone fractures
Otolaryngology surgeon	Surgeon skilled in the surgery of the ear, nose, throat and sinuses; also known as ENT surgeon
Paediatric surgeon	Surgeon who specializes in surgery on infants and children
Plastic surgeon	Surgeon skilled in reconstructive surgery to correct or improve the shape and appearance of body or facial structures (also known as a cosmetic surgeon)
Vascular surgeon	Surgeon skilled in the surgery of disorders and diseases of the blood vessels, such as varicose veins

Conventional treatments

Treatments of many illnesses involve a multidisciplinary approach. It helps to understand what each specialist does and what modalities are used. Conventional medical treatment could involve one or more of the following depending on the condition: physical therapies, osteopathy and chiropractic, drugs, chemotherapy, radiotherapy and surgery.

PHYSIOTHERAPY

A trained physiotherapist can manipulate damaged or injured parts of the body, such as joints, so function can be restored. The techniques are gentle and are built upon week by week so that the healing body is not put under unnecessary stress.

PHYSICAL THERAPIES

A physiotherapist may work with various doctors and specialists in order to help ease damaged joints or muscles, while an exercise physiologist can guide you with a safe programme for aerobic activity. And, in addition, therapists trained in various different massage techniques can stimulate circulation and tone muscle.

Fixing your body

A trained physiotherapist corrects or anticipates problems that arise from the body being put under pressure. Sports injuries, pregnancy and stroke are all areas of interest to a physiotherapist as are children suffering from cystic fibrosis or mobility disorders and women with stress incontinence.

A physiotherapist knows the way the structures of the body are supposed to work and has various techniques to either prevent or treat known disorders. The understanding of the vital role the muscles play in a women's reproductive system has helped the development of urogynaecology. For example, a pregnant woman, a new mother and a menopausal woman may all be referred by their doctor or by a hospital to a gynaecological physiotherapist for exercises to help improve the tone of pelvic floor muscles and stop bladder leakage.

Physiotherapists mainly work via manipulation (passive exercise) and take the patient through exercises they can do at home. Parents of children with cystic fibrosis will be taught by a therapist how to clear their child's lungs of accumulating mucus, as will people with respiratory problems, such as chronic bronchitis or emphysema. In stroke treatment and hip or knee replacement the early involvement

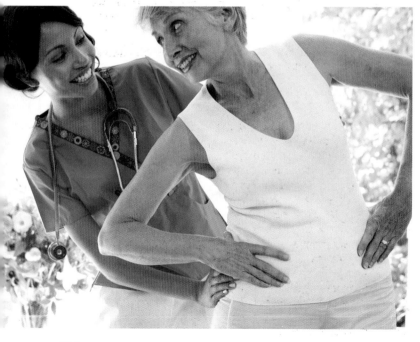

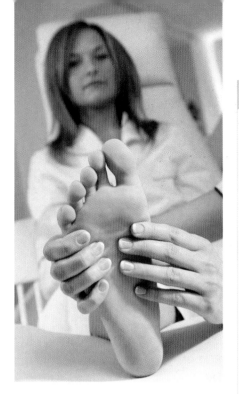

PURE BLISS
Massage of the feet is gentle and has the benefit of relaxing the whole body.

of a physiotherapist is essential, since this therapy is used post-operatively to help restore normal body function.

Other treatments include heat or ultrasound applied to damaged tissues such as strained ligaments, cold packs to reduce inflammation, and hydrotherapy in which patients with back or limb problems may move or be manipulated in a pool of warm water. Such therapy puts less pressure on their joints and supports their weight, thus making movement and manipulation easier.

Using exercise to stay healthy

While a physiotherapist will treat sports injuries, an exercise physiologist aims to prevent their occurrence through the safe prescription of aerobic activity. A physiologist devises and supervises exercise regimes that meet the needs of the person–to lose weight, tone muscles, build stamina, for example–without causing harm. A physiologist will teach a variety of warm-up and cool-down stretches in order to prepare the body for any activities and to prevent lactic acid, a by-product of exercise, from accumulating in the muscles after you stop your workout.

NINE WAYS TO FEEL GOOD

All types of massage involve the application of physical forces such as pressure and manipulation to your body. The massage targets particular tissues, such as muscles, tendons and joints, relieving tension and inducing a feeling of wellbeing.

Hellerwork
Of U.S. origin, it uses manipulation and movement re-education to release tension, restore balance and improve vitality.

Indian head massage
Gentle treatment on upper back and arms, shoulders, neck, face and head; it improves hair and scalp condition and relieves tension.

Looyenwork
Deep precise pressure is used to stretch and lengthen muscles, allowing the body to return to its natural balanced state.

Rolfing
Originating in the United States, it improves posture by stretching and pressing connective tissue and muscles; it can be quite intense.

Shiatsu
Japanese holistic massage applies pressure to points along the body's energy meridians. It is also called acupuncture without needles.

Swedish massage
Classic Western massage was developed in Sweden during the 19th century. It is therapeutic and good for relieving stiffness and tension.

Thai (marma)
Rigorous treatment with the therapist applying pressure with hands, elbows, knees and feet.

Trager
A Western body-work system using stretching, compression and rocking to release deep-seated emotional and physical tension.

Tui na
Intense massage of neck, arms, hands or back from Chinese medicine; good for neck, shoulder and back pain and migraine.

Massage

As an adjunct to conventional medicine or an exercise regime, massage has a slew of physical benefits. Massage therapists study anatomy and physiology as part of their training and use a range of hand movements to improve the circulation and flow of lymph. Their specialized techniques can aid the immune system, tone muscles and smooth out knots in connective tissue. The main purpose is therapeutic, to encourage self-healing. It is relaxing and comforting and eases tension. The different types of massage are described in the box above.

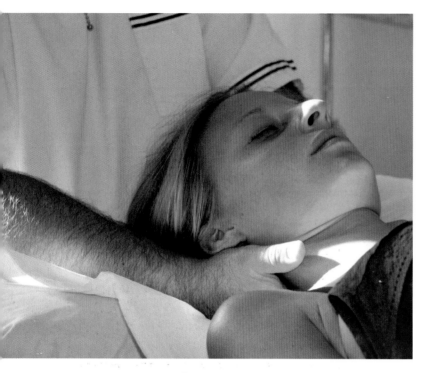

GENTLE MANIPULATION
An osteopath's treatment is based on massaging deep muscle tissue with the hands and fingers and manipulating the joints that are not working as well as they should.

OSTEOPATHY AND CHIROPRACTIC

Osteopathy and chiropractic therapies concentrate on the musculoskeletal system but use different methods to relieve problems related to the spine, joints and muscles. Both techniques may be used in conjunction with conventional treatment.

Osteopaths and chiropractors believe that bones can move out of position through misuse or injury. As a result of ageing or because we do not use our bodies enough, muscles and connective tissue (ligaments and tendons) can become weak or inflexible, upsetting the skeletal system. The most immediate effect is pain, as the muscles try to compensate and the nerves are irritated. However, because the proper working of our body depends on the supportive framework provided by bones, the effects of these problems can be much more widespread.

Although both of these therapies can help conditions seemingly unrelated to the musculoskeletal system, most people choose them for the relief of back and neck pain.

Choosing a practitioner

Osteopaths and chiropractors must have professional qualifications to practise. An osteopath is a medical doctor. A chiropractor is not. They diagnose as well as treat–which means that if they don't think they can help you and you would be better off with a different sort of practitioner, they will say so. Although treatment is purely manual–meaning no drugs or surgery are involved–some of the diagnostic techniques are similar to those of a conventional doctor. You should advise your primary care doctor if you are interested in being treated by an osteopath or chiropractor and discuss any possible risks.

Osteopathy

This treatment was developed in the U.S. at the end of the 19th century. Practitioners use various techniques of which the most important is deep tissue massage. This can be combined with manipulation and "thrusts"–sudden movements that click bones back into place. It should not be painful although you may feel stiff for a time after a session. Another gentle technique, cranial osteopathy (*see* box, right), is used on children or people who are frail.

Osteopaths can treat soreness and stiffness as well as severe pain, and acute as well as chronic cases. You can also see an osteopath for a regular check-up. It is a recognized therapy, and your doctor can refer you. Even if an osteopath can't cure a problem (for example, rheumatoid arthritis, which is a disease of the immune system) osteopathic treatment may reduce pain and, in time, increase your range of movement.

As well as the back and neck, osteopaths treat other areas of the body such as the feet, knees, hips, hands and arms. For example, they will try to relieve the pain of tennis elbow or repetitive strain injury and advise on preventing recurrence. They will treat acute injuries such as those from sports or car accidents (such as whiplash). Headaches may be helped, particularly if they result from muscular tension and bad posture. Pregnancy, childbirth and carrying around a baby or toddler can place a lot of strain on the back and joints, and osteopathy can be beneficial. In addition, osteopaths say a range of other problems may respond to osteopathy treatment: premenstrual syndrome (PMS), dizziness, recurrent sinusitis, asthma and digestive problems.

Chiropractic

Unlike osteopathy, chiropractic treatment largely concentrates on the spine and makes greater use of manipulation and thrusts to bring the body back to its proper balance. Chiropractors must complete a five-year training before they can practise.

They use conventional diagnostic techniques, and many have X-ray machines on site (although X-rays are not taken if a woman is pregnant). Visits tend to be short (45 minutes for a first visit, 20 minutes for later ones), and treatment may not begin until the second appointment. Basic to treatment is the chiropractic couch, which can be placed at different angles to increase the effectiveness of treatment. The practitioner will decide how many treatments will be needed; the average is five.

What you can expect

At your first visit you will be asked about your symptoms and medical history, as well as details of your daily life– whether you drive a lot or sit at a desk all day, how much you exercise, and so on. The practitioner will want to see the way you stand and move and may test some of your reflexes. An important part of the diagnosis is examination by touch–feeling your muscles, ligaments and range of movement. An X-ray, blood test or urine analysis may be suggested. You may be asked to undress down to your underwear, but a gown should be offered. You may feel sore or stiff after a session as parts of the body are brought back into use, and you may find that pain increases for a day or two. In acute cases you may need several weekly sessions, and you may be given exercises to do between treatments.

RELATED PHYSICAL TREATMENTS

There are other types of physical manipulation or massage that may help with different conditions. You should check the qualifications of any practitioner with your primary care physician before agreeing to a course of therapy.

Bowen technique
A modern therapy developed by an Australian osteopath that uses rolling-type moves with fingers and thumbs to work on the body's soft tissue (muscles, ligaments) and the energy pathways. It is fast acting. Therapists may treat respiratory conditions, chronic fatigue, hayfever, headaches, kidney problems and musculoskeletal problems. Also, lymphatic drainage can be improved by this technique.

Cranial osteopathy
A combination of extremely gentle touches and massage on the bones of the skull that can be used in conjunction with osteopathy.

McTimoney and McTimoney-Corley
Gentle, more holistic forms of chiropractic, McTimoney and McTimoney-Corley are named after their British originators and treat the whole body, using light, rapid tapping movements instead of manipulation. X-rays are not used as part of the therapy.

Polarity therapy
An amalgam of Ayurvedic and Western ideas, using manipulation, touch, stretching postures, diet and counselling. It is a gentle therapy,

Sacrocranial osteopathy
The therapist focuses on the pulsations within the fluid that cushions the brain and spinal cord, feeling for them and working on them by placing the hands on or just above the surface of your body. It is good for sensitive or painful conditions.

Zero balancing
A deeply relaxing technique developed by an osteopath/ acupuncturist that uses gentle finger pressure and stretches to enable you to release physical and emotional tension.

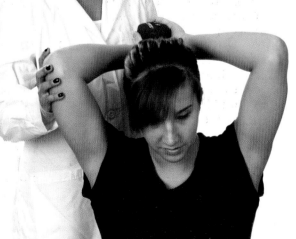

IS IT A HEALTHY SPINE?
Chances are that it is. Paediatricians and school nurses check our spines when we're young; primary care physicians double-check as we reach adulthood.

DRUGS FOR SPECIFIC CONDITIONS

On these charts you'll find drugs grouped into main categories along with their possible side effects and when they should not be taken (contraindications). The names given are generic; they refer to a drug's official name rather than a proprietary brand name. The list is not exhaustive: it would be virtually impossible to include all drugs available for prescription or over the counter in pharmacies.

Three things to remember: First, make sure you ask your doctor about anything he or she prescribes, and read any information provided by the drug company. Second, take drugs precisely as directed, and report any side effects to your doctor immediately. Finally, over-the-counter drugs are also labelled with information on their ingredients, usage and side effects. Make sure that you read and understand the labels.

Drug	Use	Action	Side effects	Contraindications
THE SKELETAL SYSTEM				
Antirheumatics: chloroquine, sodium aurothiomalate, mesalazine, methotrexate, non-steroidal anti-inflammatories (NSAIDs)	Rheumatoid arthritis, juvenile arthritis, systemic lupus erythematosus	Modifies disease process, reduces inflammation	Nausea, vomiting, diarrhoea, skin rashes, blood disorders, mouth ulcers, eye damage	Kidney and liver disorders, pregnancy
Hormone therapy: oestrogens, SERMS (raloxifene)	Osteoporosis for which other drugs don't work; short-term use for menopausal symptoms	Maintains the level of oestrogen	Nausea, weight changes, oedema, depression, headaches, rashes, breast cancer	Pregnancy, oestrogen-dependent cancer, thromboses (DVTs)
Immunosuppressives: azathioprine, prednisone, sulfasalazine	Rheumatoid arthritis, psoriatic arthritis, systemic lupus erythematosus	Suppresses the immune system; reduces inflammation	Kidney damage, changes in blood pressure, nausea, susceptibility to infections	Kidney disease, pregnancy, high blood pressure, infectious disease
Muscle relaxants: baclofen, dantrolene, diazepam, quinine	Damaged spinal cord, muscle spasm, cramp	Reduces muscle tone either systemically, centrally or locally	Drowsiness, nausea, lethargy, dry mouth, blurred vision	Peptic ulcer, liver damage, cerebrovascular disease, psychiatric problems
Bisphosphonates: etidronate disodium, tiludronate disodium	Osteoporosis	Inhibits osteoclast (breakdown of bone) activity	Nausea, diarrhoea	Renal disorders, pregnancy, breastfeeding
THE NERVOUS SYSTEM				
Muscle relaxants: baclofen, dantrolene, diazepam	Multiple sclerosis	Reduces muscle tone either systemically, centrally or locally	Drowsiness, nausea, lethargy, dry mouth, blurred vision	Peptic ulcer, liver damage, cerebrovascular disease, psychiatric problems

CA=Canadian drug name

Drug	Use	Action	Side effects	Contraindications
THE NERVOUS SYSTEM *(continued)*				
Anticonvulsants: carbamazepine, phenytoin, sodium valproate	Epilepsy, some mood disorders such as manic depression	Decreases the excitability of the brain	Drowsiness, liver damage	Liver disorders, bone marrow dysfunction, porphyria
Tricyclic antidepressants: amitriptyline, desipramine, doxepin, imipramine, nortriptyline	Depression (some tricyclic antidepressants also have sedative properties)	Believed to increase brain levels of adrenaline, noradrenaline and mood-enhancing serotonin	Dry mouth, constipation, blurred vision, drowsiness, drop in blood pressure when changing position	Recent heart attack, irregular heartbeat, severe liver disease, suicidal tendencies
Selective serotonin reuptake inhibitors: fluoxetine, paroxetine	Depression (when sedation not required)	Increases serotonin levels by inhibiting it being taken back into nerve endings	Nausea, vomiting, diarrhoea, weight loss, headache, suicide	Mania, epilepsy, liver and kidney problems
Monoamine oxidase inhibitors: isocarboxazid, phenelzine	Depression, especially with hysteria and hypochondria; if other drugs not effective	Causes increase in levels of neurotransmitters in brain	Low blood pressure, dizziness, fatigue, dry mouth, constipation, weight gain	Liver disease, cerebrovascular problems, rise in blood pressure (due to food)
Lithium carbonate	Bipolar disorder, recurrent depression	Stabilizes mood	Nausea, diarrhea, weight gain, thyroid disorder	Kidney and heart disorders
Anticholinergics: orphenadrine, trihexphenidyl	Parkinson's disease	Reduces tremor in Parkinson's disease	Dry mouth, vision problems, difficulty in passing urine	Glaucoma
Antipsychotics: flupenthixol, pimozide, sulpiride; atypical antipsychotics: olanzapine, risperidone	Schizophrenia, bipolar disorder, delusion	Reduces the excitability of nerve pathways in the brain	Drowsiness, dry mouth, Parkinson's-like symptoms, weight gain, dizziness	Bone marrow disorders, liver disease, Parkinson's disease, cardiovascular disease, epilepsy, pregnancy
Hypnotics: diazepam, nitrazepam	Insomnia, stress, anxiety, senile dementia	Affects the part of the brain controlling wakefulness	Drowsiness, confusion, dependence	Respiratory, liver and psychiatric problems
Donepezil, rivastigmine	Alzheimer's, dementia	Inhibits the enzyme acetylcholinesterase, which increases brain alertness	Diarrhoea, nausea, fatigue, cramps, peptic ulcers	Pregnancy, breastfeeding
THE ENDOCRINE SYSTEM				
Hormone therapy: oestrogens, progestogens	Menopausal symptoms	Maintains the level of oestrogen	Nausea, weight changes, oedema, depression, headache, rashes, breast cancer	Pregnancy, oestrogen-dependent cancer, thromboses (DVTs)

(continued)

Drug	Use	Action	Side effects	Contraindications
THE ENDOCRINE SYSTEM (*continued*)				
Hormone: insulin	Diabetes	Ensures glucose enters the cells, so restoring fat and carbohydrate metabolism	Hypoglycaemia—too much insulin, hyperglycaemia—too little insulin	None
Antithyroid drug: carbimazole	Hyperthyroidism, thyrotoxicosis, goitre, exophthalmus	Decreases the production of thyroxine by the thyroid gland	Enlarged thyroid gland, headache, nausea, hair loss, low immunity, loss of thyroxine production	Low white blood count, infectious disease
Hormone: thyroxine	Hypothyroidism (myxoedema), cretinism, thyroid cancer	Replaces missing production of thyroxine hormone by thyroid gland	Weight loss, angina, arrhythmias, cramps, headache, restlessness, sweating	Cardiovascular disorders, adrenal gland disorders
Corticosteroids: beclomethasone, betamethasone, dexamethasone, fludrocortisone, hydrocortisone, prednisone	Addison's disease, adrenalectomy, inflammatory disorders, asthma, eczema	Inhibits the body's reaction to damage or disease, thus reducing inflammation	Long-term treatment—fluid retention, hypertension, Cushing's syndrome, osteoporosis, depression, diabetes; sudden cessation—rapid fall in blood pressure; topical use (on skin)—thinning of skin, worsening of infection	Systemic steroids (requires careful monitoring)—exposure to chickenpox; topical and inhaled steroids—rosacea, acne, skin infections, psoriasis, tuberculosis
THE BLOOD AND CIRCULATORY SYSTEM				
ACE (angiotensin-converting enzyme) inhibitors: captopril, enalapril	Heart failure, high blood pressure	Dilates arteries and veins and reduces the amount of fluid in the circulation	Dizziness, hypotension, skin rashes, impaired renal function, cough	Pregnancy, renal problems, aortic stenosis (narrowing)
Antiarrhythmics: adenosine, lidocaine, verapamil	Restores an irregular heartbeat to normal	Slows down the transmission of electrical impulses within the heart	Dizziness, confusion, constipation, breathing difficulties	Cardiac or respiratory failure, porphyria
Anticoagulants: heparin, warfarin	Internal blood clots—pulmonary embolus, cerebral or coronary infarcts, deep vein thrombosis	Decreases the clotting factors in the blood	Bleeding of the gastrointestinal tract and kidneys, bruising of the skin	Haemophilia, high blood pressure, cerebral haemorrhage, peptic ulcers, kidney or liver failure
Antihypertensives: hydralazine, methyldopa, prazosin	High blood pressure	Dilates blood vessels; partially blocks adrenaline and noradrenaline	Palpitations, oedema, dizziness, headache	Rapid heartbeat, congestive heart failure, aneurysm, depression

Drug	Use	Action	Side effects	Contraindications
THE BLOOD AND CIRCULATORY SYSTEM (*continued*)				
Beta-blockers: acebutolol, atenolol, celiprolol, metoprolol, propranolol	High blood pressure, angina, heart attacks, arrhythmias	Slows heart and lowers blood pressure by blocking adrenaline production	Cold extremities, general malaise, sleep disturbances, nightmares	Asthma, chronic bronchitis, emphysema, diabetes, later stages of pregnancy
Calcium channel blockers: amlodipine, diltiazem, nicardipine, nifedipine, nimodipine, verapamil	High blood pressure, angina, arrhythmias, subarachnoid haemorrhage	Relaxes the muscles of the heart and arteries	Headache, oedema, fatigue, nausea, flushing, dizziness, constipation	Heart failure, liver failure, pregnancy, heart attack, on beta-blockers
Diuretics: furosemide (frusemide AUS), mannitol, spironolactone, thiazides	High blood pressure, congestive heart failure, cerebral oedema	Causes the kidneys to excrete water and salts	Gout, impotence, potassium deficiency	Renal failure, pregnancy, breastfeeding, diabetes, Addison's disease
Nitrates: glyceryl trinitrate, isosorbide dinitrate, isosorbide mononitrate	Angina, left ventricular failure	Widens the coronary arteries and reduces blood flow into the heart	Headache, flushing, dizziness	Hypotension, narrowing of aorta, cerebral haemorrhage, head injury, glaucoma
Statins: atorvastatin, fluvastatin, simvastatin	High cholesterol levels, slow coronary atherosclerosis, reduces risk of strokes	Blocks production of cholesterol and use of circulating cholesterol	Nausea, insomnia, stomach pain, muscle pain, headache	Liver disease, pregnancy, breastfeeding
Cardiac glycosides: digoxin	Congestive cardiac failure, atrial fibrillation	Makes heartbeat stronger; restores normal beat	Visual problems, weakness, headache, depression	Complete heart blockage, arrhythmia
Aspirin	Prevention of blood clots	Reduces platelet stickiness	Gastric bleeding	Peptic ulcer, allergy to aspirin
THE RESPIRATORY SYSTEM				
Decongestants, antitussives: dextromethorphan, menthol, triprolidine	Coughs, bronchial secretions	Dries up secretions; reduces coughing	Insomnia, tachycardia (heartbeat irregularity), restlessness, anxiety with overuse	High blood pressure, diabetes
Anticholinergics: ipratropium, oxitropium	Asthma	Relaxes muscles of the bronchii	Dry mouth, constipation, difficulty in passing urine	Glaucoma
Antihistamines: acrivastine, cetirizine, chlorpheniramine, cyclizine, loratidine, promethazine	Allergies: hayfever	Reduces action of histamine in the body—which dilates small blood vessels and tightens the bronchioles	Drowsiness, rashes, dry mouth, blurred vision, palpitations	Epilepsy, liver and kidney disorders, glaucoma, porphyria

(continued)

Drug	Use	Action	Side effects	Contraindications
THE RESPIRATORY SYSTEM (*continued*)				
Bronchodilators: fenoterol, salbutamol, salmeterol, terbutaline	Chronic obstructive pulmonary disease, asthma	Relaxes the muscles of the bronchioles	Shaking hands, headache, nervous tension, flushes, palpitations	Hyperthyroidism, high blood pressure, arrhythmias
Corticosteroids: beclomethasone, budesonide, fluticasone, hydrocortisone, prednisone	Chronic respiratory disease, asthma	Inhibits the body's reaction to damage or disease, thus reducing inflammation	Long-term treatment—fluid retention, high blood pressure, osteoporosis, depression, diabetes; sudden cessation—rapid fall in blood pressure, shock	Systemic steroids (requires careful monitoring)—avoid exposure to chickenpox; inhaled steroids—oral thrush
Montelukast, zafirlukast	Asthma	Blocks leukotriene receptors	Gastrointestinal rashes	Liver failure
Decongestants: ephedrine, xylometazoline	Hayfever, common cold	Reduces inflammation in the nasal passages and the production of mucus	Nose dryness and irritation	High blood pressure
THE DIGESTIVE SYSTEM				
Antacids: magnesium carbonate, magnesium trisilicate, sodium bicarbonate; alginates	Peptic ulcers, hiatal hernia, indigestion	Neutralizes the acid in the stomach and gut, reducing inflammation	Rare, but overuse may disturb body's fluid balance	Antacids neutralize or react with other medications
Anticholinergics: hyoscine, dicycloverine (not AUS)	Irritable bowel syndrome, peptic ulcers	Relaxes muscles of the gut, reduces gastric secretions	Dry mouth, vision problems, difficulty in passing urine	Glaucoma
Antidiarrhoeals: subsalicylate, codeine phosphate, kaolin (not AUS), loperamide	Diarrhoea	Slows down passage of faeces; reduces loss of water and salts from bowel	Constipation, bowel obstruction	Bowel infections, inflammatory bowel disease, kidney and liver disorders
Antiemetics: cyclizine, metoclopramide, promethazine	Vomiting, severe nausea, motion sickness	Inhibits the vomit reflex at the base of the brain	Drowsiness, dry mouth, involuntary twitches	Kidney and liver disorders, dehydration, glaucoma
Appetite suppressants, anti-obesity agents: methycellulose, orlistat, phentermine	Gross obesity	Gives a feeling of fullness; dampens the appetite centre in the brain; prevents absorption of fat	Constipation, flatulence, diarrhoea, drowsiness, dizziness, anxiety, depression	Psychiatric disorders, drug abuse, personality disorders, pregnancy, breastfeeding, epilepsy, glaucoma
Immunosuppressants: sulfasalazine	Ulcerative colitis	Suppresses immune system; reduces inflammation	Headache, rash, nausea, fever, hypersensitivity	Blood dyscrasias, sensitivity to sulphonamides

Drug	Use	Action	Side effects	Contraindications
THE DIGESTIVE SYSTEM *(continued)*				
Laxatives: bisacodyl, bran, lactulose, magnesium hydroxide, methycellulose, psyllium, senna	Constipation, expulsion of parasites	Increases the water content of the faeces; stimulates the colonic muscles to contract	Diarrhoea, flatulence, bloating, colic	Intestinal obstruction
Replacement salts: glucose, potassium chloride, sodium chloride	Fluid and electrolyte replacement during diarrhoea	Replaces salts and fluids	Oedema	Kidney and cardiovascular disorders, high blood pressure
Corticosteroids: budesonide, dexamethasone, hydrocortisone, prednisone	Crohn's disease	Inhibits the body's reaction to damage or disease, reducing inflammation	Fluid retention, high blood pressure, osteoporosis, depression, diabetes; sudden cessation—fall in blood pressure, shock	Use of systemic steroids requires careful monitoring; avoid exposure to chickenpox
H$_2$ receptor blockers: cimetidine, nizatidine, ranitidine	Peptic ulcers, protects stomach against NSAID damage, reflux oesophagitis	Reduces gastric acid output as a result of histamine H$_2$ blockade	Diarrhoea, rash, dizziness	Some drug interactions
Proton-pump inhibitors: lansoprazole, omeprazole	Peptic ulcers, given with NSAIDS to prevent gastric side effects	Inhibits gastric acid formation	Diarrhoea, nausea, rash, constipation, headache	Intestinal obstruction
THE URINARY SYSTEM				
Diuretics: furosemide (frusemide AUS), mannitol, spironolactone, thiazides	Fluid retention, cirrhosis, kidney disorders	Causes the kidneys to excrete water and salts	Gout, impotence, potassium deficiency	Renal failure, pregnancy, diabetes, Addison's disease
Alkalinizing agents: potassium citrate	Cystitis	Decreases acidity of urine	Gastric irritation, diarrhoea	Bowel ulceration, renal malfunction, late pregnancy
THE REPRODUCTIVE SYSTEM				
Beta-2 agonists: salbutamol, terbutaline	Premature labour	Relaxes uterine muscles	Shaky hands, headache, nervous tension, flushes, palpitations	Hyperthyroidism, high blood pressure, arrhythmias
Antifungals: econazole, ketoconazole, miconazole, nystatin	Yeast infection (candidiasis)	Attacks fungi	Orally—nausea, vomiting; secondary bacterial infections; severe liver problems possible with ketoconazole	Orally—liver disease
Gonadotrophins and gonadotrophin-releasing hormone analogues: buserelin, goserelin, menotrophin	Endometriosis, infertility, excessive menstrual bleeding, PMS, uterine fibroids	Stimulates the release of gonadotrophin	Overstimulation of the ovaries, possible multiple pregnancy, allergic reactions	Pregnancy, ovarian cyst, unexplained vaginal bleeding

(continued)

Drug	Use	Action	Side effects	Contraindications
THE REPRODUCTIVE SYSTEM (continued)				
Hormone replacement therapy: oestrogens, progestogens	Menopause	Maintains the level of oestrogen	Nausea, weight changes, oedema, depression, headache, rash	Pregnancy, oestrogen-dependent cancer, deep vein thromboses (DVTs)
Hormone: progestogens	Painful/heavy menstruation, endometriosis, breast cancer	Increases the level of progesterone in the body	Nausea, fluid retention, weight gain	Pregnancy, liver disorders, arterial disease, porphyria
THE IMMUNE SYSTEM				
Antihistamines: acrivastine, chlorpheniramine, cyclizine, loratadine, promethazine	Allergies: hay fever, urticaria (hives), insect stings, drug allergy	Reduces the action of histamine in the body—which dilates small blood vessels and tightens the bronchioles	Drowsiness, rashes, dry mouth, blurred vision, palpitations	Epilepsy, liver and kidney disorders, glaucoma, porphyria
Immunosuppressants: azathioprine, ciclosporin (cyclosporin AUS), tacrolimus	Organ transplant	Suppresses the immune system; reduces possibility of rejection of transplanted tissue	Kidney damage, hirsutism, high or low blood pressure, nausea, susceptibility to infections	Kidney disease (ciclosporin), pregnancy, high blood pressure, infectious disease
THE SKIN AND THE SENSES				
Antifungals: amorolfine, econazole, ketoconazole, miconazole, nystatin, terbinafine	Ringworm, athlete's foot, fungal nail infections	Attacks fungi	Severe liver problems possible with ketoconazole; orally—nausea, vomiting, secondary bacterial infections	Orally—liver disease
Corticosteroids: betamethasone, hydrocortisone, triamcinolone	Allergies, eczema-type disorders	Inhibits the body's reaction to damage or disease, reducing inflammation	Thinning of skin, worsening of infection	Rosacea, acne, skin infections, psoriasis
Decongestants: ephedrine, pseudoephedrine, xylometazoline	Middle ear infections	Dries up mucous secretions	Nose dryness and irritation	High blood pressure

DRUGS WITH SEVERAL USES

Certain drugs are not formulated for a specific illness or condition but are used to treat a variety of disorders. Painkillers are the most commonly used drugs in this category. Antibiotics and antivirals are also used for a wide variety of infections to help the body's immune system fight the disease.

Drug	Use	Action	Side effects	Contraindications
PAINKILLERS				
Simple analgesics: paracetamol	Mild to moderate pain, fever	Reduces the body's ability to appreciate pain; not an anti-inflammatory	Mild skin rashes; overdose—severe liver and kidney damage	Liver and kidney disorders

Drug	Use	Action	Side effects	Contraindications
PAINKILLERS				
Opiate analgesics: codeine, meperidine, methadone, morphine	Severe, acute and chronic pain—heart attack, labour, cancer, kidney stones, gallstones; moderate pain relief (for example, codeine)	Reduces the perception of pain and induces euphoria and drowsiness	Constipation, slows breathing, nausea, lowered blood pressure, addiction	Raised intracranial pressure, head injuries
Non-steroidal anti-inflammatories (NSAIDs): aspirin, fenoprofen, ibuprofen, indomethacin, naproxen	Moderate pain, rheumatoid arthritis, osteoarthritis, musculoskeletal problems, gout, dysmenorrhoea, fever, headache	Inhibits inflammation, which irritates nerve endings and thus causes pain	Gastrointestinal disturbances, nausea, liver and kidney damage, headache, peptic ulcers	Peptic ulcer, asthma, blood-clotting disorders, pregnancy, breastfeeding
Fever reducers: aspirin, paracetamol	High temperature	Lowers the body temperature by blocking the inflammatory effect of prostaglandins	Nausea, indigestion, peptic ulcers; aspirin may cause Reye's syndrome—do not give to children under 12 years	Allergy to aspirin, liver and kidney disease, peptic ulcer, pregnancy
ANTIBIOTICS				
Aminoglycosides, cephalosporins, metronidazole, penicillins, sulphonamides, tetracyclines	Bacterial infections	Finds and destroys particular bacteria	Nausea, vomiting, diarrhoea, allergic response, skin rash, teeth stains	Kidney problems, alcohol abuse, allergic reaction to a specific antibiotic, pregnancy (aminoglycosides, sulphonamides, tetracyclines)
ANTIMALARIALS				
Chloroquine, halofantrine, mefloquine, proguanil, pyrimethamine, quinine	Prevention and treatment of malaria	Seems to prevent the malaria-carrying parasite from reproducing	Headache, eye damage, ringing in ears; mefloquine: rarely, headache, visual, psychiatric and neurological disturbances	Epilepsy, early pregnancy, breastfeeding, liver and kidney disorders
ANTIVIRALS				
Aciclovir, amantadine, zidovudine	Cold sores, genital herpes, shingles, chickenpox, HIV, AIDS, influenza A	Prevents the virus from multiplying	Use on skin—slight dryness, stinging; orally—nausea, headache, anaemia, insomnia, fatigue	Anaemia, kidney and liver disorders, epilepsy, peptic ulcer
CHEMOTHERAPY				
Cyclophosphamide, doxorubicin, etoposide, fluorouracil, ifosfamide, vincristine	Cancers, malignancies	Destroys cancer cells and inhibits their division; normal cells also affected	Nausea, vomiting, hair loss, low immunity, bone marrow disturbance, sterility, life-threatening toxicity	Pregnancy; when cancer is severe, toxic effects will not prolong or improve quality of life

Having cancer and being treated for it are difficult. But there is much that you can do to help yourself—not only to cope with cancer but to put yourself in the best physical and mental shape to treat it. Here are some suggestions:

- Hang out with friends, but be careful not to exhaust yourself.
- Remember that cancer can be treated.
- Practise relaxation techniques, such as deep breathing, meditation or visualization.
- Learn to say no to protect your energy levels.
- Continue to work if possible—or negotiate part-time hours for the course of your treatment.
- Make time for your family, partner and friends.
- Join a support group.
- Avoid taking vitamins and drugs without your doctor's knowledge; some may weaken your response to chemotherapy.

CHEMOTHERAPY

Cancer cells divide rapidly and spread to other areas of the body via the bloodstream or lymphatic system. Chemotherapy aims to prevent this, employing "cytotoxic"–poisonous to cells–drugs that damage or kill cancerous cells. Chemotherapy may result in either a complete cure or a remission. Since cytotoxic drugs are not specific to cancer cells and may affect non-cancerous cells, you need to know what to expect from a course of chemotherapy and how to deal with it.

Cancer cells are not the only fast-growing cells in your body. The cells of the blood-producing tissues in the bone marrow, the hair follicles, the digestive tract and the reproductive system all multiply rapidly. Most of the side effects of chemotherapy are caused by damage to cells in these areas. Other, less common, side effects may include diarrhoea, constipation, neuropathy, and kidney and bladder problems. The side effects, however, diminish over time after treatments are complete.

What to expect

Since chemotherapy has to be planned carefully so that it progressively destroys the cancer, but not the normal cells and tissue, the drugs are given over several weeks, with breaks between. Depending on the drug or drugs chosen, treatment will be divided into sessions, and each one can last from a few hours to a few days. Sometimes a hospital stay of one or more nights is necessary.

During this extended period, it is important to try to minimize the disruption to your life and give yourself the best possible chance for treatment to succeed. To contend with fatigue and feelings of lethargy and weakness–all common side effects–make sure you have plenty of rest at night, take time for short naps during the day and have a regular walking regime at a time of day when your energy level is at its highest. Arrange for help with household chores and childcare, and cut back on activities that could tire you.

You may feel faint and weak because chemotherapy reduces the production of red blood cells in the bone marrow that transport oxygen. A lack of these cells results in anaemia and low blood pressure. Make sure that your bath or shower is not too hot, and get in and out of it slowly. Take your time when getting up from a chair or out of bed.

Nausea and vomiting are the most common side effects of chemotherapy, and your doctor may prescribe antinausea pills to minimize them. Although you may not feel like eating, your body needs the nourishment of a balanced diet, rich in fresh fruit, vegetables and iron. Eat small amounts throughout the day rather than large meals and avoid fast food or foods that are spicy or fatty. Drink plenty of fluids but not at the same time as eating. Don't eat before treatment.

If, after a session, you have an attack of vomiting, don't eat for a few hours and instead drink plenty of fluids in small amounts. Stay away from places where odours are strong–restaurants and perfume counters, for example–and use relaxation techniques to ease the effects of treatments on your body.

Protect your immune system

Chemotherapy drugs interfere with the production of the body's infection-fighting white cells. Your blood is monitored during treatment and if your white blood cell count falls too low, chemotherapy may be suspended or reduced for a time to allow the bone marrow to recover.

Help your immune system by maintaining strict personal hygiene, and avoid animals, crowds and people who are ill with colds or flu or who have recently been immunized. You should report any sign of an infection to your doctor immediately–fever, sweating, inflammation of the skin, sore throat, cough, vaginal discharge or itching. Cuts and abrasions are sites for infection so wear protective gloves when doing dirty chores, housework or gardening to prevent damage to your skin. The drugs can make your skin sensitive to sunlight, so cover up well.

Your mouth, gums and throat can be susceptible to sores that can become infected and bleed. Your mouth may feel dry, and there is an increased risk that your teeth may develop cavities. Be strict with teeth cleaning, using a very soft toothbrush, and avoid commercial mouthwashes–many contain alcohol that makes the mouth even drier. Speak to your doctor regarding the best options to keep your mouth moist.

Cut your hair

Certain anticancer drugs can temporarily damage the hair follicles, causing hair loss all over the body. The colour and structure of your hair may also change. Before treatment starts, have your hair cut short so it is easier to manage. Use a soft brush and mild shampoos to prevent scalp damage, avoid heated curlers and use your hairdryer on its lowest setting. Your hair will grow back eventually, but in the meantime, you can disguise its absence with a wig, hat or scarf.

What to watch for

Some chemotherapy drugs affect the bone marrow's ability to make platelets, the cells that help the blood to clot. During treatment you may bruise easily, and a small cut may bleed profusely. Report to your doctor immediately signs such as nosebleeds that will not stop,

a black colouring to the stools, blood in the urine or red spots under the skin. A blood transfusion may be needed if the platelet count drops too low. Do not take any over-the-counter medicines without checking with your doctor–many, such as aspirin, ibuprofen and paracetamol affect platelet function.

Fertility issues

Many chemotherapy drugs can cause infertility in men and women. In women, they can damage the ovaries and affect the menstrual cycle. Fertility may return to normal after the treatment is stopped, but it may not. Before treatment starts, you should know your options–for example, storing your eggs if you and your partner want to have a child after you have recovered. If you are receiving infertility treatment, it should be postponed until the chemotherapy course is completed. The drugs can also cause menopausal symptoms, such as hot flushes and vaginal dryness.

Anticancer drugs are also unsafe for a developing fetus. Ensure you always use contraception during chemotherapy. If you are pregnant when diagnosed, you will want to know what the implications are before starting chemotherapy, and what postponement might mean.

How it works

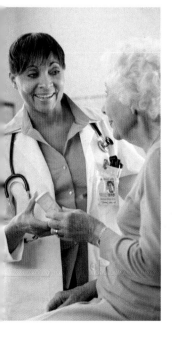

Chemotherapy uses cytotoxic drugs to prevent cancerous cells from growing or multiplying. Drugs are given in various ways: intravenously (injected into a vein), directly into a specific area through a catheter (a fixed line) or orally (as pills, although not all drugs have an oral form).

The method chosen depends on many factors including the type and stage of cancer, the drugs you have been prescribed, your age and your general health. If you are not given oral drugs to be taken at home, you may have to attend a special outpatient clinic, or go into hospital if you need intensive treatment. The treatment is usually given in bursts to minimize the side effects. Also,

since normal cells recuperate more quickly than cancerous cells, intermittent courses of cytotoxic drugs allow normal cells such recovery time.

The best outcomes (treatment success rates and happy patients) are generally found at centres that specialize in cancer treatment, rather than at general hospitals where doctors may treat only a few cancer cases a year.

The duration of treatment, time between treatments and the dosages vary from person to person. An oral course may last from one to two weeks, while intravenous injections may be given once every three to four weeks.

RADIOTHERAPY

Radiotherapy uses high-energy radiation (radioactivity) to attack and kill malignant growths. Unlike treatment with drugs (chemotherapy) that affects the whole body, radiotherapy is a precise form of treatment that can be aimed specifically at the growth. Today radiotherapy is more specialized and encompasses electron-beam therapy and neutron therapy.

How it works

Radiation is used to kill cancer cells while causing as little damage as possible to neighbouring normal cells. Cancer cells are particularly sensitive to radiation because they divide and grow quickly and, while normal cells are also affected by it, they have greater recuperative powers, so that many are able to recover between treatments. Nevertheless, the damage inflicted on normal cells causes side effects, although the treatment itself is completely painless.

Radiotherapy is often used in conjunction with chemotherapy or surgery. It may be used before surgery or chemotherapy to shrink a tumour so that surgery can be of a less radical nature and chemotherapy more effective. After surgery or chemotherapy, it may be used to destroy any cancer cells that remain. You may be given radiotherapy during an operation or while receiving chemotherapy. Radiation may also be given to ease the symptoms of advanced cancer, such as pain. Exactly how radiation is used depends on the assessment of your condition and the treatment plan.

What to expect from a course of radiotherapy

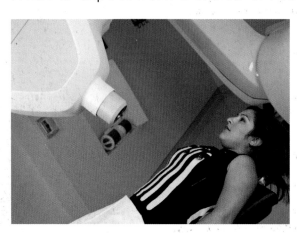

A specialist doctor—a radiologist or radiation oncologist—decides on the type and dose of radiation and the precise area of the body to be treated. Most patients receive external radiation therapy: the waves of radiation are emitted from a machine and pass through the skin to the site of the tumour. In some cases, an implant of radioactive material is positioned at the site of the tumour, or you may be given a course of external radiation and then an implant.

External radiation

The first phase is a pretreatment session, which can last anywhere from 30 minutes to three hours. The medical team works out exactly at what point, or port, the beam of radiation should enter the body, at what depth and for how long. Each port is recorded on your skin with an indelible marker, and sometimes a cast is made so that your body is in exactly the same position for each treatment session.

Treatment is usually given as an outpatient, every day for six to eight weeks, except weekends when the normal cells are left to recover. Shorter, more intensive courses, however, have been tested recently and found to be equally effective in some tumours. Some areas of your body may be covered with protective shields. The session lasts up to an hour, although the radiation beam is only on for a few minutes.

Internal implant radiation

Implant therapy allows a high dose of radiation to be given to a limited area in a shorter time. Radioactive material is implanted, under general anaesthetic, into or close to the tumour. Sometimes, a radioactive substance is injected into the bloodstream or a body cavity. While radiation is emitted, you have to stay in a single room in the hospital so that other people are not exposed to it. However, the stay lasts for only a few days, since the implant gradually loses its potency.

A radioactive implant may be kept in place for a few minutes up to a few days. Smaller implants may be left in place after you leave the hospital.

Side effects

The side effects of radiotherapy vary from person to person and also depend on which area is being treated: they can range from the mild to the acutely unpleasant. The most common are fatigue, loss of appetite, skin irritation over the treatment area and emotional stress. There may also be local side effects: for example, radiation to the head may cause hair loss on the scalp, but it will not cause other body hair to fall out; and treatment for breast cancer can cause a stiff shoulder, breast and nipple soreness and either an increase or decrease in breast size.

Dealing with fatigue

Most radiotherapy patients experience tiredness and a lack of energy. During therapy, the body uses energy in the attempt to fight off the radiation and heal itself. At the same time, symptoms of the cancer, such as pain, a loss of appetite and stress compound the problem. However, much of the feeling of exhaustion fades at the end of treatment.

To help matters, have plenty of rest night and day. Cut out household chores. Ask for and accept help from friends and family. Engage in moderate exercise. Accept only those social engagements that you want to. Inform your employer of your treatment and choose whether to work full- or part-time or to take time off.

Treat skin gently

External radiation can make the skin red and sore as if sunburned. After a few treatments, it can feel dry and itchy. Any moistness should be reported to the medical team, because open sores could develop without treatment. You will be given guidelines about skin care, and it is important that you follow these, because the skin becomes sensitive and fragile and susceptible to damage and infection.

Ask your doctor which products–talc, creams, sunblock and so on–you can use. Avoid stiff, tight clothing; soft, loose cotton is best. Do not scrub, scratch, rub or put a plaster on the affected area. Bathe in lukewarm water and avoid extremes of heat or cold. Keep the area out of the sun–wear a loose scarf or soft-based wig over the head. Continue with

EAT WELL, HEAL WELL

People undergoing radiotherapy tend to lose their appetite, resulting in a significant loss of weight each week. Cancers of the digestive system may make it difficult to chew, swallow or digest food, aggravating the problem. Your weight will be monitored during treatment and any problems with eating, or nausea, vomiting, constipation or diarrhoea should be reported to the medical team. Studies show that people who maintain an adequate intake of food cope better with both the cancer and its treatment. These tips will help:

- Eat small amounts often throughout the day rather than just at mealtimes.
- Maintain a well-balanced, varied diet—the dietitian will tell you if you need to follow a special one.
- Add extra cream, cheese and butter to your food.
- Liquidize your food if swallowing is hard.
- Buy liquid diet supplements to increase your protein intake.
- Cook and store meals in the freezer (or get others to do so for you) so that you can eat whenever hunger strikes.
- Keep snacks by your side—while watching television, for example.
- Cheer up meals with a glass of wine, but only with your doctor's permission.

the same skin care regime after the end of treatment until your doctor tells you that you can change.

Beat the fear

Being given a diagnosis of cancer and undergoing therapy is frightening because you have to face the unpleasant side effects of treatment, the symptoms of the cancer itself and fear of the unknown. Make sure you keep informed about the nature of your disease, your treatment and its progress. Write down any questions that you want answered and take the list with you to all your medical appointments. Regular sessions with a psychologist may be useful, and you may find it helpful to practise relaxation techniques. Join a self-help group of cancer sufferers to talk over concerns with people you can trust.

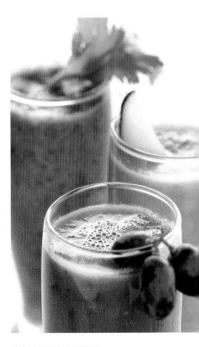

HEALTHY EATING
If swallowing is painful, liquidize fresh fruit and vegetables to make a delicious and revitalizing drink that you can sip. Take care to thoroughly wash all raw fruits and vegetables to avoid infection during this period.

SURGERY

There can be multiple indications for a surgical procedure: to repair or rebuild something that's damaged or broken, remove something that shouldn't be in your body, transplant tissue, implant electronic or mechanical devices, reposition something that's no longer where it should be, help your doctor diagnose a problem, prevent a disease from spreading, or relieve discomfort.

Sometimes surgery is a cure and makes you feel better. And sometimes it simply answers questions. Whatever its final outcome, however, it has risks and benefits just like any other treatment.

Who is involved in your care?
Your primary care doctor, surgeon and anaesthetist work together as a team when preparing for your surgery. This team can help you figure out the risks and benefits of your specific procedure. If you are not fully confident that surgery is the best treatment, you may want to seek a second opinion. If you do so, make sure that the surgeon you consult has sound knowledge of your condition and plenty of experience and expertise in treating it.

Your surgeon should be certified by a national organization of surgical professionals, such as the Royal College of Surgeons in the UK or the Royal Australasian College of Surgeons in Australia. Your surgeon should also be certified by a national medical specialty board that checks to make sure he or she is qualified to perform specific types of surgery relevant to your particular problem. UK surgeons with the initials FRCS or MRCS after their names have had their training and skills evaluated and approved by the Royal College of Surgeons. Australian surgeons who have undergone a similar evaluation at the Australian college are able to use the qualification FRACS.

Emergency surgery
If you're lying in Accident and Emergency and the emergency physician tells you that immediate surgery is necessary to save your life, you're not going to be in a position to do much

checking. You'll meet with the surgeon on call who will discuss the risks and benefits. You'll also involve and discuss the surgery with your family or friends.

Common types of emergency surgery include those for automobile injuries, gunshot wounds, burns, heart attacks, cardiac arrhythmias, aneurysms, brain injuries and appendicitis.

What to expect on the day of surgery?
If you're having inpatient surgery, once you've signed all the paperwork that hospitals invariably require before a procedure, you'll receive a wristband with your name on it and be sent to the ward assigned for your stay. There you'll swap your clothes for a hospital gown, and will be asked to remove any contact lenses, glasses, hearing aids, dentures and make-up. A hospital representative will guide you on the hospital policy about where and how to manage your personal belongings.

You'll be asked to empty your bladder, and a nurse will give you medication to help you relax. Your nurse may insert an intravenous (IV) catheter into a vein to be used to deliver fluids and medication.

When it is time for you to have your surgery, you'll be taken to the operating room on a trolley–a padded table with wheels. Depending on hospital policy, your family may wait on the ward or in a small waiting area next to the operating theatre.

Once in the operating theatre, a nurse will carefully check your wristband against his or her chart to confirm who you are and the specific surgery you're having done. Anaesthesia, which the anaesthetist will have discussed with you prior to the surgery, will be administered, and you'll be hooked up to various monitors that will measure your blood oxygen level, blood pressure, pulse, temperature, breathing, heartbeat and level of consciousness during and after surgery.

Once the surgery is over, you'll be taken to a recovery room where you will be monitored until you wake up from the anaesthesia. Once you're awake and the surgeon is comfortable you're in good shape, you'll be returned to your ward.

ASK THE RIGHT QUESTIONS

Prior to surgery, you should have time to do a bit of research, ask some searching questions, and think long and hard about the procedure you're considering. Here are some questions that should be answered before you head into an operating theatre:

- Is this surgery really necessary?
- What are the alternatives?
- Is there a less invasive procedure available?
- What will happen if I don't have the surgery?
- What are the risks and benefits?
- How many of these surgeries has the surgeon performed?
- How many in the past month?
- What were the outcomes and survival rates of the surgery?
- What type of anaesthesia will be used?
- What are my other options?

CONSIDERATIONS BEFORE AND AFTER SURGERY

Surgery may be an emotional and stressful experience. To make the process as stress-free as possible, it is important to feel prepared before the procedure and to feel well informed about the outcome while you recuperate. Your doctor should advise you before you have surgery of the risks and benefits. The table below highlights some other medical and practical considerations before, immediately after and in the longer term following your operation.

YOUR MEDICAL HISTORY If the answer is yes to any of the below, inform your doctor before surgery.

- Do you have any drug or food allergies?
- Has your general health been good?
- Do you have a fever, cold or rash?
- Do you take any over-the counter drugs? If you do, give full details to your doctor
- Do you take blood thinners?
- Could you be pregnant?
- Do you use alcohol, tobacco or illegal drugs?
- Do you have diabetes, high blood pressure or any form of heart disease?

YOUR ROLE IN PREPARING FOR SURGERY

- Quit or cut down on smoking before surgery
- If you are taking any medication, ask your doctor whether you should stop taking it
- Arrange for someone to drive you to and from the hospital
- It is important that you stop drinking alcohol at least two days prior to the procedure
- Inform your doctor immediately if you are feeling unwell or have developed a rash

THE EVENING PRIOR TO AND THE MORNING OF YOUR PROCEDURE

- On the night before your morning surgery, do not eat or drink anything after midnight
- When brushing your teeth, rinse and spit—do not swallow
- Do not chew gum
- Take any medication (if your doctor agrees) with only a very small sip of water
- If you are an insulin-dependent diabetic, ask your doctor about whether or not to inject insulin
- Shower or bathe as advised
- Wear loose, comfortable clothing
- Remove makeup, lipstick and nail polish

WHAT TO BRING

- A copy of your doctor's orders for surgery or any paperwork given to you by your doctor to bring to the hospital
- A list of all your medications or your medication containers
- Formal ID, such as a legal ID card, a student ID or a driver's license
- Insurance cards and forms
- A parent or legal guardian if you are under the age of 18
- A case or box with your name on it for personal items

THINGS TO BE CLEAR ABOUT FOLLOWING SURGERY

- Medications that are prescribed to you
- Stitches, staples or incision care
- Bathing and showering
- Pain—what to expect and how to control it
- Physical activity, including housework
- What to eat
- Driving
- When to resume sexual relations

SIGNS AND SYMPTOMS FOLLOWING SURGERY THAT REQUIRE A DOCTOR'S ATTENTION

- Fever
- Unrelieved or prolonged pain
- Undue nausea or vomiting
- Pain, redness, heat or oozing from your suture, staple or incision line
- Inability to urinate or have a bowel movement

Complementary and Alternative Treatments

Complementary and alternative treatments involve botanicals, massage, acupuncture, dietary modalities, mind-body modalities or whole medical systems such as Ayurveda, and Traditional Chinese Medicine. Complementary treatments are treatments used in addition to conventional medical treatment, while alternative treatments are used in place of conventional treatment. A recent U.S. survey revealed that 38 percent of adults use complementary or alternative treatments.

THE OLDEST MEDICINE
Herbs have been used medicinally from ancient times and are still the primary source of medicine in many parts of the world.

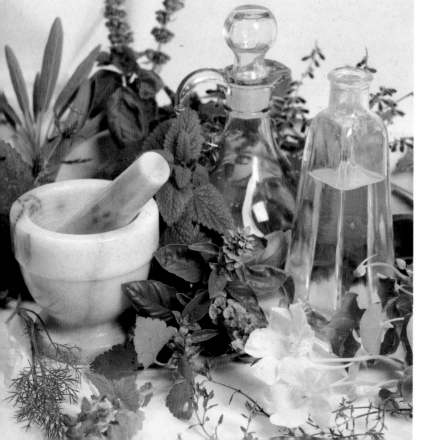

BOTANICAL MEDICINE

Botanical or herbal medicine is the oldest form of medicine known. More than 80 percent of the population has used herbs for health. Unfortunately, it is often not known why a particular herb produces its effect. You should consult your doctor as well as a herbalist before trying herbs—and no herb should be used during pregnancy, while breastfeeding, or given to children without a doctor's specific approval.

Herbal medicine uses plant material from around the world to treat ailments. All parts of the plant—stems, leaves, roots and seeds—may be used by herbal practitioners, who regard the active ingredients of each as useful in preventing or treating illness. Medical herbalists always look at the patient's habits, lifestyle and overall wellbeing—not just the symptoms—to find and treat the underlying cause of any problem. Remedies are tailored to the individual, so no two are likely to be the same.

Mother Nature's approach

Although many pharmaceutical drugs are extracted from plants or contain synthesized versions of substances found in plants, herbalists believe that giving the whole plant is safer and more effective than an isolated chemical.

Plants contain other substances apart from the active one, and these can sometimes enhance its action or prevent side effects, herbalists explain. For example, the drug ephedrine, used to treat asthma in conventional medicine, also raises blood pressure. But the plant it comes from contains a substance that prevents a rise in blood pressure.

Unfortunately, some plants such as rhubarb have one part that heals and another that is toxic. That is why it is always best to consult a herbalist who has a degree in botany, plant pharmaceuticals, or other related field.

What they're used to treat

Herbs are used to treat almost any condition, acute or chronic. Complaints commonly taken to herbalists include skin problems such as psoriasis, acne and eczema, and digestive problems such as ulcers, colitis, irritable bowel syndrome (IBS) and indigestion.

Although they are not medical doctors, herbalists also treat hormonal and gynaecological disorders–premenstrual syndrome (PMS), endometriosis, infertility, problems connected with the menopause and postnatal depression– and circulation disorders such as varicose veins and hypertension. Other conditions herbalists may help include arthritis, migraine, headaches, hay fever, asthma, insomnia and stress, and infections such as flu and tonsillitis. Be careful about what you take since some herbs interact with medications.

The first visit

Your first visit to a herbalist may take at least an hour. The therapist will want to find out about your symptoms and state of mind as well as what you eat and the sort of life you lead. You may also be given a physical examination, similar to that conducted by a family doctor, to obtain a blood pressure reading, to test your reflexes or to assess the condition

STOP AND SMELL THE FLOWERS

"Flower remedies" are diluted infusions of wild plants for the self-treatment of emotional symptoms. Although evidence to support their efficacy is slim, you will find them in natural health stores.

There are now some two dozen remedy producers worldwide, but the original and best-known remedies are those developed by the English doctor and homeopath Edward Bach (pronounced batch) in the 1930s. The following are examples of Bach Flower Remedies:

Rescue Remedy A combination of five remedies to treat shock or to comfort at times of stress (also available as cream).

Clematis For inattention, dreaminess, absentmindedness or mental escapism.

Elm For when you feel overwhelmed by inadequacy and responsibility.

Larch For lack of self-confidence, feelings of inferiority and fear of failure.

Walnut Assists in adjusting to change such as the menopause or divorce.

of your heart or lungs. Treatment can take a variety of forms. The most common is a tincture, which is an herbal extract preserved in alcohol that you take as drops. You may be given dried herbs that you brew in the same way as tea to make an infusion, or you may be asked to make a decoction, in which you boil tough material such as roots and bark and then strain and drink the liquid. Infusions and decoctions can taste very strange. Tablets, suppositories, creams or ointments may also be prescribed.

Work as a team

You may be asked to change your diet or to make some small adjustments to your lifestyle, such as getting more exercise or giving yourself time to relax. As with all alternative medicine, healing is a matter of teamwork between you, the therapist and the treatment. The aim is to restore the body's natural balance, which is called homeostasis.

The follow-up appointment will be shorter and may occur two weeks later, with further monthly visits if necessary. You can often combine herbal treatment with conventional drugs, but you must ensure that both your doctor and your herbalist know that you are doing this.

CLEMATIS CURE
Clematis vitalba, also known as wild clematis or Traveller's joy, is one of the ingredients in the Bach Flower Remedy for absentmindedness. Be sure to use prepared remedies only, since parts of the plant are poisonous.

MIND-BODY TREATMENTS

There may be a need, at different times and stages of your life, to discover ways of getting in touch with the inner person, to be able to use the strength of your mind to improve your physical health and wellbeing. Relaxation and yoga are two techniques that may help you.

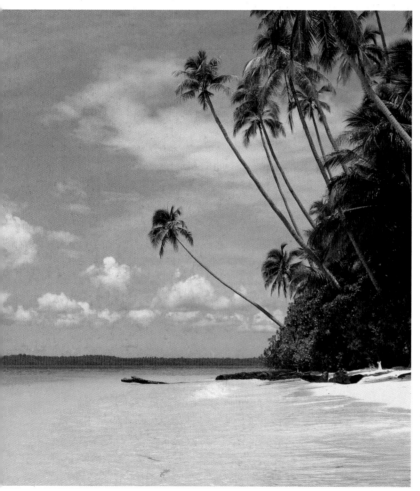

LETTING GO
Try to relax by imagining you are in a beautiful place, such as a tropical beach; absorb the sights, sounds and smells you find there. Although this technique needs practice, it can be very therapeutic.

Relaxation and guided imagery
Together, relaxation and guided imagery help you calm tension in your body while you conjure up attractive images to still worries in your mind. Once learned, these techniques enable you to counter the stress you feel, get things back in proportion and remain confident despite setbacks. They are "mindful" techniques that stop you from carrying tension without realizing it. They help you to be more aware of the present and the pleasures it holds.

Relaxation is an acquired skill that you can call on in any situation that stresses you. The methods you use will be the ones you find the easiest to do. You may try breath focus, for example, in which you pay attention to your breathing while concentrating on muscle tension in those parts of the body where stress shows–such as the forehead, jaw, neck, back, shoulders and stomach. Think of the muscle as you inhale, let go of the tension in it as you exhale. As frown lines go, the jaw unclenches, the neck relaxes and you start to feel the effects. It may be something to practise as you go to sleep.

Progressive muscle relaxation (PMR) is similar, but you increase the degree of muscular tension before you relax and let go. It is particularly helpful for those women who have hyperactive minds and who are showing stress from too much happening in their lives. But you need to take time to practise it. Following a few minutes of deep breathing, you focus on each muscle in your body, starting from the top and working down (or down, and working up if you prefer) and force yourself to stay there mentally until you feel relaxed in that part. It may be a way to prepare yourself for meditation that can lead to a profound sense of calmness in mind and body.

Body-oriented methods of relaxation might not suit women with eating disorders or with chronic pain (from endometriosis, migraine or skeletal problems), as they focus your attention too closely on the source of the pain or physical distress and therefore may be counterproductive.

Instead, guided imagery may provide the answer. It involves imagining yourself in an imaginary place and paying attention to sights, sounds and colours you experience there. You can feel the warmth on your skin, smell the sea or flowers, appreciate the hues of a sunset or the gentle lapping of waves on the sand. You close your eyes, see the image and become calm.

Another image encourages you to see your medication at work in the body destroying a disease–acting like a machine gun on a tumour, for example, or imagining the drug as an army attacking a mass of abnormal cells.

Yoga

A gentle, noncompetitive form of physical and mental exercise that is suitable for all ages and levels of fitness, yoga originated in India at the same time as Ayurvedic medicine. Yoga has many strands–Hatha, Raja, Ashtanga, Tantric, Kundalini–all of which encourage full use of your lungs so that energy, vitality and blood circulation are improved. The form of yoga that is best known in the West is Hatha, which consists of asayanas (physical postures), pranayamas (breathing techniques) and relaxation or meditation that leaves you feeling revitalized. It works on every single part of the body, including internal organs, and aims to create suppleness rather than stamina and promote a balanced mental outlook.

It's ideal for people already suffering from physical problems or just starting to exercise, as each individual works at her own pace and the postures range from the extremely simple to the more demanding. With your doctor's consent, it is perfectly safe in pregnancy; in fact, in the third trimester it may be of great use in cases where the baby is breech, because it encourages flexibility in the muscles and relaxation in the mother so the baby may find the room to turn. The breathing learned in yoga classes helps to prepare the body for pain control during contractions in labour and in addition keeps muscles toned for pelvic floor exercises after birth.

Get expert help It is best to learn yoga from an experienced teacher initially as it can be difficult to make sense of the postures from a book. A teacher will be able to gauge your level of fitness and stop you from undertaking anything that might cause a strain. It is important to learn to relax properly at the end of a session, which is something you might be tempted to skip unless you understand more fully what yoga is all about. To gain the full benefits of yoga, it is best to practise a little at least every other day, but if you don't have the time even a class once a week can make a big difference to your body.

No special clothes are needed, but it is important to wear something you can bend and stretch in, such as leggings and a T-shirt. A mat is necessary; special nonslip yoga mats are available, but a rug or blanket is fine to start with. Leave an hour or two between a meal and starting a yoga session and don't drink anything immediately beforehand.

LISTEN TO YOUR BODY

In the technique of biofeedback, a person with an illness is linked to monitors that translate her heart rate, blood pressure, muscle tension or brainwave activity into sounds or video images that can be easily interpreted. A trained therapist teaches you to use mental means to gain some degree of control over previously unconscious processes. The therapist does this by helping you recognize the subtle shifts in heart rate and electrical activity on the skin. This technique is especially useful in relaxation training. Biofeedback sessions may benefit a range of people, including those with eating disorders, hypertension, migraine headaches, addictions related to anxiety and spinal injuries.

STILLNESS HEALS
Breathing techniques combined with meditation help you move into deep relaxation, stilling your mind, encouraging mental balance and blocking disease-enhancing stress chemicals.

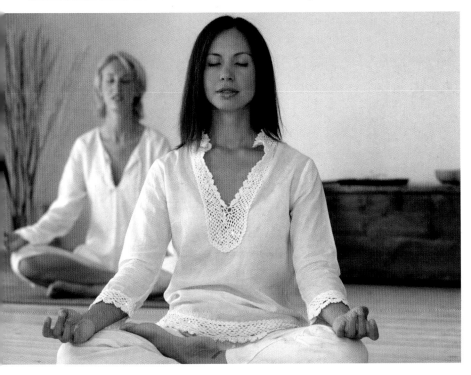

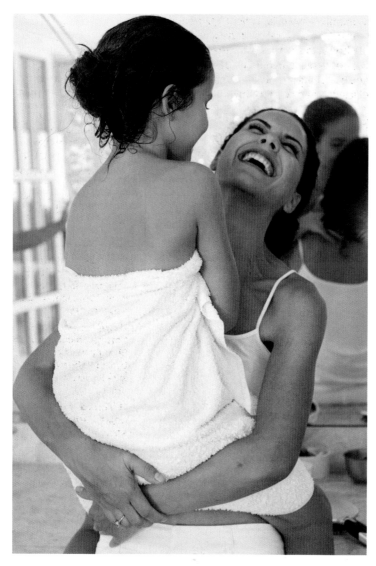

PROTECT YOUR BACK
Even young, fit people can get aches and pains from lifting and bending incorrectly. The trick is to keep your back straight while the push is exerted through your legs. This is especially important when lifting something relatively heavy, such as a child.

POSTURAL TREATMENTS

The Alexander Technique, the Feldenkrais Method and Pilates are therapies concerned with posture. Often recommended by doctors for people with bad backs, these therapies are also excellent for proper body mechanics.

The Alexander Technique

This therapy teaches people to be aware of the way they use or misuse their bodies so that they can avoid habitual tension and eventually move in an effortless, graceful way.

Frederick Alexander, an Australian actor, suddenly started to lose his voice during performances. When doctors were unable to uncover the cause, he decided to observe himself in the mirror while reciting and noticed that he habitually tensed his neck muscles. This affected his breathing and consequently his voice. By constantly checking and correcting himself, he was able to perform in a more natural way, and began to teach others to do the same.

We develop physical tension for several reasons. As children we pick up bad postural habits from slouching or from sitting for long periods at badly designed desks. We breathe shallowly, rather than using the entire extent of our lungs. Many of us have jobs that force us to spend hour after hour in positions contrary to the natural shape and movement of the body. As a result, it is easy to lose touch with our bodies, and we often fail to recognize the stress we are placing on them.

Get needs assessed In an Alexander Technique lesson your teacher assesses how you are misusing your body and will gently encourage it to assume the correct position. At first you may find the natural position much more difficult to sustain than the tense one. Among our common bad habits is tilting one way or the other, or holding the head too far forwards. As the teacher corrects this you may feel you have tilted the other way or that your head is thrust back. You are in the process of being re-educated. Emphasis is placed on the position of the head, neck and spine as Alexander felt that once these were positioned correctly, everything else would follow naturally.

Re-educating the body can take time. The recommended number of Alexander Technique lessons is at least 10 and preferably as many as 30. Lessons are one-to-one and last about 45 minutes. They start with simple movements, such as walking, sitting and lying down and progress to more complicated ones.

Instruction is a combination of demonstration by the teacher of what you are doing, discussion between the two of you and gentle guidance by the teacher with his or her hands. You remain fully clothed but take your shoes off. You should wear your normal clothes because this gives the teacher the most accurate picture of your everyday range and type of movement.

Lose excess tension Anyone can benefit from Alexander Technique lessons, since we all hold tension in our bodies, even if we think we have good posture. Being tense uses up energy, and releasing tension can give you new vitality and a sense of lightness.

Many people find they grow taller as they stop "crunching" their spines, or wider as their shoulders stop hunching forwards and their rib cage expands to its proper shape. The technique is popular with musicians, actors and athletes for enhancing performance and reducing fatigue. Musicians, in particular, have to spend many hours with their bodies twisted out of alignment as they play their instruments and can be shown ways of minimizing this distortion and restoring their posture. Singers and actors who have to project their voices need to feel that their chests and neck muscles are relaxed rather than tense.

Lifelong cure Alexander Technique is best known as a cure for back and neck pain but can help other joint pain, headaches and migraine. People with respiratory disorders, such as asthma, digestive disorders, such as irritable bowel syndrome, and high blood pressure may benefit from a course of Alexander lessons. The Alexander Technique does not aim to be a quick fix. The intention is to give you good habits to last a lifetime.

The Feldenkrais Method

Moshe Feldenkrais was a physicist and judo expert who taught himself to walk again after crippling knee injuries. His experience led him to develop a method to help with movement difficulties. While the Alexander Technique employs an external ideal of posture, the Feldenkrais Method puts you in touch with your nervous system to find your best posture. It does not emphasize the head/neck/spine relationship of the Alexander Technique but seeks to discover the imbalance upsetting the rest of the body and teaching you how to adapt.

As with the Alexander Technique, Feldenkrais is helpful for joint pain but can also be effective in dealing with central nervous system conditions such as multiple sclerosis, cerebral palsy and stroke. The purpose of training in this method is to show you how to expand your options, to find new ways of moving and breathing so you can live more fully, efficiently and comfortably.

Pilates

Pilates grows ever more popular because its exercises help you develop a leaner, longer line by strengthening the deep postural, abdominal muscles. The exercises are performed following the six principles of concentration, breathing, control, centering, flowing movement and precision. As with the Alexander Technique, Pilates is very popular with dancers because it promotes graceful and balanced movement.

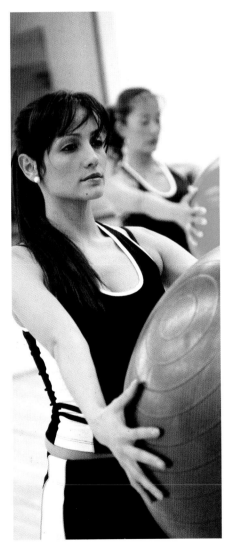

PILATES EXERCISES
Most of the exercises involve bending and stretching slowly and rhythmically, with calm concentration. The whole of your body should be aligned and controlled throughout, with the effort performed on each exhalation of breath.

BUILD A BETTER BODY

- If you have to stand for long periods of time, position one leg behind the other with the feet at about 45 degrees to each other and your body weight resting mostly on the rear leg.

- When sitting, keep your feet in contact with the ground. If you have to lean forwards, do it from the hips so that your back and shoulders are straight. To get up, bring your buttocks to the edge of the chair so that your body weight is over your feet before you stand up.

- Get up from time to time and move around. Shrug your shoulders, turn your head from side to side several times.

- When lifting a heavy object, bend at the knees as well as the hips so that, as you come up again, the muscles of your thighs take the strain, not your back.

- Change position frequently.

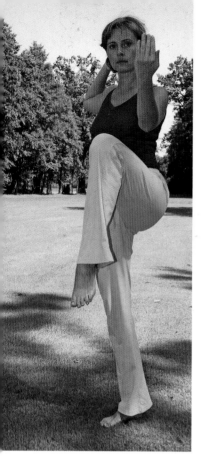

SERENE MOVEMENT
The focused movements of t'ai chi help to improve balance and encourage a sense of peace.

MOVEMENT THERAPIES

Movement-related mind-body treatments such as t'ai chi chu'an and qigong from Traditional Chinese Medicine work on your "vital energy"–qi–and its pathways in your body, seeking to find natural harmony around and within you and harnessing it. Other movement-related therapies from the Western world can help women with medical conditions express emotions such as anger, which can aid the healing process. These therapies do not need any knowledge of dance and can be adapted to varying levels of fitness or special needs. All movement therapies seek to release stress and harmonize mind and body.

T'ai chi chu'an

More commonly known as t'ai chi (pronounced tie chee), this therapy consists of a series of movements linked together into one flowing sequence. It can be performed by people of all ages and levels of fitness.

T'ai chi was originally developed in China in the 11th century to mitigate the aggressive nature of martial arts. It aims to harmonize your yin and yang (feminine and masculine qualities) and balance the flow of energy through the body. The graceful actions do not require strength and are performed fairly slowly. This, combined with the concentration needed to remember each movement, helps take your mind off your problems. It is a calming antidote to stress and stress-related illness, helping to clear mental blocks.

You need to learn t'ai chi in a class. It may take six months of classes to learn the movements, but you will start to feel the benefits immediately because the sequences affect every muscle, tendon and joint. You should practise for at least 10 minutes a day at home. It does not increase your heart rate or make you breathless, but you may sweat from the heat your qi is generating. You will feel your posture, balance, breathing and circulation improve.

Qigong

Sometimes written as "chi kung," the term qigong describes another ancient practice based on Traditional Chinese Medicine. The technique involves many exercises, all of which involve meditation, controlled breathing (*see* box, opposite), deceptively simple postures and movements and visualization of qi as it moves in the body. It was developed specifically for healing and in China today is often included in hospital aftercare to speed recovery and to help patients whose illnesses may not have responded to other forms of medicine.

Dance

Dance movement is a nonverbal form of psychotherapy that helps a wide variety of people, some who are simply interested in self-development, others who are emotionally disturbed or who have physical or mental illness. The therapy can work on an individual or group level; either way you will probably see the therapist on your own to start with. Therapists work both privately and within health, education and social services departments.

Dance movement therapy is particularly helpful for people with severe behavioural problems or for those whose feelings are too complicated or deep to put into words. It can be useful for individuals who are blind or deaf or have learning disabilities. It may also be a beneficial therapy for stress-related physical illness.

Gabrielle Roth's five rhythms

Working in the United States, Gabrielle Roth is a proponent of experimental dance and theatre. The key to her work is spontaneity–in workshops using her methods, you are encouraged to express yourself freely through dance. The goal of her technique is to put you back in touch with your body and to liberate your natural creativity and joy.

The technique is named after the five different types of music or rhythms that are used. These are flowing, staccato, chaotic, lyrical and still. Gabrielle Roth workshops may last for one day or may consist of a course performed in groups. Additional workshops may offer poetry writing, painting or drama–all of a spontaneous nature.

Biodanza

This dance therapy from South America was developed by a professor of medicine to help people emotionally and physically. It is held in groups because improving your relationship with other people is part of the therapy. Dance exercises focus on five modes of living: your integrity and vitality; sensuality and sexuality; creativity and your ability to change; affectivity or your capacity to love; and transcendence–the expansion of consciousness and sense of ecstasy.

Medau

This dance therapy aims to produce a strong, lithe body in harmony and at ease with itself. Movements are rhythmic and dynamic, without jerky repetitions or overstretching. It has been adapted to help problems such as back pain, high blood pressure, arthritis, Parkinson's disease and psychiatric disorders.

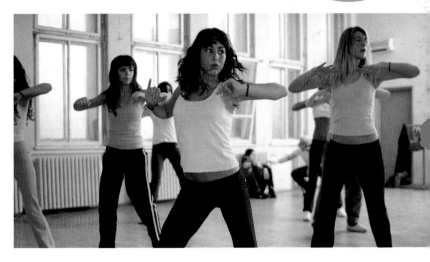

LET GO!
The rhythm of music can unlock energy while stimulating and balancing the body. Dance movement therapy is a valuable treatment for a range of conditions, physical or mental, and can provide relaxation for women of all ages.

The heart of qigong

Standing with good, relaxed posture is at the heart of qigong. By "centering" your weight on your frame and calming yourself with breathing, you won't waste any energy by holding unnecessary tension inside. Once learned, the technique helps you carry out actions using energy economically while gaining access to the unlimited source of energy within. Begin by doing the exercise for a few minutes at a time.

Imagine you are hanging from the crown of your head like a puppet on a string and that all your tension is sinking downwards and going out through your feet. Concentrate on each of the elements shown at right until they become second nature.

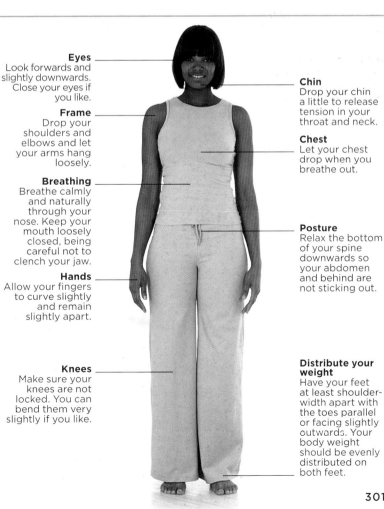

Eyes
Look forwards and slightly downwards. Close your eyes if you like.

Frame
Drop your shoulders and elbows and let your arms hang loosely.

Breathing
Breathe calmly and naturally through your nose. Keep your mouth loosely closed, being careful not to clench your jaw.

Hands
Allow your fingers to curve slightly and remain slightly apart.

Knees
Make sure your knees are not locked. You can bend them very slightly if you like.

Chin
Drop your chin a little to release tension in your throat and neck.

Chest
Let your chest drop when you breathe out.

Posture
Relax the bottom of your spine downwards so your abdomen and behind are not sticking out.

Distribute your weight
Have your feet at least shoulder-width apart with the toes parallel or facing slightly outwards. Your body weight should be evenly distributed on both feet.

Whole Medical Systems

Whole medical systems are entire systems of theory and practice that have evolved independently from conventional medicine. Homeopathic medicine and Traditional Chinese Medicine (TCM) are examples. Often, these systems have evolved earlier than the conventional medical approach.

HOMEOPATHY

In use for more than 200 years, homeopathy uses a holistic approach. It is based on the principle that "like cures like"–something that causes symptoms in a well person can also cure the same symptoms in someone who is sick. This is somewhat similar to the principle behind vaccinations, but because of the way they are prepared, homeopathic remedies are so greatly diluted they contain no chemical trace of the active substance and are therefore safe. They were developed at the end of the 18th century by a German doctor, Samuel Hahnemann, after he became disillusioned with the medical practices of his time. Today homeopathic practitioners are rarely medical doctors.

Homeopathic remedies

Remedies are prepared from plants, minerals and animal substances (such as snake venom). The substances are steeped in liquid that is then drained off and diluted many times until there is so little left of the original substance that it is not detectable scientifically. With each dilution the liquid is "succussed", or shaken vigorously, which causes an "energy imprint" of the original substance to be left in it. This imprint works on the body's own energy system, boosting its natural healing responses.

There are about 3,000 remedies, and finding the correct one is complicated. Remedies are chosen because the substances in large doses would cause the symptoms from which you are suffering. The practitioner, who is not a medical doctor, will need to take into account the nature of all your symptoms,

The Medicine Chest

These mineral salts, found naturally in the human body, may be prescribed by homeopaths, naturopaths and herbalists to correct a disease caused by deficiency of one of them. For instance, lack of calc phos can manifest itself as teeth problems or an inability to absorb nutrients. There are 12 biochemical tissue salts, taken in highly diluted combinations of two or more.

Calc Fluor
(calcium fluoride)

Calc Phos
(calcerea phosphorica)

Calc Sulph
(calcium sulfate)

Ferr Phos
(iron phosphate)

Kali Mur
(potassium chloride)

Kali Phos
(potassium phosphate)

kali Sulph
(potassium sulfate)

Mag Phos
(magnesium phosphate)

Nat Rur
(natrium muriaticum/sodium chloride)

Nat Phos
(natrium/sodium phosphate)

Nat Sulph
(natrium/sodium sulfate)

Silicea (silica)

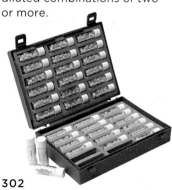

physical and emotional. He or she will also need to find out all about you and your personality and may prescribe a "constitutional" remedy, geared to your particular physical and mental constitution and designed to give you an overall boost. A homeopath usually prescribes one remedy at a time.

What to expect

Remedies are generally given as pills that you dissolve on or under the tongue. You should not touch them with your fingers but put directly on your tongue from the packet or tip into your mouth from the lid and suck. You should not eat or drink for 15 minutes before and after taking the remedies. Sometimes your symptoms will worsen for a short time when you start the remedies. In homeopathic terms, this indicates that your body's defences are being stimulated. Homeopathy works from the inside out, and often external symptoms, such as a skin complaint, can be the last to clear up. You may find that your symptoms reverse. For example, if your hay fever started as itchy eyes, proceeded to sneezing and then attacked your chest, the symptoms may recur in reverse order as you start to get better.

If you are taking any conventional medicine, tell your doctor and your homeopath in case of interactions.

A HOMEOPATHIC PHARMACY

Homeopaths maintain special pharmacies that provide over-the-counter remedies to help people with certain symptoms. In homeopathy, symptom analysis is key to a prescription. Talk with the homeopathic pharmacist about your choices and the dilutions recommended, and follow instructions precisely.

SYMPTOMS	REMEDY
OBESITY	
Fearful and depressed, slightly obsessional, cold but sweaty, lack of energy, indigestion, recurrent infections	Calcerea
Moody, anxious, depressed, tendency to wake and worry in the early hours of the morning	Kali phos
Constant eating but never feel satisfied, talk too much but do too little, diarrhoea, indigestion, flatulence	Sulphur
SMOKING	
Dry smoker's cough, usually worse in morning	Bryonia
Trying to quit smoking	Tabacum
Restlessness, low body weight, pale, chest weakness	Tuberculinum
CYSTITIS	
Continuous passing of urine	Belladonna
Urine feels hot and is passed in drops with violent burning pain	Cantharis

SYMPTOMS	REMEDY
COLDS AND HAY FEVER	
Violent sneezing, dry cough	Aconite
Throbbing headache, obstructed nose, pain in throat	Chamomile
Sore runny nose, mouth dry, eyes irritated, feverish	Arsenicum album
Much sneezing, runny nose, dry hacking cough	Allium cepa
Eyes worse than nose, sneezing with streaming eyes first thing in morning	Euphrasia
Nose blocked at night, sneezing in morning, sensitivity to light, itching in ears	Nux vomica
MENSTRUAL PROBLEMS	
Irregular periods, heavy, painful periods coming on too soon	Belladonna
Painful periods	Mag phos
Irregular periods, spasmodic period pains especially in lower back, irritability	Nux vomica
Irregular or absent periods, heavy or late periods with pain on left	Pulsatilla

AYURVEDA

Ayurveda (which means "science of life") is a complete health care system that originated in India about 3,000 years ago. There, and in Sri Lanka, it is a mainstream form of treatment that is practised alongside Western-style medicine. It is rapidly gaining popularity in the Western world.

According to Ayurveda, the world is composed of five elements: space, air, fire, water and earth. Existence is governed by three "doshas" (energies), each made up of two of the elements. Health in general consists of finding a balance between these three energies. Each person tends to be dominated by one dosha and needs to work with this energy to find the lifestyle uniquely suited to her.

Ayurvedic medicine recognizes six stages of disease and aims to intervene at the first stage, when the doshas first get out of balance. Western medicine tends to intervene only at the third or fourth, when marked symptoms appear. Health

is a dynamic process that needs to take into account not just a person's age and constitution but also the seasons and climate, even the movements of the planets. Treatment is wide ranging and may include massage, self-massage, detoxification (for example, saunas, enemas or laxatives), diet, herbal and other remedies, surgery, counselling, meditation, yoga, crystals and astrology.

Some methods of treatment are unique to Ayurvedic medicine. For instance, medicines for the head are sometimes administered through the nose. Herbal remedies, minerals, metals and some animal substances are prescribed. Dietary recommendations cover not simply what you eat but when and how the food is prepared. Cooking ingredients are important not only for their nutritional value but also for their taste because different tastes have different effects on the doshas. Crystals are used for spiritual healing to focus the mind and spirit, and astrology helps people view their lives in a wider, more cosmic, context.

SOOTHING A COLD
Part of Ayurvedic medicine treats an imbalance with its opposite in order to restore mental and physical well-being. For example, a cold may be soothed with warmth by slowly dripping warm oil onto the forehead.

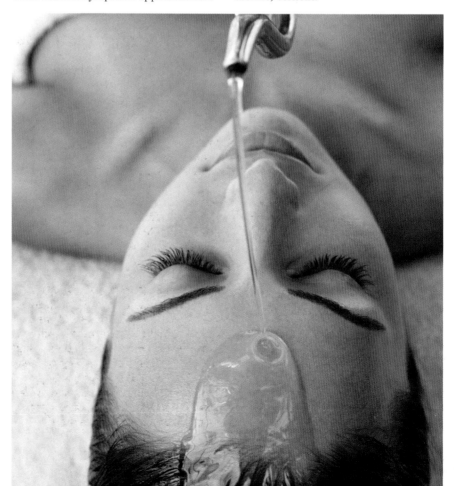

THE DOSHAS

Ayurvedic practitioners believe there are three kinds of energy in the body that are called doshas, and our constitutions are characterized by the relationships between these. One or two of these doshas will usually be dominant, and each person can be described as a pitta type or a vátha/kapha type, for example. You are born with your doshas in balance, but they may need readjusting throughout life.

ELEMENTS	MENTAL	PHYSICAL	MENTAL EFFECTS OF IMBALANCE	PHYSICAL EFFECTS OF IMBALANCE
VÁTHA				
Air Space	Creativity, energy	Nervous system	Confusion, loss of energy, insomnia, anxiety	Constipation, weight loss, sensitivity to cold
PITTA				
Fire Water	Confidence, courage	Memory, heat regulation, digestion, vision	Irritability, anger, dullness	Digestive disorders, impaired vision, acne, skin rashes, premature greying
KAPHA				
Earth Water	Tolerance, centredness, compassion	Structure of body, growth, weight	Intolerance, insecurity, jealousy	Weight gain, mucus and congestion, achy joints

The six stages of disease

The relative amounts of doshas that make up your type are inherited from your parents; you are born with them in a state of balance that is right for you– these are called "prakruthi". What you eat is the basis of prakruthi, as different sorts of foods are more suited to different dosha types. Through stress, the wrong diet or injury, your constitution can become unbalanced, and you enter a state called vikruthi. Practitioners do not aim to change the constitution you inherited, but they try to restore its original balance.

According to Ayurvedic medicine, a disease builds up gradually through six stages from a mild version to the full-blown condition:

Accumulation Excess dosha accumulates in its natural sites in the body, causing only minor discomfort. Ayurvedic practitioners aim to intervene at this stage.

Aggravation Accumulated dosha becomes irritated, producing more specific symptoms.

Dispersion Aggravated dosha spills out into the rest of the body, causing much more widespread symptoms.

Relocation Clear signs of dysfunction appear in both the original site and other parts of the body. This stage corresponds with the time people in the Western world generally seek medical attention.

Manifestation The symptoms can be grouped into the specific diseases recognized by Western medicine.

Maturation The disease is fully developed. There still exists a possibility of a cure, but it becomes chronic or fatal if left untreated.

How to choose a practitioner

Training in Ayurvedic medicine includes five years in medical school and one in hospital practice. There are currently only a few schools outside India offering the full training and not enough trained practitioners to meet demands. To try this healing system, you can locate your nearest practitioner by contacting your local professional Ayurveda society.

TRADITIONAL CHINESE MEDICINE (TCM)

As in Ayurvedic medicine, Traditional Chinese Medicine is a whole medical system that is practised alongside conventional medicine in China and in many parts of the West.

TCM has components that include herbal medicine, massage, acupuncture and movement based on mind-body modalities. Proponents say that the best results come from using two or more of the components at the same time.

As with Ayurvedic medicine, TCM's theoretical basis is completely different from that of Western science. In holistic terms, illness of all kinds, whether physical, emotional, mental or spiritual, is the result of an imbalance in our vital energy–called "qi" (pronounced chee, sometimes written as "chi"). An imbalance can be caused by internal factors, such as heredity, and emotions and by external factors, such as weather, pollution, infection, injury and drugs. TCM aims to restore this balance.

The flow of energy

Qi, the source of all the body's activity and maintenance, is in a constant state of flux. It is divided into complementary forces called yin and yang and is manifested in five interrelated elements: wood, fire, earth, metal and water. These elements both nourish and control each other–for example, water nourishes wood (trees) but controls fire.

These forces and elements are related to parts of the body, functions and emotions, and the practitioner uses these connections to assess exactly where an imbalance might be and what is causing it.

In TCM, prevention is as important as a cure and is recommended as a way of maintaining equilibrium–called homeostasis. Balance is particularly important at times of change or stress, as well as for a wide variety of conditions, both physical and mental.

Yin and yang

The balance of yin and yang is key to the flow of qi and so to health and wellbeing in TCM. Traditionally, yin is associated

The flow of qi

The channels along which the energy called qi flows are known as meridians. The meridians correspond to yin and yang organs:

- Arm tai yin (lung, or Lu)
- Leg tai yin (spleen, or Sp)
- Arm shao yin (heart, or He)
- Leg shao yin (kidney, or Kid)
- Arm jue yin (pericardium, or Per)
- Leg jue yin (liver, or Liv)
- Arm yang ming (large intestine, or LI)
- Leg yang ming (stomach, or St)
- Arm tai yang (small intestine, or SI)
- Leg tai yang (bladder, or Bl)
- Arm shao yang (san jiao, or SJ)
- Leg shao yang (gallbladder, or GB)

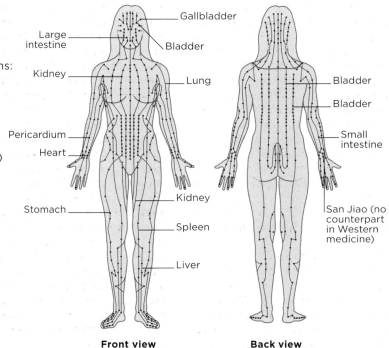

Front view

Back view

Front view labels: Gallbladder, Bladder, Large intestine, Kidney, Lung, Pericardium, Heart, Kidney, Stomach, Spleen, Liver

Back view labels: Bladder, Bladder, Small intestine, San Jiao (no counterpart in Western medicine)

THE FIVE ELEMENTS

The ideas behind Chinese medicine have grown out of close observation of the natural world. In the philosophy of TCM, the ways in which nature deals with or meets changes—called dynamic processes—are translated to the functioning of the body. The five elements have individual characteristics. Wood is growing, flexible, rooted. Fire is dry, hot, ascending, moving. Earth is productive, fertile, has potential for growth. Metal is cutting, hard, conducting. Water is wet, cool, descending, flowing, yielding. All have yin and yang aspects, and all five elements support each other. The aim of TCM is to apply the elements to the health of the body and to discover what it is that is causing disharmony.

	PARTS OF THE BODY	SENSE ORGAN	EMOTION	TISSUE
WOOD				
	Liver, gallbladder	Eyes	Anger	Tendon
FIRE				
	Heart, small intestine	Tongue	Joy	Blood vessel
EARTH				
	Spleen, stomach	Mouth	Worry	Muscle
METAL				
	Lungs, large intestine	Nose	Grief, melancholy	Skin
WATER				
	Kidney, bladder	Ears	Fear	Bone

with female characteristics, and with shade, passivity and softness. Yin governs the front of the body, the interior organs and the muscles. Yang is associated with masculine traits, with the sun and vitality, and governs the back of the body and the skin.

An imbalance of too much yin can lead to physical symptoms of chronic disease, diarrhoea and to feeling cold and sleepy. Mental symptoms include being too submissive, impractical, overly sensitive and lacking conviction. Too much yang leads to the opposite: acute disease, constipation and feeling hot and restless. Mentally, an imbalance of yang makes people domineering, insensitive, dogmatic and overly materialistic.

What you can expect

As in Ayurvedic medicine, detailed advice on diet and lifestyle is an integral part of the treatment. You will be asked when and how you eat, the taste of the food, the time you get up or go to bed, about how much you exercise–since all are deemed relevant to your health and wellbeing. As well as finding out all about you and your life, in much the same way as a Western doctor does, a practitioner of TCM will take your pulse in six places on each wrist and also examine the state of your tongue, nails, skin and hair.

Remedies may contain animal parts, such as powdered deer horn or insect skin. If you do not want these particular remedies because you suspect that they may be prepared from endangered species or for any other reason, you should say so, and the practitioner can take steps to avoid them.

Make sure you see a reputable practitioner who uses a proper supplier because standards on imported herbal remedies are not as stringent as those on ones that are produced domestically. Practitioners should be registered so you should ensure this is the case before embarking on any treatment. Also be sure to check that language is not likely to be a barrier to communication with your practitioner.

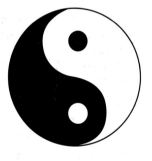

YIN AND YANG
The t'ai chi symbol illustrates how yin and yang are balanced and interlinked but opposite.

ACUPUNCTURE

The philosophy behind Traditional Chinese Medicine is to enhance wellbeing, keep illness and disability at bay and to lead a healthy and fulfilling life. Acupuncture–the use of needles to stimulate the flow of qi (energy) in the body–is as much a method of achieving these ends as is the use of herbal remedies. Its practice has evolved over many thousands of years, and today in Western countries qualified and experienced practitioners offer acupuncture treatment for a variety of different conditions.

Fully registered acupuncturists have completed a recognized training in Chinese medicine, meet the Western

Studies show that both acupuncture and acupressure can help to relieve physical pain.

standards of anatomy, physiology and pathology, and understand conditions in the same terms as a conventional doctor, although they do not offer treatment in that way. They should belong to a professional body such as BAcC (in the UK) or AACMA (in Australia).

In acupuncture terms, an illness shows that there is disharmony in the body caused by a deficiency or excess of the yin and/or yang energy or the presence of pathology, which may be either superficial or has penetrated internal tissue. Other considerations are how long the pathology has been there and what it may have affected during that time.

Even if you feel wary about the use of needles, it is completely safe because strict hygiene is standard practice, with rigorous infection control procedures. Made of stainless steel (some have copper-coil handles), the needles vary in length and thickness–the most common are fine–between 1.25 cm (½ in) and 7.5 cm (3 in) long. Most acupuncturists today use disposable needles.

What to expect

In a typical first session, which may last from 30 minutes to an hour, an acupuncturist will take a personal history, in a similar way to a conventional doctor. He or she will ask you to describe in your own words the problem you have. After this, diagnosis is made on the basis of four examinations.

The first part of the examination called looking, is an assessment of your physical appearance, your skin colour and tone, and your tongue. The second, hearing and smelling, may be done so discreetly that it may not even be obvious to you. The intention is to find clues of deficiency or excess. Next comes questioning, when the acupuncturist seeks more information about you that may have a bearing on the fuller picture of your disharmony. The final part is touching, during which the practitioner will gain understanding of your painful areas by feeling your skin to assess its temperature and condition, and taking your pulse in more than one place (the wrist and neck, for example).

The information gathered enables the acupuncturist to identify the type of disharmony you have and how it is affecting you before deciding on and explaining the treatment. It is rare that one treatment will resolve a problem; many over several months may be needed for chronic and longstanding conditions. Progress may be slow if acupuncture is sought as a last resort, as it commonly is.

Acupuncture is contraindicated in someone with low blood counts, high fever or a severe psychotic condition. It is sometimes used during pregnancy in the third trimester when the fetus is breech, or for labour pains. Moxabustion (the burning of small mugwort cones) may be recommended by a midwife.

A treatment should not be given if you have recently been drinking alcohol or taken drugs (although acupuncture is known for its successful use in alcohol and drug rehabilitation). When trying to quit smoking, acupuncture can help withdrawal symptoms and can be used at the same time as using nicotine patches or gum.

Needles and finger pressure

The 14 meridians of the body, known as energy pathways, have over 350 acupoints that acupuncturists categorize according to the effects they are believed to have on the body's organs. The acupuncturist will insert needles to stimulate or calm, or use acupressure–fingertip or nail massage–on those acupoints related to your condition. The insertion and manipulation of needles to achieve the desired therapeutic effect usually causes little pain, although there may be a heavy sensation. This is called "deqi", literally meaning acquiring the qi (energy).

Acupuncturists may also use moxabustion, the application of heat above an acupoint. The heat comes from tiny cones of smouldering mugwort leaves (*Artemisia vulgaris*, known as moxa), that burn down until the skin turns red. The musky odour of moxa may remain on clothing and hair for a time after the session. Moxa may be used with needles on an acupuncture point or in a special box that allows a larger area–such as the kidneys–to be warmed. To turn a baby from its breech position, a cone is burned on the little toe, on alternate sides, until the heat is felt. The number of sessions needed varies.

Acupoints and pain relief

There is much documentation to show that acupuncture and acupressure can relieve physical pain–they release the body's natural painkillers, endorphins and other neurotransmitters. Both may provide symptomatic relief in stroke rehabilitation and in relieving nausea, for example.

PLACING THE NEEDLES
The acupuncturist treats conditions by placing needles so that harmony is restored to the body. The needles do not hurt but may sometimes cause a heavy feeling.

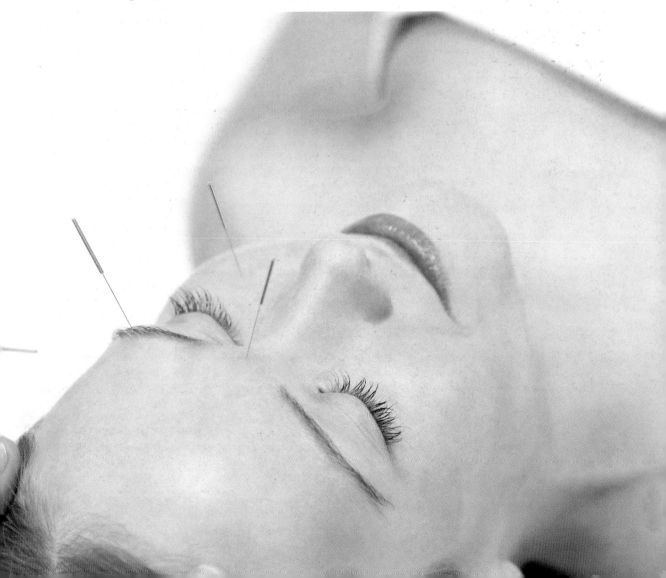

NATUROPATHY

Naturopaths are the family doctors of holistic medicine, and the practice goes back to ancient times. To them, disease is something that happens when an organism is not functioning as it should. The goal of a naturopath is to discover the best way of fighting disease and restoring homeostasis. He or she will use a variety of therapies to support the body's own natural healing powers to restore wellness.

The principles of naturopathy maintain that the body has the ability to heal itself, and that symptoms of disease are the body's attempts to right itself and should not be suppressed. Treatment should not inflict further harm and is tailored to the individual not the disease. The long-term aim of treatment is to re-educate patients so they can take care of their health for themselves.

How it works

According to naturopaths, the fundamental requirements for good health are fresh air, clean water, gentle exercise, relaxation and a good diet. The causes of disease can be chemical, mechanical or psychological.

A naturopath may use therapies such as iridology (study of the iris, *see* box below) and acupuncture to provide further insight and manage your problem. Two treatments commonly used by naturopaths are hydrotherapy and nutritional therapy. Nutritional therapy uses fasting, special diets, the elimination of certain foods, and infusions that together allow the body to rest and detoxify. These measures are only temporary, but long-term dietary changes may be recommended, too. Nutritional supplements and herbal or homeopathic remedies may also be prescribed.

Naturopaths treat physical and mobility problems using therapies such as osteopathy, chiropractic and the Alexander Technique. They are skilled in special soft-tissue techniques that can relieve muscular tension, decongest and free movement in any part of the body, not just the joints. They may advise you on exercises to do at home. Counselling may be given or meditation and relaxation techniques taught to help your psychological outlook.

What to expect

Naturopaths use conventional medical techniques for diagnosis, such as blood and urine tests, and alternative ones.

In addition, like all alternative medicine practitioners, they will want details of your medical history, an in-depth view of your lifestyle and an understanding of your state of mind.

During treatment you may undergo a "healing crisis", which makes your symptoms temporarily worsen. In naturopathic terms, this is a good sign because it shows that the treatment is working. You may also find that old symptoms return, usually in the reverse order of their appearance.

As you get better, the symptoms should progress from the deeper tissues to the more superficial and from the more vital organs to the less vital.

Naturopathy can benefit anyone, whatever their age and complaint and can also be used preventively. It is worth considering for helping chronic conditions such as chronic fatigue syndrome, allergies, hay fever, asthma and migraine and can speed recovery from an infection or injury.

Iridology

Practitioners feel that this therapy may be used in conjunction with others to detect a tendency to disease that can be seen in the iris. Practitioners look for a range of signs that indicate poor health by studying the colour, texture and markings of the iris. There is, however, currently no scientific proof that this technique produces accurate results.

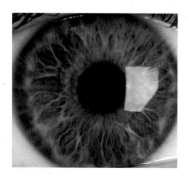

A MAP OF THE BODY
Iridologists believe that the iris maps the human glands, organs and body systems, so that flecks, streaks or other marks in the eye all have a counterpart in different areas or functions of the body. A special magnifying camera can make a slide for enlarged viewing and assessing.

HYDROTHERAPY

The medium of water, used either at different temperatures or with added minerals or herbs, may heal all kinds of disease. It is sometimes employed by osteopaths and physiotherapists and is a staple of naturopathy.

Modern hydrotherapy started in the 18th and 19th centuries in Germany and led to the establishment in Europe of hydrotherapy hotels or "hydros", many of which are still in existence and offer a wide range of healing and treatments. Similarly, "spas" use naturally warm mineral-rich spring waters for internal and external medical treatment. Thalassotherapy involves the use of seawater in the same way.

How it works

Hot water brings blood to the skin and takes it away from internal organs. This has a sedative effect on the body as a whole, relieves pain and stimulates the elimination of toxins through sweat. Cold water has the opposite effect. It increases blood flow to internal organs thereby stimulating the body as a whole, and it reduces inflammation in outer organs. Water sprays and jets massage the body and may give pain relief by stimulating nerves.

Other water therapies

Water is also used in a variety of other therapies:

Colonic irrigation A stream of fresh water is passed around the colon through the rectum for about 30 minutes to clean out accumulated waste matter. Usually several treatments are needed. Colonic practitioners believe that a modern diet high in processed foods damages the health of the intestines, which leads to toxins accumulating rather than being broken down and eliminated. These are then reabsorbed by the body and can lead to a range of health problems. However, this treatment may be harmful if it is done too often, so proceed with caution.

Water birth Being in warm water during labour is relaxing and can help to relieve pain. Many believe it is also a more soothing way for the baby to

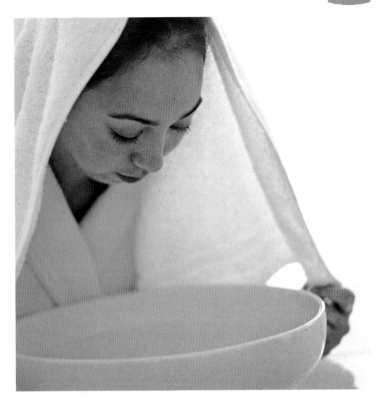

be born, as long as care is taken and proper professional guidance given on safety and scrupulous hygiene. Some hospitals have birthing pools, or you may be able to rent one.

Flotation This involves floating in warm water filled with mineral salts to make you completely buoyant in an enclosed compartment. In the darkness and silence, with no need to use your muscles, you reach a state of profound relaxation. The therapy is thought to help ease pain or stress-related conditions, as well as strengthen the immune system. Some centres even offer movies or music to aid the relaxation experience.

Sprays and affusions (pouring) These combine jets of hot or cold water directed at parts of the body to ease pain and to aid relaxation.

WRAPPING OR SWATHING
Damp sheets or towels are used to wrap the whole body or parts of it to help eliminate toxins.

STEAMING
Steam-bath cabinets enclose the entire body except the head and cause profuse sweating. Saunas are less humid. At home, a towel over a bowl of hot water can direct steam to the head or elsewhere.

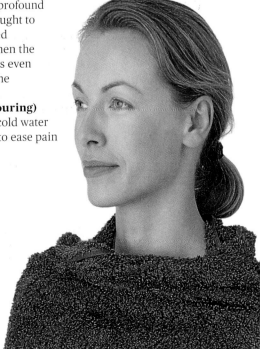

WHO CAN HELP?

If you feel nutritional therapy would benefit you, ask your doctor to recommend a nutritionist with a Ph.D. in nutritional science from a reputable college or university, or a registered dietitian. The assistant in your local natural foods' store does not qualify.

NUTRITIONAL THERAPY

A carefully worked out combination of special diets and nutritional supplements is used by nutritional therapists to treat an enormous number of ailments. Nutritional therapists consider many of today's diseases to be the result of poor nutrition or improperly absorbed nutrients as a result of bad eating habits, apathy, lack of money, lack of time or constant dieting. As well as nutritional deficiencies, food allergies and toxic overload can cause persistent tiredness and lead to long-term disease besides such dramatic and immediate symptoms as vomiting.

Pollutants in food, water and the environment increase our need for nutrients. Yet we now get fewer nutrients from food due to the modern chemical methods of growing and processing often used. Over time, environmental stress and malnutrition can damage your ability to absorb food, creating a vicious circle of ill health.

Whom it can help

Nutritional therapists treat problems clearly connected to food such as weight, adult-onset diabetes, food allergies or intolerances, and digestive disorders. The therapy may help with hormonal problems such as PMS or polycystic ovaries and with menopausal symptoms.

Nutritional therapy may be used preventively to reduce the risk of heart disease, cancer, adult-onset diabetes or osteoporosis occurring later in life. Preconceptional nutritional therapy for both partners may reduce the risk of miscarriage and birth defects and may help prevent your children from developing allergies.

What to expect

Therapists start by taking a detailed medical history. They will ask about your everyday diet and habits such as drinking alcohol and smoking. They also discuss what your exercise routine is, your emotional state and what medication, if any, you are on and any side effects you are experiencing. Your therapist may also use specialized blood tests to assess the general state of health of your body.

A nutritional therapist may prescribe an array of supplements—vitamins, minerals, enzymes, amino acids, essential fatty acids and fibre—depending on the person's needs. Diets are short term, and advice is given on menu planning and food preparation. A basic diagnostic diet, which usually lasts for two weeks, may be prescribed in order to exclude those foods that most commonly cause allergies.

Nutritional therapists recommend a varied wholefood diet of fresh food and

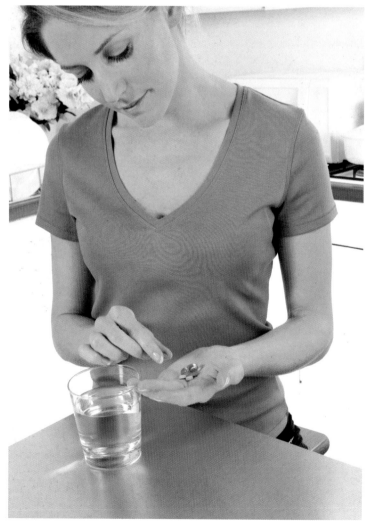

TAKING VITAMINS
A basic vitamin regime consists of a multivitamin, calcium, vitamin D and omega-3 fatty acids. These should be taken every day.

a minimum quantity of animal fats and protein. They encourage exercise and relaxation to restore a normal eating pattern again.

Understanding blood sugar

Maintaining a stable level of blood sugar is important to health. Foods are turned into sugar at different speeds. To find the correct balance for your needs, use the glycaemic index. Foods that are digested rapidly have a very high or high index; those that are digested slowly have a moderate to very low index.

Indications of low blood sugar are fluctuating energy, fatigue (especially upon waking and mid-afternoon), cravings for sweet foods such as cakes, irritability and lack of concentration. You may feel weak, light-headed or irritable if you skip or delay a meal.

Combating low blood sugar

If you have symptoms of low blood sugar levels, you should eat mostly foods with a low glycaemic index. Avoid high index foods since they tend to cause low blood sugar, even if you have an initial burst of energy after eating. Combine a high index food with one of a lower rating: for example, a baked potato with cheese, vegetables or chicken. Eat regularly, little and often, with no more than three to four hours between food. Snack on fresh fruit rather than biscuits between meals. Other healthy snacks based on natural foods include unsalted and unsweetened popcorn, plain yogurt, crackers, nuts, raw vegetable sticks and dried fruit such as apricots or figs.

Starchy foods can encourage the body to produce hormones that make you sleepy. This can account for a mid-afternoon slump, especially if your lunch consists of a sandwich, pasta salad, baked potato or french fries. Try instead to lunch on a salad with protein such as hard-boiled eggs, chicken or fish, or a sustaining and nutritious soup, and save your carbohydrate-based meals for breakfast or the evening.

Dehydration prevents the body from absorbing essential nutrients and energy. So drink plenty of water, especially if you are in the habit of drinking copious cups of strong coffee and tea.

GLYCAEMIC INDEX

Foods with a high glycaemic index may give an initial surge of energy, but this is often followed by a slump. Foods low on the index release energy slowly.

VERY HIGH

Cornflakes, glucose, maltose, puffed rice, rice cakes, white bread*

HIGH

Bananas, brown rice, carrots, corn, corn chips, mangoes, muesli, oat bran, parsnips, potatoes, raisins, rye crackers, white rice, wholegrain bread

MODERATE

Kidney beans (cooked or canned), lactose, oranges, peas, potato chips, pumpernickel bread, sucrose, white and wholewheat pasta

LOW

Apples, barley, chickpeas, lentils, milk, peaches, pears, wholegrain rye bread, yogurt

VERY LOW

Fish, fructose, grapefruit, green vegetables, meat, peanuts, plums, seafood, soya beans

*Foods with a high glycaemic index are generally those that are high in refined carbohydrates and sugar.

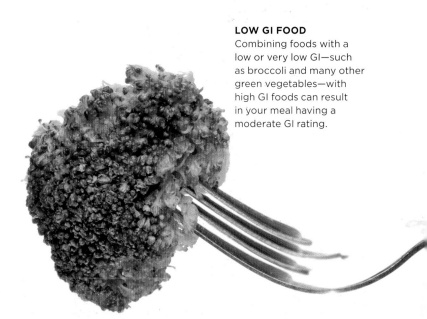

LOW GI FOOD
Combining foods with a low or very low GI—such as broccoli and many other green vegetables—with high GI foods can result in your meal having a moderate GI rating.

Index

Acknowledgements

The publisher would like to thank the following for their kind permission to reproduce their photographs:

Pages: 1 Shutterstock/Monkey Business Images; **2** Shutterstock/Ersler Dmitry; **3l** Shutterstock/Monkey Business Images; **3c** Shutterstock/Studio 1One; **3r** Shutterstock/Absolut; **6** iStock/Jacomstephens; **7** Shutterstock/Monkey Business Images; **8** Shutterstock/Stephen Coburn; **9l** Shutterstock/Diana Lundin; **9r** Shutterstock/Monkey Business Images; **10** iStock/Andresr; **12** Shutterstock/Rick Becker-Leckrone; **13br** Shutterstock/Lev Dolgachov; **13tr** iStock; **14** iStock/Ana Abejon; **14b & 15tr** Shutterstock/Monkey Business Images; **15b** Shutterstock/Carme Balcells; **16** iStock/Dmitry Galanternik; **18 & 20** Laura Wickenden; **21** iStock/Li Kim Goh; **23l** Shutterstock/Andresr; **23c** Fotolia/GOL; **23r** Fotolia/Moodboard; **24** Shutterstock/Monkey Business Images; **26** Laura Wickenden; **27tl** Shutterstock/Michelangelo Gratton; **27tr** Shutterstock/János Gehring; **27bl** Shutterstock/Monkey Business Images; **27br** Shutterstock/Absolut; **28** iStock/Paul Kooi; **29t** Shutterstock/Monkey Business Images; **37** Shutterstock/Bliznetsov; **44–45** Shutterstock/CURA Photography; **48** Laura Wickenden; **49** Science Photo Library/Mehau Kulyk; **50l** Laura Wickenden; **50c** Shutterstock/Supri Suharjoto; **50r** Alamy/Chris Rout; **51** iStock/Pamela Burley; **52** Alamy/Moodboard; **53** Jacob Hutchings Photography; **54 & 56** Paul Forrester; **58l** Science Photo Library/Steve Gschmeissner; **58r** Science Photo Library/Dee Breger; **59** Science Photo Library/Zephyr; **60** Science Photo Library; **61** Shutterstock/Francesco Carta Fotografo; **62** Science Photo Library/National Cancer Institute; **63** Paul Forrester; **65tl** iStock/Eric Hood; **65tc** iStock/Digitalskillet; **65tr** iStock/Absolut 100; **65b** Science Photo Library/Matt Meadows; **66t** Science Photo Library/Geoff Tompkinson; **66b** Science Photo Library/Sovereign ISM; **69** Paul Forrester; **70t** Shutterstock/Monkey Business Images; **70b** Shutterstock/Monkey Business Images; **73bl** iStock/Amanda Rohde; **73bcl** Shutterstock/Vgstudio; **73bcr** Shutterstock/Monkey Business Images; **73br** iStock/Michael Krinke; **78** Shutterstock/Wolfgang Amri; **80bl** iStock/Jacom Stephens; **80bcl** Shutterstock/Monkey Business Images; **80bcr** Shutterstock/Junial Enterprises; **80br** iStock/Digitalskillet; **81b** Science Photo Library/AJ Photo; **81t** Science Photo Library/AJ Photo; **83tl** iStock/Aldo Murillo; **83tc** Shutterstock/Dean Mitchell; **83tr** Shutterstock/Martina Ebel; **84** Shutterstock/Mircea Bezergheanu; **86** Shutterstock/Monkey Business Images; **87** Laura Wickenden; **88** Shutterstock/Monkey Business Images; **94** Science Photo Library/Steve Gschmeissner; **96** Paul Forrester; **97** Laura Wickenden; **100l** Shutterstock/Demid; **100r** iStock/Ekaterina Monakhova; **102** Shutterstock/Monkey Business Images; **105** Paul Forrester; **107** Shutterstock/Johnny Lye; **110** Science Photo Library/Dr Robert Friedland; **114** Science Photo Library/Biophoto Associates; **115** Alamy/Bubbles Photolibrary; **116** Shutterstock/Vera Bogaerts; **117** Science Photo Library/Eye of Science; **118** Science Photo Library; **119** Science Photo Library/Zephyr; **121** iStock/Christopher Bernard; **123** Paul Forrester; **127** iStock/See Hear Media, Inc; **130** Laura Wickenden; **131** iStock/Rob Hadfield; **134bl** Science Photo Library/Tony McConnell; **134bcl** Science Photo Library/Dr P Marazzi; **134bcr** Science Photo Library/Dr P Marazzi; **134br** Science Photo Library/Prof. P H Franceschini/CNRI; **135** Science Photo Library/Dr P Marazzi; **136** iStock/Ersler; **137** Laura Wickenden; **138bl** Science Photo Library/Dr P Marazzi; **138bc** Science Photo Library/Dr P Marazzi; **138br** Science Photo Library/CNRI; **139** Alamy/Jan Halaska; **140** iStock/J Horrocks; **141** iStock/Starush; **142l** iStock/Digitalskillet; **142r & 143l** Shutterstock/Monkey Business Images; **143c** Shutterstock/Strawberrystock; **143r** iStock/Ranplett; **146–147** Shutterstock/Monkey Business Images; **148** Shutterstock/Monkey Business Images; **149** Shutterstock/Diego Cervo; **150** Shutterstock/Amrita; **151** Shutterstock/Michelangelo Gratton; **153** Shutterstock/Galina Barskaya; **155** Chas Wilder; **156** Getty/Flying Colours; **158** Paul Forrester; **161** Shutterstock/Drazen Vukelic; **162l** iStock/Digitalskillet; **162c** Shutterstock/Monkey Business Images; **162r** Shutterstock/AVAVA; **164** Shutterstock/Yuri Arcurs; **165** Laura Wickenden; **166** Shutterstock/Kirill Vorobyev; **167** Corbis/LWA-Dann Tardif; **168** Shutterstock/Anton Gvozdikov; **170** Shutterstock/Philip Date; **172** Andrew Sydenham; **173** Shutterstock/Valua Vitaly; **174** Paul Forrester; **175** iStock/Galina Photo; **177** Shutterstock/John Bailey; **178** Alamy/Media Color's; **179t** Shutterstock/AVAVA; **179b** Shutterstock/Viki2win; **180–181** Shutterstock/Dmitriy Shironosov; **182, 185 & 186** Laura Wickenden; **188** Shutterstock/Monkey Business Images; **192** iStock/Leigh Schindler; **193t** Science Photo Library/AJ Photo; **193b** Science Photo Library/Marco Ansaloni/Eurelios; **194** Science Photo Library/Zephyr; **195** iStock/Pgiam; **200** iStock/Gansovsky Vladislav; **205** Shutterstock/Studio 1One; **206** Shutterstock/Karen H Ilagan; **217** iStock/Michael Krinke; **217** iStock/James Peragine; **217** Shutterstock/Simone van den Berg; **217** iStock/Digitalskillet; **220** Science Photo Library/Mauro Fermariello; **221** Science Photo Library/Dr E Walker; **231** Science Photo Library/TEK IMAGE; **232** Corbis/C. Devan; **234** iStock/Neustockimages; **234** Shutterstock/MalibuBooks; **234** iStock/Anne Clark; **234** iStock/Sheryl Griffin; **235** Shutterstock/Luba V Nel; **236** Shutterstock/Ersler Dmitry; **237** Corbis/Jason Horowitz; **239** Shutterstock/Monkey Business Images; **243** Shutterstock/Vgstudio; **249** Corbis/John Henley; **250** iStock/Katrina Brown; **252** Alamy/Angela Hampton Picture Library; **252** Science Photo Library/Gustoimages; **254** Shutterstock/Niderlander; **255** Shutterstock/Vgstudio; **268** Shutterstock/Yuri Arcurs; **276** Corbis/Brooke Fasani; **277** Shutterstock/Tomasz Markowski; **278** iStock/Claus Mikosch; **279** Fotolia/Aceshot; **289** Alamy/George Chamberlain; **290** iStock/Mark Kostich; **291** Shutterstock/Liv Friis-Larsen; **294** iStock/Robert Pears; **295** Alamy/Frank Blackburn; **296** Shutterstock/Javarman; **297** Shutterstock/Michelangelo Gratton; **298** Getty/John-Francis Bourke; **299** Shutterstock/Andresr; **300** Fotolia/Wojciech Gajda; **301** Shutterstock/Andresr; **301** DorlingKindersley/Russell Sadur; **304** Getty/Brooke Slezak; **309** Shutterstock/Yuri Arcurs; **310** Shutterstock/T-Design; **311** Getty/Russell Sadur; **312** Alamy/Foodfolio; **313** Shutterstock/Rob Byron